METHODS IN MOLECULAR BIOLOGY

Series Editor
John M. Walker
School of Life and Medical Sciences
University of Hertfordshire
Hatfield, Hertfordshire, AL10 9AB, UK

For further volumes:
http://www.springer.com/series/7651

Preeclampsia

Methods and Protocols

Edited by

Padma Murthi

Monash Medical Centre, Monash University, Clayton, VIC, Australia

Cathy Vaillancourt

INRS-Institut Armand-Frappier, Laval, QC, Canada

Humana Press

Editors
Padma Murthi
Monash Medical Centre
Monash University
Clayton, VIC, Australia

Cathy Vaillancourt
INRS-Institut Armand-Frappier
Laval, QC, Canada

ISSN 1064-3745 ISSN 1940-6029 (electronic)
Methods in Molecular Biology
ISBN 978-1-4939-7497-9 ISBN 978-1-4939-7498-6 (eBook)
https://doi.org/10.1007/978-1-4939-7498-6

Library of Congress Control Number: 2017957846

Cover illustration: Human chorionic villi from the intervillous space © UMR-S 1139 INSERM, University of Paris Descartes; Pathophysiology and Pharmacotoxicology of the Human Placenta and Cellular and Molecular Imaging Facility, Inserm US 25, CNRS UMS 3612, Faculty of Pharmacy of Paris, 4 avenue de l'Observatoire. 75006 Paris, France

Printed on acid-free paper

This Humana Press imprint is published by Springer Nature
The registered company is Springer Science+Business Media, LLC
The registered company address is: 233 Spring Street, New York, NY 10013, U.S.A.

Preface

> *Hippocrates wrote in one of his Aphorisms that "convulsions take place from either repletion or depletion." He was then, the first to describe pre-eclampsia, and the sudden and unexpected appearance of maternal "grand-mal seizure" which occur when the disease progresses to eclampsia (from the Greek "lightning")* [1]

The aim of this volume on *Preeclampsia: Methods and Protocols* is to present the latest developments in the methodologies for the study the physiopathology, the diagnosis of the pathogenesis, as well as the treatment of preeclampsia (PE).

Preeclampsia is the most common serious medical disorder of human pregnancy. The disease is almost exclusive to humans and delivery of the pregnancy continues to be the only effective treatment. Particularly in their first pregnancy, pregnant women can suffer from high blood pressure; kidney dysfunction leading to leakage of protein into the urine; swelling of the hands, feet, and face; and, in severe cases, dizziness, headaches, and difficulties with vision. This condition is called preeclampsia. If left untreated, it can lead to convulsions (eclampsia) and other life-threatening problems for both mother and baby. Preeclampsia only occurs when a woman is pregnant, and currently, the only cure for it is to end the pregnancy, even if the baby is not yet ready for birth. PE and complications associated with this condition account for 15% of direct maternal mortality and 10% of perinatal mortality. Preeclampsia is the indication for 20% of labor inductions and 15% of caesarean. It also accounts for 5–10% of preterm deliveries. Preeclampsia is a major cause of maternal morbidity and mortality in both Western and developing countries affecting some 2–10% of all pregnancies. There is now evidence that women who have preeclampsia have a greater risk of developing cardiovascular disease later in life. Despite this, our understanding of the underlying causes of preeclampsia is limited. The field remains in desperate need of innovative modeling approaches and new insights into understanding the pathophysiology of preeclampsia.

Despite the publication of over 25,000 articles on the etiology, prediction, diagnosis, and treatment of preeclampsia, many basic questions to critically identify the key pathogenesis of preeclampsia still remain. Can we accurately predict those women who will manifest preeclampsia by using a single set of parameters/biomarkers? If diagnosed early enough, can the disorder be prevented? If so, what will an effective prevention strategy entail? Can we reverse a process that might begin with alteration of trophoblast invasion at its earliest stages? Many models have been developed to address these questions, but many others must be developed before we have the necessary tools to fully understand this complex disorder. The chapters included in this book, we have carefully included the laboratory-based methodologies that are currently in use by researchers to model the placental and vascular pathology of preeclampsia, as well as targeting vascular abnormalities of preeclampsia with the focus of emerging therapies.

In this book, we have included the key protocols to study placental function using in vitro and ex vivo model systems, comprehensive genetic analysis of preeclampsia to date, identification of critical angiogenic factors associated with the development of preeclampsia, and finally pilot studies on randomized controlled trial to investigate targeted therapy for preeclampsia. In developing each of the sections of the chapters included in this book, we encountered the difficulty to choose which subjects should be included and how to organize the 28 chapters that spend from fundamental studies to clinical diagnosis and then to the potential treatment of preeclampsia. Our decision was to start with the diagnosis methods, followed by the in vitro aspect of the physiopathology and then treatment protocols in trial. We hope the reader will find this volume useful and reader-friendly.

A key aspect of this book is that it is written by established and early career investigators who have developed and used the techniques extensively; each protocol includes tips on avoiding pitfalls, notes on the method's advantages and disadvantages, and a critical survey of the literature. Each chapter follows the successful Methods in Molecular Biology™ series format, each offering step-by-step laboratory instruction, an introduction outlining the principles behind the technique, lists of the necessary equipment and reagents, and notes designed to help the reader perform the experiments without difficulty. Also, illustrations highlight particular techniques as well as expected outcomes.

We will be negligent not to take this opportunity to thank the contributions of the many individuals who make this volume possible. We wish to express our gratitude to the contributing authors for their time and their willingness to share their knowledge and expertise. Our deep appreciation and gratefulness go to Laetitia Laurent (postdoctoral researcher) and Andrée-Anne Hudon Thibeault (PhD student) for their dedicated efforts and help in the revision, editing, and organization of the chapter manuscripts. Our acknowledgment also goes to the publisher who provided us with helpful guidance and instruction crucial for the realization of this volume.

Comprehensive and state-of-the-art, *Preeclampsia: Methods in Molecular Biology* provides both fundamental and clinical researchers as well as postdoctoral researchers and graduate students a firm foundation for successful analysis of placentation and placental function and a description of the limitations and advantages of the techniques proposed. We hope that it will be useful to all of those who have an interest in unraveling the critical role of the placenta in the maternal-fetal crosstalk. We believe you will find in this reference book the most recent and detailed protocol of the experiment that will prove or disprove your wildest hypothesis.

Cathy Vaillancourt
Padma Murthi

Aphorism XXXI 507 in the Coan Prognosis state: "…a headache accompanied by heaviness and convulsions during pregnancy is considered bad" (Hippocrates, 400 BCE/1950) [1].

Reference

1. Chadwick J, Mann WN, translators (1950) Hippocrates. The medical works of Hippocrates. England: Blackwell Scientific Publications, England. Original work published fifth century BC

Contents

Contributors

MOHAMED H. ABUMAREE • *Stem Cells and Regenerative Medicine Department, King Abdullah International Medical Research Center, College of Science and Health Professions, King Saud Bin Abdulaziz University for Health Sciences, King Abdulaziz Medical City, National Guard Health Affairs, Riyadh, Kingdom of Saudi Arabia*

NADIA ALFAIDY • *Institut National de la Santé et de la Recherche Médicale, Unité 1036, Grenoble, France; University of Grenoble-Alpes, Grenoble, France; Commissariat à l'Energie Atomique (CEA), BIG-Biology of Cancer and Infection, Grenoble, France*

GAAYATHRI ARIYAKUMAR • *Division of Perinatal Medicine, Kolling Institute, Northern Sydney Local Health District, St. Leonards, NSW, Australia; Sydney Medical School Northern, University of Sydney, St. Leonards, NSW, Australia*

ANTHONY W. ASHTON • *Division of Perinatal Research, Kolling Institute, Northern Sydney Local Health District, St. Leonards, NSW, Australia; Sydney Medical School Northern, University of Sydney, Sydney, NSW, Australia*

MOHAMED BENHAROUGA • *University of Grenoble-Alpes, Grenoble, France; Commissariat à l'Energie Atomique (CEA), BIG-Biology of Cancer and Infection, Grenoble, France; Unite Mixte de Recherche, Laboratoire de Chimie et Biologie des Metaux, Centre National de la Recherche Scientifique, Grenoble, France*

JOSIANNE BIENVENUE-PARISEAULT • *INRS-Institut Armand-Frappier, Laval, QC, Canada; BioMed Research Centre, Laval, QC, Canada; Center for Interdisciplinary Research on Well-Being, Health, Society and Environment, Université du Québec à Montréal, Montréal, QC, Canada*

CARIN BLACK • *Department of Obstetrics and Gynaecology, University of Melbourne, Melbourne, VIC, Australia*

SHAUN P. BRENNECKE • *Department of Maternal-Fetal Medicine Pregnancy Research Centre, The Royal Women's Hospital, Melbourne, VIC, Australia; Department of Obstetrics and Gynaecology, The University of Melbourne, Melbourne, VIC, Australia*

SOPHIE BROUILLET • *Institut National de la Santé et de la Recherche Médicale, Unité 1036, Grenoble, France; University of Grenoble-Alpes, Grenoble, France; Commissariat à l'Energie Atomique (CEA), BIG-Biology of Cancer and Infection, Grenoble, France; Department of Obstetrics and Gynecology, et Laboratoire d' Aide à la Procreation-CECOS La Tronche, University Hospital of Grenoble, Grenoble, France*

PAUL BROWNBILL • *Maternal and Fetal Health Research Centre, Division of Developmental Biology and Medicine, School of Medical Sciences, Faculty of Biology, Medicine and Healthy, University of Manchester, Manchester Academic Health Science Centre, Manchester, UK; St. Mary's Hospital, Central Manchester University Hospitals NHS Foundation Trust, Manchester Academic Health Science Centre, Manchester, UK*

EVANGELINA CAPOBIANCO • *Laboratory of Reproduction and Metabolism, CEFYBO, CONICET, School of Medicine, University of Buenos Aires, Buenos Aires, Argentina*

LAWRENCE W. CHAMLEY • *Department of Obstetrics and Gynaecology, Faculty of Medical and Health Sciences, The University of Auckland, Auckland, New Zealand*

TEJASVY CHOLLANGI • *Department of Maternal-Fetal Medicine, Pregnancy Research Centre, The Royal Women's Hospital, Parkville, VIC, Australia; Department of Obstetrics and Gynaecology, The University of Melbourne, Parkville, VIC, Australia*

SIMON CHU • *Hudson Institution of Medical Research, Monash University, Clayton, VIC, Australia; Department of Molecular and Translational Research, Monash University, Clayton, VIC, Australia*

HÉLÈNE CLABAULT • *INRS-Institut Armand-Frappier, Laval, QC, Canada; BioMed Research Centre, Laval, QC, Canada; Center for Interdisciplinary Research on Well-Being, Health, Society and Environment, Université du Québec à Montréal, Montréal, QC, Canada*

FABRICIO DA SILVA COSTA • *Monash Ultrasound for Women, Clayton, VIC, Australia; Department of Obstetrics and Gynaecology, Monash University, Clayton, VIC, Australia*

SEVERINE A. DEGRELLE • *Faculté de Pharmacie de Paris, INSERM, UMR-S1139, Paris, France; Université Paris Descartes, Sorbonne Paris Cité, Paris, France; Fondation PremUp, Paris, France*

GUILLAUME DESPAROIS • *Laboratoire de Physiologie Materno-Foetale, Centre de Recherche BioMed, Université du Québec à Montréal, Montréal, QC, Canada*

EVEMIE DUBÉ • *Laboratoire de Physiologie Materno-Foetale, Centre de Recherche BioMed, Université du Québec à Montréal, Montréal, QC, Canada*

OMAR ELFEKY • *Exosome Biology Laboratory, Centre for Clinical Diagnostics, University of Queensland Centre for Clinical Research, Royal Brisbane and Women's Hospital, The University of Queensland, Brisbane, QLD, Australia*

STACEY ELLERY • *The Ritchie Centre, Hudson Institute of Medical Research, Clayton, VIC, Australia; The Department of Obstetrics and Gynecology, School of Clinical Sciences, Monash University, Clayton, VIC, Australia*

THIERRY FOURNIER • *Faculté de Pharmacie de Paris, INSERM, UMR-S1139, Paris, France; Université Paris Descartes, Sorbonne Paris Cité, Paris, France; Fondation PremUp, Paris, France*

DOMINIC GUANZON • *Exosome Biology Laboratory, Centre for Clinical Diagnostics, University of Queensland Centre for Clinical Research, Royal Brisbane and Women's Hospital, The University of Queensland, Brisbane, QLD, Australia*

SESHINI GURUSINGHE • *Maternal Fetal Medicine Unit, Department of Obstetrics and Gynaecology, Monash Medical Centre, Monash Health and Monash University, Clayton, VIC, Australia; Hudson Institute of Medical Research, Clayton, VIC, Australia*

SEBASTIAN R. HOBSON • *Maternal Fetal Medicine Unit, Department of Obstetrics and Gynaecology, Monash Medical Centre, Monash Health and Monash University, Clayton, VIC, Australia*

RYAN J. HODGES • *Maternal Fetal Medicine Unit, Department of Obstetrics and Gynecology, Monash Medical Centre, Monash Health and Monash University, Clayton, VIC, Australia*

JUVITA DELANCY ILJAS • *Exosome Biology Laboratory, Centre for Clinical Diagnostics, University of Queensland Centre for Clinical Research, Royal Brisbane and Women's Hospital, The University of Queensland, Brisbane, QLD, Australia*

EDWARD ARAUJO JÙNIOR • *Department of Obstetrics, Paulista School of Medicine, Federal University of São Paulo (EPM-UNIFESP), São Paulo, SP, Brazil*

BILL KALIONIS • *Department of Obstetrics and Gynaecology, Royal Women's Hospital, University of Melbourne, Parkville, VIC, Australia; Department of Maternal-Fetal Medicine Pregnancy Research Centre, Royal Women's Hospital, Parkville, VIC, Australia*

STEFAN C. KANE • *Department of Obstetrics and Gynaecology, The Royal Women's Hospital, The University of Melbourne, Parkville, VIC, Australia; Department of Maternal Fetal Medicine, Pregnancy Research Centre, The Royal Women's Hospital, Parkville, VIC, Australia*

SU LYNN KHONG • *Department of Maternal Fetal Medicine, Sunshine Hospital, Western Health, St. Albans, VIC, Australia*

JOHN C. KINGDOM • *Maternal Fetal Medicine Division, Department of Obstetrics and Gynaecology, Mount Sinai Hospital and University of Toronto, ON, Canada*

VYJAYANTHI KINHAL • *Exosome Biology Laboratory, Centre for Clinical Diagnostics and Clinical Research, Royal Brisbane and Women's Hospital, University of Queensland, Brisbane, QLD, Australia*

GINA D. KUSUMA • *Department of Obstetrics and Gynaecology, Royal Woman's Hospital, University of Melbourne, Parkville, VIC, Australia; Department of Maternal-Fetal Medicine Pregnancy Research Centre, Royal Women's Hospital, Parkville, VIC, Australia*

JULIE LAFOND • *Laboratoire de Physiologie Materno-Foetale, Centre de Recherche BioMed, Université du Québec à Montréal, Montréal, QC, Canada*

ANDREW LAI • *Exosome Biology Laboratory, Centre for Clinical Diagnostics, University of Queensland Centre for Clinical Research, Royal Brisbane and Women's Hospital, The University of Queensland, Brisbane, QLD, Australia*

LAETITIA LAURENT • *INRS-Institut Armand-Frappier, Laval, QC, Canada; BioMed Research Centre, Laval, QC, Canada; Center for Interdisciplinary Research on Well-Being, Health, Society and Environment, Université du Québec à Montréal, Montréal, QC, Canada*

BRYAN LEAW • *Hudson Institute of Medical Research, Clayton, VIC, Australia*

DILYS T.H. LEUNG • *Hudson Institution of Medical Research, Monash University, Clayton, VIC, Australia; Department of Molecular and Translational Research, Monash University, Clayton, VIC, Australia*

REBECCA LIM • *Maternal Fetal Medicine Unit, Department of Obstetrics and Gynaecology, Monash Medical Centre, Monash Health and Monash University, Clayton, VIC, Australia*

NORA MARTINEZ • *Laboratory of Biology of Reproduction, IFIBIO, CONICET, School of Medicine, University of Buenos Aires, Buenos Aires, Argentina*

SHARON A. MCCRACKEN • *Division of Perinatal Medicine, Kolling Institute, Northern Sydney Local Health District, St. Leonards, NSW, Australia; Sydney Medical School Northern, University of Sydney, St. Leonards, NSW, Australia*

ERIN V. MCGILLICK • *The Ritchie Centre, Hudson Institute of Medical Research, Clayton, VIC, Australia; The Department of Obstetrics and Gynecology, School of Clinical Sciences, Monash University, Clayton, VIC, Australia*

KELLY J. MCKELVEY • *Division of Perinatal Medicine, Kolling Institute, Northern Sydney Local Health District, St. Leonards, NSW, Australia; Sydney Medical School Northern, University of Sydney, St. Leonards, NSW, Australia*

ELLEN MENKHORST • *Centre for Reproductive Health, Hudson Institute of Medical Research, Clayton, VIC, Australia*

RAMKUMAR MENON • *Division of Maternal-Fetal Medicine and Perinatal Research, Department of Obstetrics and Gynecology, The University of Texas Medical Branch at Galveston, Galveston, TX, USA; Department of Biochemistry and Molecular Biology, The University of Texas Medical Branch at Galveston, Galveston, TX, USA*

JOANNE C. MOCKLER • *Maternal Fetal Medicine Unit, Department of Obstetrics and Gynaecology, Monash Medical Centre, Monash Health and Monash University, Clayton, VIC, Australia*

ERIC K. MOSES • *Centre for Genetic Origins of Health and Disease, The University of Western Australia, Perth, Australia*

PADMA MURTHI • *Department of Medicine, School of Clinical Sciences, Monash University, Clayton, VIC, Australia; Department of Obstetrics and Gynaecology, School of Clinical Sciences, Monash University, Clayton, VIC, Australia; The Ritchie Centre, Hudson Institute of Medical Research, Clayton, VIC, Australia*

LUCIANO MARCONDES MACHADO NARDOZZA • *Department of Obstetrics, Paulista School of Medicine, Federal University of São Paulo (EPM-UNIFESP), São Paulo, SP, Brazil*

ROLAND ABI NAHED • *Institut National de la Santé et de la Recherche Médicale, Unité 1036, Grenoble, France; University of Grenoble-Alpes, Grenoble, France; Commissariat à l'Energie Atomique (CEA), BIG-Biology of Cancer and Infection, Grenoble, France*

SHAGUN NARULA • *The Ritchie Centre, Hudson Institute of Medical Research, Clayton, VIC, Australia*

ZARIN NUZHAT • *Exosome Biology Laboratory, Centre for Clinical Diagnostics and Clinical Research, Royal Brisbane and Women's Hospital, University of Queensland, Brisbane, QLD, Australia*

KIRSTEN PALMER • *Department of Obstetrics and Gynecology, School of Clinical Sciences, Monash University, Clayton, VIC, Australia*

PRIYADARSHINI PANTHAM • *Carl R. Woese Institute for Genomic Biology, University of Illinois at Urbana-Champaign, Urbana, IL, USA*

MARK D. PERTILE • *Victorian Clinical Genetics Services, Murdoch Children's Research Institute, Royal Children's Hospital, Parkville, VIC, Australia; Department of Paediatrics, Royal Children's Hospital, University of Melbourne, Parkville, VIC, Australia*

ALBERTO BORGES PEIXOTO • *Department of Obstetrics, Paulista School of Medicine, Federal University of São Paulo (EPM-UNIFESP), São Paulo, SP, Brazil; Mario Palmério University Hospital – University of Uberaba (UNIUBE), Uberaba, MG, Brazil*

KATIE L. POWELL • *Division of Perinatal Research, Kolling Institute, Northern Sydney Local Health District, St. Leonards, NSW, Australia; Sydney Medical School Northern, University of Sydney, Sydney, NSW, Australia; Pathology North, NSW Health Pathology, Royal North Shore Hospital, St. Leonards, NSW, Australia*

DÉBORAH REYNAUD • *Institut National de la Santé et de la Recherche Médicale, Unité 1036, Grenoble, France; University of Grenoble-Alpes, Grenoble, France; Commissariat à l'Energie Atomique (CEA), BIG-Biology of Cancer and Infection, Grenoble, France*

GREGORY E. RICE • *Exosome Biology Laboratory, Centre for Clinical Diagnostics, University of Queensland Centre for Clinical Research, Royal Brisbane and Women's Hospital, The University of Queensland, Brisbane, QLD, Australia; Maternal-Fetal Medicine, Department of Obstetrics and Gynecology, Ochsner Clinic Foundation, New Orleans, LA, USA*

LILIAM CRISTINE ROLO • *Department of Obstetrics, Paulista School of Medicine, Federal University of São Paulo (EPM-UNIFESP), São Paulo, SP, Brazil*

LUCAS SAGRILLO-FAGUNDES • *INRS-Institut Armand-Frappier, Laval, QC, Canada; BioMed Research Centre, Laval, QC, Canada; Center for Interdisciplinary Research on Well-Being, Health, Society and Environment, Université du Québec à Montréal, Montréal, QC, Canada*

CARLOS SALOMON • *Exosome Biology Laboratory, Centre for Clinical Diagnostics, University of Queensland Centre for Clinical Research, Royal Brisbane and Women's Hospital, The University of Queensland, Brisbane, QLD, Australia; Maternal-Fetal Medicine, Department of Obstetrics and Gynecology, Ochsner Clinic Foundation, New Orleans, LA, USA; Department of Clinical Biochemistry and Immunology, Faculty of Pharmacy, University of Concepción, Concepción, Chile*

J. THOMAS SANDERSON • *INRS-Institut Armand-Frappier, Laval, QC, Canada*

KATHERIN SCHOLZ-ROMERO • *Exosome Biology Laboratory, Centre for Clinical Diagnostics, University of Queensland Centre for Clinical Research, Royal Brisbane and Women's Hospital, The University of Queensland, Brisbane, QLD, Australia*

NEIL SEBIRE • *Institute of Child Health, University College London, London, UK*

FRÉDÉRIC SERGENT • *Institut National de la Santé et de la Recherche Médicale, Unité 1036, Grenoble, France; University of Grenoble-Alpes, Grenoble, France; Commissariat à l'Energie Atomique (CEA), BIG-Biology of Cancer and Infection, Grenoble, France*

SHAYNA SHARMA • *Exosome Biology Laboratory, Centre for Clinical Diagnostics, University of Queensland Centre for Clinical Research, Royal Brisbane and Women's Hospital, The University of Queensland, Brisbane, QLD, Australia*

ANDRÉE-ANNE HUDON THIBEAULT • *INRS-Institut Armand-Frappier, Laval, QC, Canada; BioMed Research Centre, Université du Québec à Montréal, Montréal, QC, Canada; Center for Interdisciplinary Research on Well-Being, Health, Society and Environment (CINBIOSE), Université du Québec à Montréal, Montréal, QC, Canada*

MANCY TONG • *Department of Obstetrics and Gynaecology, Faculty of Medical and Health Sciences, The University of Auckland, Auckland, New Zealand*

CATHY VAILLANCOURT • *INRS-Institut Armand-Frappier, Laval, QC, Canada; BioMed Research Centre, Laval, QC, Canada; Center for Interdisciplinary Research on Well-Being, Health, Society and Environment, Université du Québec à Montréal, Montréal, QC, Canada*

EUAN M. WALLACE • *Maternal Fetal Medicine Unit, Department of Obstetrics and Gynaecology, Monash Medical Centre, Monash Health and Monash University, Clayton, VIC, Australia*

HANNAH E.J. YONG • *Department of Maternal-Fetal Medicine Pregnancy Research Centre, The Royal Women's Hospital, Melbourne, VIC, Australia; Department of Obstetrics and Gynaecology, The University of Melbourne, Melbourne, VIC, Australia; Centre for Trophoblast Research, Department of Physiology, Development and Neuroscience, The University of Cambridge, Cambridge, UK*

Chapter 1

Diagnostic Imaging: Ultrasound

Stefan C. Kane, Su Lynn Khong, and Fabricio da Silva Costa

Abstract

Diagnostic ultrasound imaging, particularly that which includes pulsed wave Doppler interrogation, is a safe, real-time modality by which the risk of developing preeclampsia can be refined, and the effects of established disease can be assessed. This chapter outlines the rationale and technique for Doppler interrogation of the maternal ophthalmic and uterine arteries and grayscale imaging of the maternal optic nerve sheath diameter.

Key words Preeclampsia, Ultrasound, Uterine artery, Doppler, Ophthalmic

1 Introduction

1.1 Ophthalmic Ultrasound

A significant proportion of the maternal mortality and morbidity associated with preeclampsia occurs as a result of its cerebral effects, in both the short and long term [1]. Although effective therapies exist to mitigate these effects, such as magnesium sulfate to prevent eclampsia [2] and antihypertensives to reduce the risk of stroke [3], clinical assessment and prediction of those patients at highest risk of these complications remains challenging [4]. In light of this, ophthalmic ultrasound has been proposed as a safe, real-time, point-of-care means by which to assess intracranial pressure and cerebrovascular hemodynamics, through assessment of the optic nerve sheath diameter [5] and Doppler properties of the ophthalmic artery [6], respectively. The ophthalmic artery represents an accessible surrogate for the smaller caliber intracerebral vessels, which is the likely level at which hemodynamic changes occur in preeclampsia. Reference ranges for a number of Doppler indices in this vessel have been published [7, 8], although it is the "peak ratio"—the ratio between the first peak diastolic velocity and the peak systolic velocity—that is considered to be the most sensitive measure of hemodynamic change in this context [7]. Further research is required to confirm the potential clinical applicability of these imaging modalities [9].

Padma Murthi and Cathy Vaillancourt (eds.), *Preeclampsia: Methods and Protocols*, Methods in Molecular Biology, vol. 1710, https://doi.org/10.1007/978-1-4939-7498-6_1, © Springer Science+Business Media LLC 2018

1.2 Uterine Artery Doppler

Uterine artery Doppler velocimetry has been utilized extensively to assess uteroplacental vascular resistance in order to predict adverse pregnancy outcomes. The parameters investigated include measurement of impedance such as an elevated pulsatility index (PI) or resistance index (RI) over 90th or 95th percentile adjusted for gestational age and waveform analysis (presence or absence of an early diastolic notch). The latter has been defined as a drop of at least a 50 cm/s from the maximum diastolic velocity but is often assessed subjectively [10].

In the first trimester, the uterine artery Doppler waveform commonly demonstrates an early diastolic notch (46–64% of normal gestations) and low end-diastolic velocities [11]. Uterine artery impedance decreases with increasing gestational age. This phenomenon is secondary to a fall in resistance in uterine vessels following trophoblastic invasion. Similarly, notching disappears between 20 and 26 weeks' gestation due to an increase in uterine artery compliance [12]. Abnormal maternal vascular tone is associated with persistent early diastolic notching in the second trimester. Despite a high negative predictive value, notching has poor reproducibility, and more objective measures such as PI are favored. Reference ranges for uterine artery Doppler parameters have been established in various populations [13–17] using the techniques described below.

2 Methods

All imaging should be performed in accordance with published safety guidelines, such as those of the British Medical Ultrasound Society [18].

2.1 Ophthalmic Ultrasound

Position the patient supine at an angle of 45° to maximize patient comfort and reduce aortocaval compression. Following the application of a small amount of transmission gel, place a high-frequency (7–15-MHz) linear array ultrasound transducer horizontally on the closed eyelid at the upper aspect of the eyeball. The examiner's hand may rest on the bridge of the patient's nose or on her forehead to control and minimize the degree of pressure on the eye. Using B-mode imaging, set the field depth to encompass the globe and the retro-orbital space, with the focus set to the latter.

2.1.1 Ophthalmic Artery Doppler Analysis (Fig. 1)

The technique for Doppler interrogation of the ophthalmic artery was originally described by Erickson et al. in 1989 [19] and has since been adopted by a majority of authors in this field.

1. Using color Doppler, identify the ophthalmic artery by its direction of flow (toward the probe) and pulsatility.

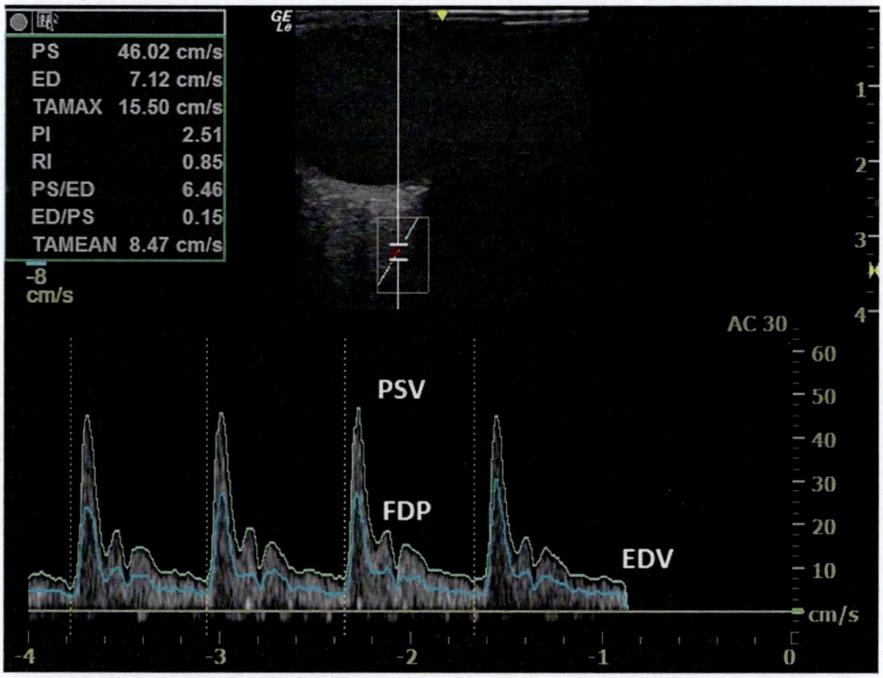

Fig. 1 The flow velocity waveform of the ophthalmic artery. PSV = peak systolic velocity, FDP = first diastolic peak velocity, EDV = end-diastolic velocity. Reproduced with permission from Kane SC et al. Ophthalmic artery Doppler analysis: A window into the cerebrovasculature of women with preeclampsia. Ultrasound Obstet Gynecol 2016 Aug 3. doi: 10.1002/uog.17209

2. Apply pulsed wave Doppler, with the sample volume placed around 15 mm behind the optic disc, medial to the optic nerve; the sample volume should be 2 mm in length.
3. Obtain 3–5 consistent cardiac cycles and store them electronically.
4. Keep the insonation angle at <20°, and set the high-pass filter to its minimum value.
5. Set the pulse repetition frequency (PRF) to 125 kHz, and adapt as necessary.

Standard Doppler indices may be calculated automatically by the ultrasound machine, although the peak ratio will require manual measurement of the first diastolic peak velocity. Measurements have been shown not to differ between the right and left eyes, validating unilateral assessment [20].

2.1.2 Optic Nerve Sheath Diameter (Fig. 2)

Use the same ultrasound probe and general approach to examination as described above. Employ B-mode imaging alone and set the field depth to 4 cm. Place electronic calipers across the optic nerve sheath 3 mm behind the globe, perpendicular to the optic

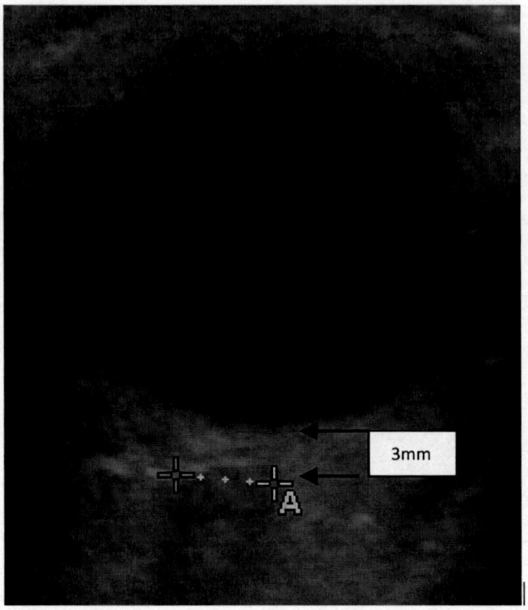

Fig. 2 The diameter of the optic nerve sheath, measured 3 mm behind the globe, perpendicular to the optic nerve. Reproduced with permission from Roque PJ et al. Optic nerve ultrasound for the detection of elevated intracranial pressure in the hypertensive patient. Am J Emerg Med. 2012 Oct; 30(8): 1357–63

nerve [21, 22]. Assess the diameter in two planes—transverse and sagittal, the latter requiring rotation of the probe by 90°. The average of the two measurements represents the mean optic nerve sheath diameter if one eye is assessed, whereas if both eyes are examined, the four measurements may be averaged for a single mean sheath diameter.

2.2 Uterine Artery Doppler Assessment

The reference ranges for uterine artery Doppler indices are different for transabdominal and transvaginal techniques, and care should be taken to ensure that the correct reference range is used. In multiple pregnancies, the uterine artery impedance measurements appear to be lower, but studies of uterine artery Doppler screening in this subgroup are limited [23, 24]. Overall, uterine artery Doppler is more accurate for prediction of preeclampsia in the second trimester than in the first, but the test does not perform adequately in isolation in any trimester to be used clinically [25, 26]. The screening performance of uterine artery Doppler analysis is improved when performed as part of a multiparametric model incorporating maternal characteristics and serum biomarkers [27–29].

2.2.1 Doppler Assessment in the First Trimester

Measurement of uterine artery impedance by Doppler can be performed via a transabdominal or transvaginal approach. The former method is preferred as it is less invasive. Doppler evaluation of

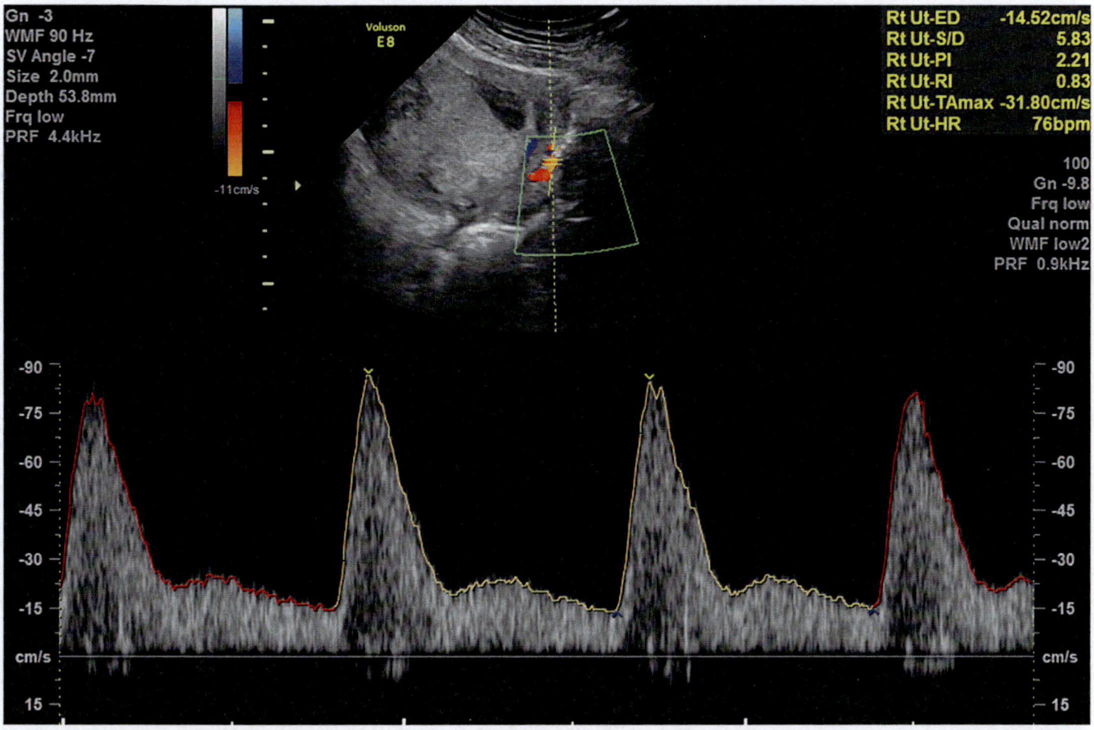

Fig. 3 Transabdominal Doppler interrogation of the uterine artery at the level of the internal cervical os. Uterine artery waveform demonstrating raised PI with an early diastolic notch (*arrow*). Reproduced under the auspices of open access from Khong SL et al. First-Trimester Uterine Artery Doppler Analysis in the Prediction of Later Pregnancy Complications. Dis Markers 2015;2015:679730. doi: 10.1155/2015/679730

uterine artery is usually performed between 11 + 0 and 13 + 6 weeks' gestation in conjunction with fetal nuchal translucency assessment.

1. Transabdominal technique (Fig. 3): Use a 5- or 3.5-MHz curvilinear transabdominal transducer. Firstly, obtain a midsagittal section of the uterus and cervical canal and move the transducer laterally until the paracervical vessels are visualized. The uterine arteries are seen as aliasing vessels along the side of the cervix when color flow Doppler is applied. Using pulsed wave Doppler, obtain flow velocity waveforms from the ascending branch of the uterine artery at the point closest to the internal os, with the Doppler sampling gate set at 2 mm. In order to achieve the highest systolic and end-diastolic velocities, use the smallest angle of insonation (<30°). Measure the PI from three similar consecutive waveforms, then repeat the process on the contralateral side. The mean PI is calculated as the average reading from each side combined.

   An alternate transabdominal technique involves Doppler insonation of the uterine artery at the level of its apparent

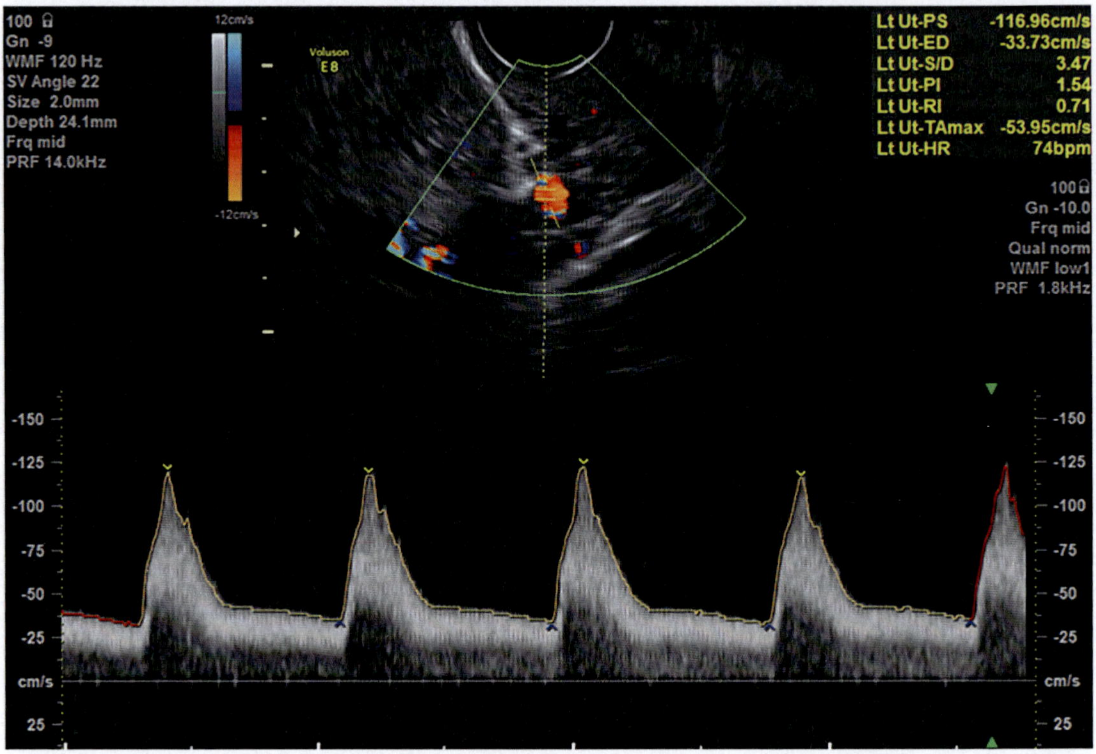

Fig. 4 Transvaginal Doppler interrogation of the uterine artery at the cervico-corporeal junction. Normal uterine artery waveforms. Reproduced under the auspices of open access from Khong SL et al. First-Trimester Uterine Artery Doppler Analysis in the Prediction of Later Pregnancy Complications. Dis Markers 2015;2015:679730. doi:10.1155/2015/679730

crossover with the external iliac artery, thus ensuring that Doppler velocities are obtained from the main uterine artery trunk. Position the transducer approximately 2–3 cm inside the iliac crests, then direct it toward the pelvis and the lateral side of the uterus. Identify each uterine artery with color flow Doppler. Apply pulsed wave Doppler approximately 1 cm above the point at which the uterine artery crosses over the external iliac artery [30].

The site of uterine artery crossover with the external iliac artery can be harder to locate with a smaller uterus in the first trimester, whereas the first technique-measuring uterine artery Doppler at the level of the internal cervical os is achievable in most cases.

2. Transvaginal technique (Fig. 4): Use a 4.6–8-MHz transvaginal transducer. Place the transducer in the anterior vaginal fornix and obtain a sagittal section of the cervix. Move the vaginal transducer laterally until the paracervical vascular plexus is

seen. Identify the uterine artery with color Doppler at the level of the cervico-corporeal junction. Take measurements with pulsed wave Doppler at this point before the uterine artery branches into the arcuate arteries [30].

2.2.2 Doppler Assessment in the Second Trimester

1. Transabdominal technique: The technique is similar to the aforementioned transabdominal method in the first trimester. Place pulsed wave Doppler 1 cm downstream from the cross-over point of the uterine artery and external iliac artery [30].
2. Transvaginal technique: Place the transducer in the lateral vaginal fornix. Using color Doppler, identify the uterine artery at the level of the internal cervical os. Take measurements as previously described [30].

References

1. Zeeman GG (2009) Neurologic complications of pre-eclampsia. Semin Perinatol 33(3):166–172. https://doi.org/10.1053/j.semperi.2009.02.003
2. Altman D, Carroli G, Duley L, Farrell B, Moodley J, Neilson J, Smith D (2002) Do women with pre-eclampsia, and their babies, benefit from magnesium sulphate? The Magpie Trial: a randomised placebo-controlled trial. Lancet 359(9321):1877–1890
3. Crovetto F, Somigliana E, Peguero A, Figueras F (2013) Stroke during pregnancy and pre-eclampsia. Curr Opin Obstet Gynecol 25(6):425–432. https://doi.org/10.1097/gco.0000000000000024
4. Kane SC, Dennis A, da Silva Costa F, Kornman L,Brennecke SP (2013) Contemporary clinical management of the cerebral complications of preeclampsia. Obstet Gynecol Int 2013:985606. https://doi.org/10.1155/2013/985606
5. Dubourg J, Javouhey E, Geeraerts T, Messerer M, Kassai B (2011) Ultrasonography of optic nerve sheath diameter for detection of raised intracranial pressure: a systematic review and meta-analysis. Intensive Care Med 37(7):1059–1068. https://doi.org/10.1007/s00134-011-2224-2
6. Diniz AL, Moron AF, dos Santos MC, Sass N, Pires CR, Debs CL (2008) Ophthalmic artery Doppler as a measure of severe pre-eclampsia. Int J Gynaecol Obstet 100(3):216–220. https://doi.org/10.1016/j.ijgo.2007.07.013
7. Carneiro RS, Sass N, Diniz AL, Souza EV, Torloni MR, Moron AF (2008) Ophthalmic artery Doppler velocimetry in healthy pregnancy. Int J Gynaecol Obstet 100(3):211–215. https://doi.org/10.1016/j.ijgo.2007.09.028
8. de Oliveira CA, de Sa RA, Velarde LG, Marchiori E, Netto HC, Ville Y (2009) Doppler velocimetry of the ophthalmic artery in normal pregnancy: reference values. J Ultrasound Med 28(5):563–569
9. Kane SC, Brennecke SP, da Silva CF (2016) Ophthalmic artery Doppler analysis: a window into the cerebrovasculature of women with pre-eclampsia. Ultrasound Obstet Gynecol. https://doi.org/10.1002/uog.17209
10. Campbell S, Bewley S, Cohen-Overbeek T (1987) Investigation of the uteroplacental circulation by Doppler ultrasound. Semin Perinatol 11(4):362–368
11. Sciscione AC, Hayes EJ (2009) Uterine artery Doppler flow studies in obstetric practice. Am J Obstet Gynecol 201(2):121–126. https://doi.org/10.1016/j.ajog.2009.03.027
12. Schulman H, Fleischer A, Farmakides G, Bracero L, Rochelson B, Grunfeld L (1986) Development of uterine artery compliance in pregnancy as detected by Doppler ultrasound. Am J Obstet Gynecol 155(5):1031–1036
13. Alves JA, Silva BY, de Sousa PC, Maia SB, Costa Fda S (2013) Reference range of uterine artery Doppler parameters between the 11th and 14th pregnancy weeks in a population sample from Northeast Brazil. Rev Bras Ginecol Obstet 35(8):357–362
14. Gómez O, Figueras F, Fernández S, Bennasar M, Martínez JM, Puerto B, Gratacós E (2008) Reference ranges for uterine artery mean pulsatility index at 11-4 1 weeks of gestation. Ultrasound Obstet Gynecol 32(2):128–132. https://doi.org/10.1002/uog.5315
15. Lefebvre J, Demers S, Bujold E, Nicolaides KH, Girard M, Brassard N, Audibert F (2012)

Comparison of two different sites of measurement for transabdominal uterine artery Doppler velocimetry at 11-13 weeks. Ultrasound Obstet Gynecol 40(3):288–292. https://doi.org/10.1002/uog.11137
16. Plasencia W, Barber MA, Alvarez EE, Segura J, Valle L, Garcia-Hernandez JA (2011) Comparative study of transabdominal and transvaginal uterine artery Doppler pulsatility indices at 11-13 + 6 weeks. Hypertens Pregnancy 30(4):414–420. https://doi.org/10.3109/10641955.2010.506232
17. Ridding G, Schluter PJ, Hyett JA, McLennan AC (2014) Uterine artery pulsatility index assessment at 11-13 weeks' gestation. Fetal Diagn Ther 36(4):299–304. https://doi.org/10.1159/000361021
18. ter Haar G (2010) The new British Medical Ultrasound Society Guidelines for the safe use of diagnostic ultrasound equipment. Ultrasound 18(2):50–51. https://doi.org/10.1258/ult.2010.100007
19. Erickson SJ, Hendrix LE, Massaro BM, Harris GJ, Lewandowski MF, Foley WD, Lawson TL (1989) Color Doppler flow imaging of the normal and abnormal orbit. Radiology 173(2):511–516. https://doi.org/10.1148/radiology.173.2.2678264
20. Correa-Silva EP, Surita FG, Barbieri C, Morais SS, Cecatti JG (2012) Reference values for Doppler velocimetry of the ophthalmic and central retinal arteries in low-risk pregnancy. Int J Gynaecol Obstet 117(3):251–256. https://doi.org/10.1016/j.ijgo.2012.01.012
21. Blaivas M, Theodoro D, Sierzenski PR (2002) A study of bedside ocular ultrasonography in the emergency department. Acad Emerg Med 9(8):791–799
22. Blaivas M, Theodoro D, Sierzenski PR (2003) Elevated intracranial pressure detected by bedside emergency ultrasonography of the optic nerve sheath. Acad Emerg Med 10(4):376–381
23. Rizzo G, Arduini D, Romanini C (1993) Uterine artery Doppler velocity waveforms in twin pregnancies. Obstet Gynecol 82(6):978–983
24. Yu CK, Papageorghiou AT, Boli A, Cacho AM, Nicolaides KH (2002) Screening for pre-eclampsia and fetal growth restriction in twin pregnancies at 23 weeks of gestation by transvaginal uterine artery Doppler. Ultrasound Obstet Gynecol 20(6):535–540. https://doi.org/10.1046/j.1469-0705.2002.00865.x
25. Stampalija T, Gyte GM, Alfirevic Z (2010) Utero-placental Doppler ultrasound for improving pregnancy outcome. Cochrane Database Syst Rev (9):CD008363. https://doi.org/10.1002/14651858.CD008363.pub2
26. Velauthar L, Plana MN, Kalidindi M, Zamora J, Thilaganathan B, Illanes SE, Khan KS, Aquilina J, Thangaratinam S (2014) First-trimester uterine artery Doppler and adverse pregnancy outcome: a meta-analysis involving 55,974 women. Ultrasound Obstet Gynecol 43(5):500–507. https://doi.org/10.1002/uog.13275
27. Cnossen JS, Morris RK, ter Riet G, Mol BWJ, van der Post JAM, Coomarasamy A, Zwinderman AH, Robson SC, Bindels PJE, Kleijnen J, Khan KS (2008) Use of uterine artery Doppler ultrasonography to predict pre-eclampsia and intrauterine growth restriction: a systematic review and bivariable meta-analysis. Can Med Assoc J 178(6):701–711. https://doi.org/10.1503/cmaj.070430
28. Kane SC, da Silva Costa F, Brennecke SP (2014) New directions in the prediction of pre-eclampsia. Aust N Z J Obstet Gynaecol 54(2):101–107. https://doi.org/10.1111/ajo.12151
29. Poon LC, Kametas NA, Maiz N, Akolekar R, Nicolaides KH (2009) First-trimester prediction of hypertensive disorders in pregnancy. Hypertension 53(5):812–818. https://doi.org/10.1161/hypertensionaha.108.127977
30. Bhide A, Acharya G, Bilardo CM, Brezinka C, Cafici D, Hernandez-Andrade E, Kalache K, Kingdom J, Kiserud T, Lee W, Lees C, Leung KY, Malinger G, Mari G, Prefumo F, Sepulveda W, Trudinger B (2013) ISUOG practice guidelines: use of Doppler ultrasonography in obstetrics. Ultrasound Obstet Gynecol 41(2):233–239. https://doi.org/10.1002/uog.12371

Chapter 2

Biomarker Immunoassays in the Diagnosis of Preeclampsia: Calculating the sFlt1/PlGF Ratio Using the Cobas® e 411 Analyser

Carin Black and Fabricio da Silva Costa

Abstract

Preeclampsia is a relatively common pregnancy-related condition associated with serious maternal and fetal morbidity and mortality. It is now well established that anti-angiogenic sFlt1 is upregulated in preeclampsia and binds PlGF and VEGF, causing an imbalance in angiogenic factors with subsequent endothelial injury and dysfunction. Measurement of placental growth factor (PlGF) and the sFlt1/PlGF ratio have both been validated in other countries for screening and diagnosis of preeclampsia and the differentiation of preeclampsia from other hypertensive disorders of pregnancy. There are several automated, commercially available immunoassays capable of measuring PlGF and the sFlt1/PlGF ratio for preeclampsia diagnosis. Here we outline the methodology for using the Roche **Cobas® e** 411 immunoassay platform to determine the sFlt1/PlGF ratio.

Key words Preeclampsia, Biomarkers, Soluble fms-like tyrosine kinase-1 (sFlt1), Placental growth factor (PlGF), Immunoassay

1 Introduction

Preeclampsia is a multisystem, pregnancy-specific disorder complicating 2–8% of pregnancies [1] and is a major cause of maternal and perinatal morbidity and mortality worldwide [2]. The diagnosis of preeclampsia is currently based on nonspecific criteria including blood pressure, proteinuria, and subjective patient symptomatology. These parameters are late, end-organ effects of disease [3–7], and they display poor test accuracy for prediction of adverse outcomes.

In 2004, it was demonstrated for the first time that increased levels of sFlt1 and decreased levels of PlGF predict the subsequent onset of preeclampsia [8]. There have been developments in the understanding of the pathophysiology of preeclampsia [9], and it is now well established that anti-angiogenic sFlt1 is upregulated [10], binding PlGF and VEGF, causing an imbalance in angiogenic

Padma Murthi and Cathy Vaillancourt (eds.), *Preeclampsia: Methods and Protocols*, Methods in Molecular Biology, vol. 1710, https://doi.org/10.1007/978-1-4939-7498-6_2,

factors [11] with subsequent endothelial injury and dysfunction. Subsequently, serum sFlt1 and PlGF have been shown to differentiate healthy women from those with preeclampsia [12]. Measurements for these biomarkers can be performed quickly allowing rapid bedside results. sFlt1, PlGF, and sFlt1/PlGF ratio have been determined valuable in the prediction and diagnosis of preeclampsia [13–16] and in the differential diagnosis of patients with hypertensive disorders of pregnancy [17–20].

There are now several commercially available automated immunoassay platforms capable of measuring both sFlt1 and PlGF, along with their ratio [17–22]. These platforms are becoming feasible to use in an everyday clinical context as part of the diagnostic workup for patients with suspected preeclampsia, given their relative ease of use and quick turnaround time for results. The platforms available have been validated in numerous studies in the diagnosis of preeclampsia [15–17, 20–23]. These studies demonstrate high sensitivity and specificity for sFlt1 and PlGF in the diagnosis of preeclampsia, particularly that of early onset [12, 24] which tends to be associated with the greatest maternal and fetal morbidity and mortality.

Here we describe the methods for testing of maternal serum for sFlt1 and PlGF, using the Roche **Cobas® e** 411 analyser [25] (*see* **Note 1**). We have used this platform within our department recently to test retrospectively collected frozen patient serum for the purpose of research into the prediction of preeclampsia at midgestation.

2 Materials

2.1 Serum Samples

1. 10 mL blood per patient (approximately).
2. Plain blood collection tubes.

2.2 Roche Cobas® e 411 Analyser and Control Unit [25]

The Roche Diagnostics **Cobas® e** 411 analyser is a fully automated, random-access, software-controlled system for immunoassay analysis (Fig. 1). The system consists of the analyser, which performs all functions required for fully automated sample and assay processing, and a control unit, which controls the analyser through the user software. It is available as both a disk system and a rack system. In this chapter we describe use of the rack system. The **Cobas® e** 411 analyser was designed for both quantitative and qualitative in vitro determination of analytes in body fluids using a wide variety of tests, with a throughput of approximately 85 tests per hour. The **Cobas® e** 411 analyser is a discrete unit, which can be placed on a benchtop in the laboratory.

All assay reagent, calibrator, and control information can be automatically entered into the software through the use of barcodes and e-barcodes. This entirely automated process begins with

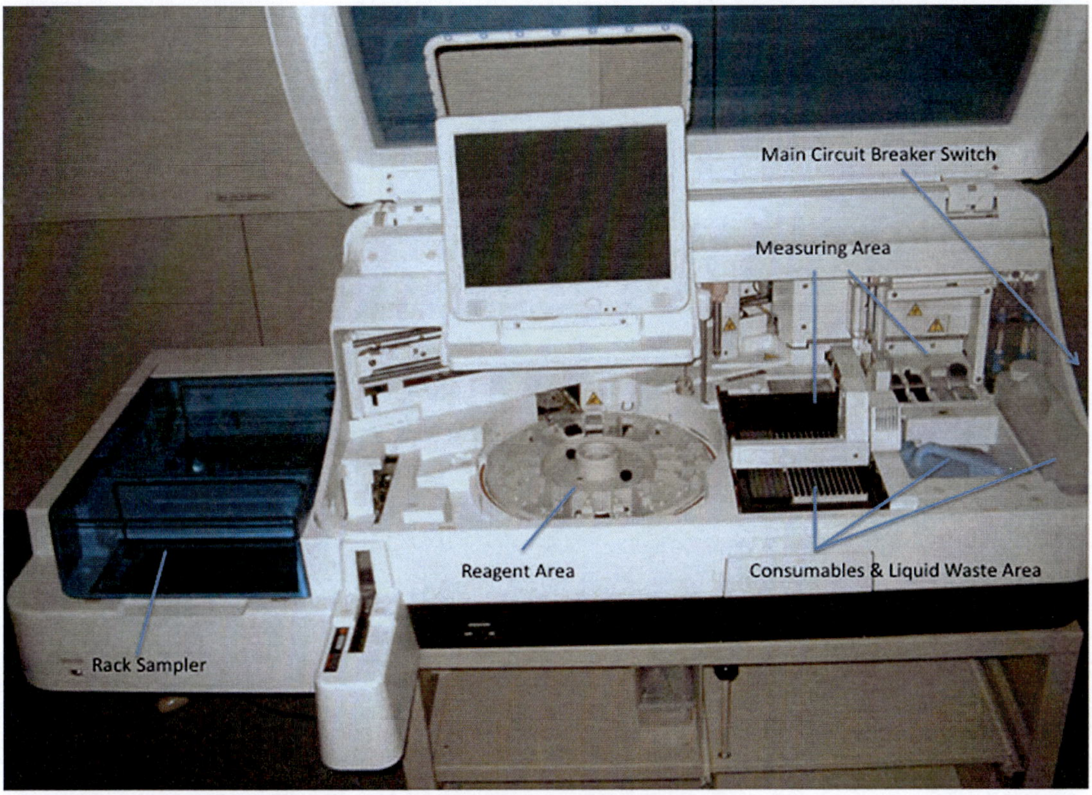

Fig. 1 Roche **Cobas® e** 411 analyser [25]

the recording of patient samples—provided that they are in barcode-labelled tubes—up to the electrochemiluminescence detection and results transmission.

Data transmission to and from the analyser, result evaluation, documentation, and quality control are performed automatically by the software. Also, the software is responsible for the management of data between a connected LIS/PSM (Pre-Analytic Systems Manager) and the **Cobas® e** 411 analyser.

2.3 Elecsys® PlGF Reagent Kits [25] Supplied by Roche Diagnostics GmbH (See Note 2)

The kit contains the following

1. Suspended paramagnetic microbeads in the form of streptavidin-coated microparticles (0.72 mg/mL, 6.5 mL per bottle) and preservative. Contained in a transparent bottle with transparent lid.
2. Biotinylated monoclonal anti-PlGF mouse antibody (0.6 mg/L, 8 mL per bottle), phosphate buffer 50 mmol/L, pH 6.0, and preservative. Contained in a black bottle with a grey lid.
3. Monoclonal anti-PlGF mouse antibody labelled with ruthenium complex (4.0 mg/L, 8 mL per bottle), phosphate buffer 50 mmol/L, pH 6.0, and preservative. Contained in a black bottle with a black lid (Fig. 2).

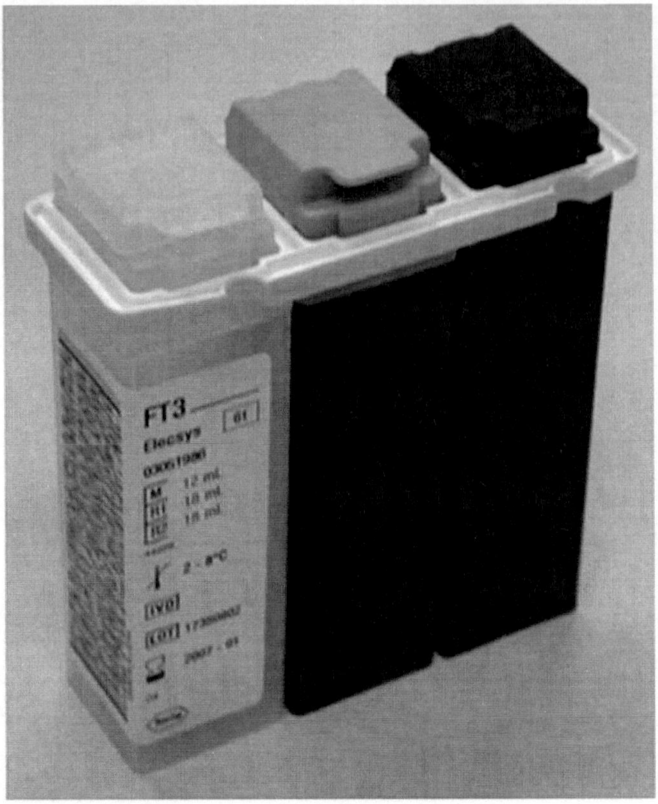

Fig. 2 Reagent pack [25]

2.4 Elecsys® sFlt1 Reagent Kits [25] Supplied by Roche Diagnostics GmbH (See Note 2)

The kit contains the following

1. Suspended paramagnetic microbeads in the form of streptavidin-coated microparticles (0.72 mg/mL, 6.5 mL per bottle) and preservative. Contained in a transparent bottle with transparent lid.
2. Biotinylated monoclonal anti-sFlt-1 mouse antibody (0.5 mg/L, 9 mL per bottle), phosphate buffer 100 mmol/L, pH 7.2, and preservative. Contained in a black bottle with a grey lid.
3. Monoclonal anti-sFlt-1 mouse antibody labeled with ruthenium complex (1.0 mg/L, 9 mL per bottle), phosphate buffer 100 mmol/L, pH 7.2, and preservative. Contained in a black bottle with a black lid (*see* **Note 3** and Fig. 2).

2.5 Elecsys® PlGF CalSet Kits [25] Supplied by Roche Diagnostics GmbH (See Note 2)

Used for calibrating the quantitative PlGF assay. Contains lyophilised buffered equine serum matrix with added recombinant (from *E. coli*) human PlGF-1 in two concentration ranges:

1. PlGF Cal1: Two bottles, each for 1.0 mL of calibrator 1 (approx 5 pg/mL).

2. PlGF Cal2: Two bottles, each for 1.0 mL of calibrator 2 (approx 1200 pg/mL).

2.6 Elecsys® sFlt1 CalSet Kits [25] Supplied by Roche Diagnostics GmbH (See Note 2)

Contains lyophilised buffered equine serum matrix with an added fragment of recombinant human sFlt-1 in two concentration ranges:

1. sFlt-1 Cal1: Two bottles, each for 1.0 mL of calibrator 1 (approx 0 pg/mL).
2. sFlt-1 Cal2: Two bottles, each for 1.0 mL of calibrator 2 (approx 15,000 pg/mL) (*see* **Notes 4** and **5**).

2.7 PreciControl Multimarker [25]

Supplied by Roche Diagnostics GmbH (*see* **Note 2**) PreciControl Multimarker is used for quality control (QC) in monitoring accuracy and precision of specified immunoassays. Contains lyophilised control serum based on an equine serum matrix in two concentration ranges:

1. PC MM1: Three bottles, each for 2.0 mL of control serum.
2. PC MM2: Three bottles, each for 2.0 mL of control serum (*see* **Note 6**).

2.8 ProCell Solution [25] Supplied by Roche Diagnostics GmbH (See Note 2)

Contains buffer solution for generating electrochemical signals. Contains phosphate buffer 300 mmol/L, tripropylamine 180 mmol/L, detergent ≤0.1%, preservative, and pH 6.8 (*see* **Notes 7** and **9**).

2.9 CleanCell [25] Supplied by Roche Diagnostics GmbH (See Note 2)

Contains solution for cleaning the measuring cell once measurement has occurred. Contains KOH 176 mmol/L (corresponds to pH 13.2) and detergent ≤1% (*see* **Notes 8** and **9**).

2.10 Elecsys SysWash [25] Supplied by Roche Diagnostics GmbH (See Note 2)

Contains synthetic biocide in the form of 2-methyl-2H-isothiazol-3-one and preservative.

2.11 Laboratory Equipment

1. AssayTips and AssayCups supplied by Roche Diagnostics GmbH.
2. Hitachi Polystyrene Sample Cups (*see* **Note 10**).

3 Methods

3.1 Samples

1. Blood collected in plain tubes and centrifuged at 1600 × *g* for 10 min at 4 °C. Following centrifugation, serum was pipetted into plain polypropylene tubes and stored at −30 °C (*see* **Note 11**).

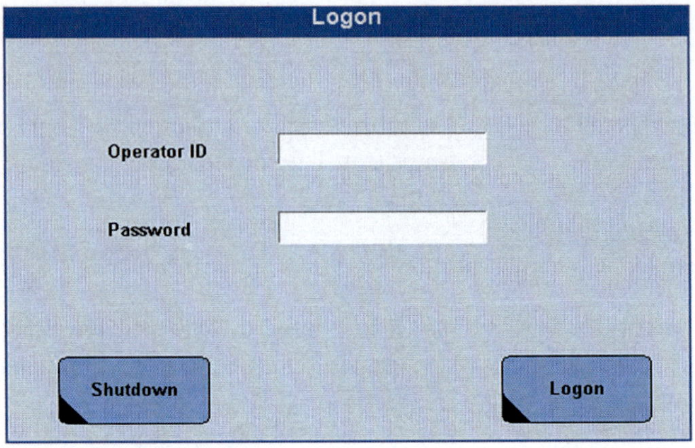

Fig. 3 Logon screen [25]

2. Prior to analysis, samples were removed from freezer and thawed to room temperature. Once thawed, samples were gently inverted several times then centrifuged for 5 min at 5000 × *g*.

3.2 Pre-start Inspection

Check the analyser for the following: (1) check for clean surfaces clear of loose articles and debris, (2) check that probes and microbead mixer paddle are in good condition and not bent, (3) check for pinched or bent tubing, (4) check that pipetter syringes and associated tubing are free of bubbles and are not leaking system water.

1. Switch on the analyser at the operation switch (*see* **Note 12**).
2. Log on to the system by typing operator ID and password into log-on window (Fig. 3).
3. Switch the printer on and check paper supply.
4. Check system alarms and remedy as instructed (*see* **Note 13**).

3.3 Pre-routine Operation

1. Navigate to the System Overview screen (*see* **Note 14** and Fig. 4).
2. Prepare reagent packs: Ensure the samples, calibrators, and controls are at 20–25 °C prior to measurement (*see* **Note 15**).
3. Replace reagent packs: Ensure that analyser is in standby mode while replacing reagents. Open the reagent rotor cover by rotating it to the left until it reaches the stop and then lift it clear. Place reagents in the reagent rotor (*see* **Notes 3** and **15**). Close the reagent rotor cover.
4. Replace system reagents: Lift the instrument cover. Open the sipper shield (*see* **Note 16**). Remove the empty PC and CC bottles and replace with a full set (*see* **Note 17**). Close the sipper shield (*see* **Notes 18** and **19**).

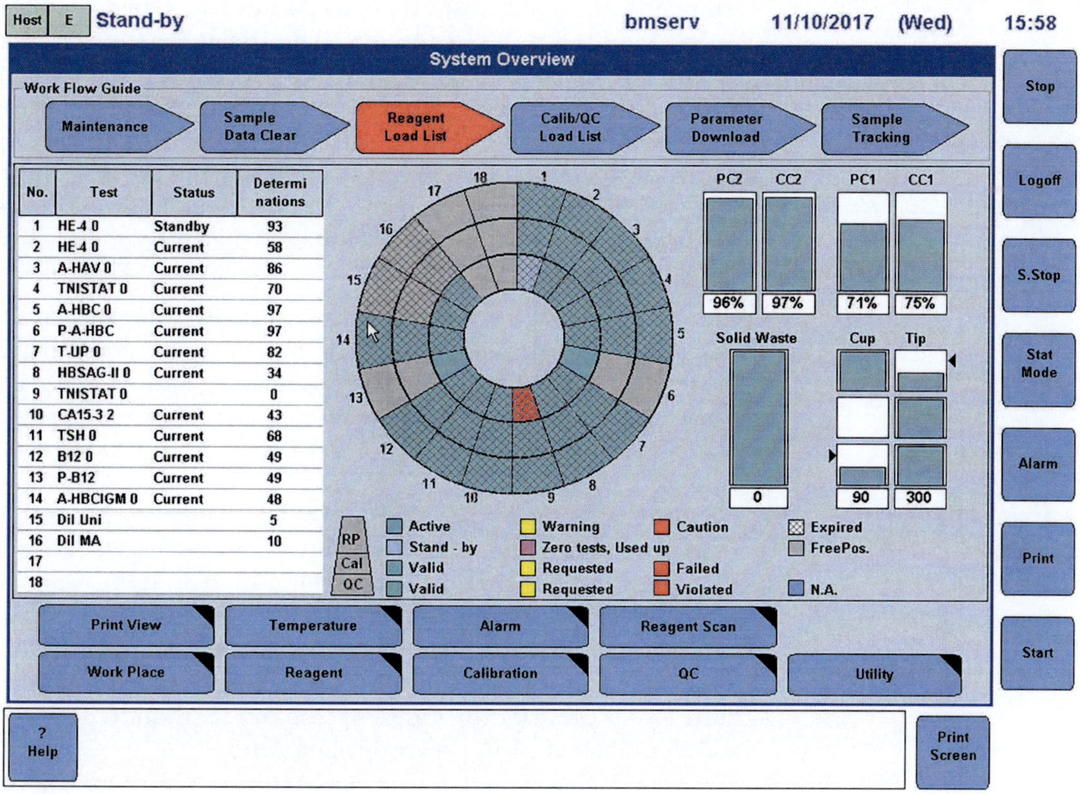

Fig. 4 System Overview screen [25]

5. Check the system water container (*see* **Note 20**): Raise and remove the system water container. Remove the cap and discard any water. Clean the container if it appears to be dirty or contaminated. Fill with distilled or deionised water up to the upper level mark. Add 35 mL of SysWash, pouring carefully to avoid creating bubbles. Dry the outside of the container with paper towels, recap, and return container to the analyser.
6. Checking the liquid waste container: Pull the liquid waste container toward you and cap it. Remove carefully, avoiding the liquid waste outlet. Place a paper towel directly under the waste outlet to avoid spillage. Empty the container and rinse with water. If the inside of the container appears to be dirty, use 70% isopropyl alcohol to rinse the container. Rinse thoroughly with water. Wipe the outside of the container and the compartment housing the container in the analyser with paper towel. Remove paper towel under the waste outlet and replace waste container. Uncap container and push forward so that container opening is under the liquid waste outlet (*see* **Note 21**).

7. Emptying the solid waste tray (*see* **Note 22**): Open the solid waste door and pull out the tray. The Clean Liner has a clear sliding lid. Slide the lid forward to close the Clean Liner. Remove the Clean Liner from the tray and dispose it according to the waste procedures in your laboratory for potentially biohazardous material. Place a fresh Clean Liner in the tray. Verify that the sliding door is open and that the opening is located at the back of the tray. Insert the tray into the analyser and close the door (*see* **Note 23**).
8. Replacing AssayCup and AssayTip trays: Replace any empty AssayCup or AssayTip trays with full ones as required (*see* **Note 24**). Once all necessary consumables and reagents are placed within analyser, close the instrument cover and perform reagent scan by selecting button on System Overview screen.

3.4 Routine Operation

1. Perform calibration with PlGF and sFlt1 CalSet (*see* **Note 25**): Dissolve the contents of both the PlGF and sFlt1 CalSet bottle by adding exactly 1.0 mL of distilled or deionised water to each and allow to stand closed for 15 min to reconstitute. Mix gently to avoid foam formation (*see* **Note 26**). Transfer aliquots of reconstituted calibrators into empty labelled Hitachi cups (*see* **Note 10**) for sampling, or freeze aliquots immediately in labelled plain polypropylene tubes at −20 °C or less. Place the reconstituted calibrators in the sample zone. Choose Start on the touchscreen monitor. Once calibration is complete, remove calibrators from the sample rack and discard appropriately. Check that calibration has been accepted before running QCs or samples (*see* **Notes 27** and **28**).
2. Perform quality control with PreciControl Multimarker (*see* **Note 29**): Dissolve the contents of one bottle by adding exactly 2.0 mL of distilled or deionised water and allow to stand closed for 30 min to reconstitute. Mix gently to avoid foam formation. Transfer the reconstituted controls into empty labelled Hitachi cups for sampling, or freeze aliquots immediately in labelled plain polypropylene tubes. Place the reconstituted QCs in the sample zone (*see* **Note 28**). Choose Start on the touchscreen monitor.
3. Validate calibration and control results: After calibrators and controls have been measured, check that results are valid prior to running any samples (*see* **Notes 27** and **29**). If there are no failed calibrations, and QCs are within the expected range (*see* **Note 29**), continue with routine sample measurement (*see* **Note 26**).

3.5 Routine Sample Measurement

Depending on whether you are using barcoded samples or not, sample tubes may need to be individually labelled and entered into the computer. Our samples were all non-barcoded samples and were manually entered into the analyser; hence, this method will be described.

1. Preparing samples for analysis: Pipette ≥220 μL of sample into corresponding Hitachi cup. Minimum volume required for each sample is as follows: dead space of Hitachi tube (150 μL) + PlGF sample (50 μL) + sFlt1 sample (20 μL) = 220 μL. From the System Overview screen, choose Workplace and then Test Selection. Select the Routine option from the sample area on the top left of the screen. A sequence number is assigned automatically. Select the sample type using the Type drop-down list. Type the rack number in the Rack No. text box. Type the position number within the rack for the sample in the Pos. text box. Type the sample ID in the Sample ID text box, if necessary. Select the test, combination of tests, or test profiles for the sample in the test key matrix (e.g., sFlt1 and PlGF for our samples). Selected tests and profile keys appear white. Choose Save to save the test selection.
2. To load patient samples: Load the racks on a tray. Place the tray on the A-Line (supply). At the same time, verify if there is a tray on the C-Line (output buffer) (Fig. 5).

   Before starting a run, ensure that all necessary samples are on board and test selections made and that position number of each sample on rack matches that entered into the analyser. Press Start. The system performs an initialisation process and then begins to process patient samples. Racks can continue to be loaded using the rack system, either by adding single racks to the A-Line or adding a loaded tray to the A-Line. Racks can

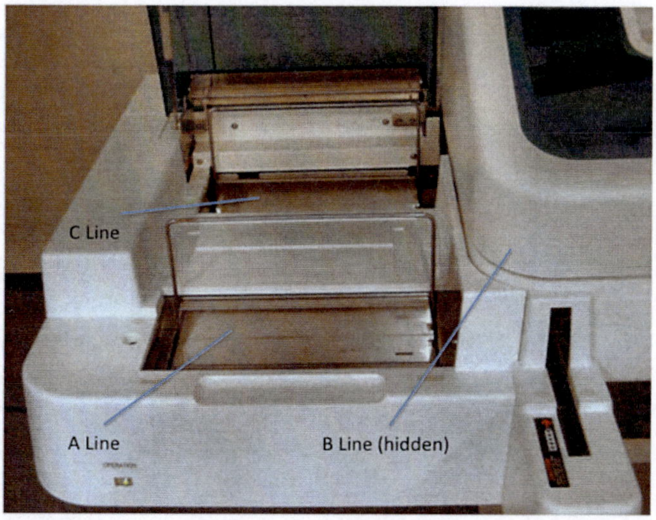

Fig. 5 Rack sampler. Load samples on the A-Line and remove analysed samples from C-Line [25]

only be loaded when the tray indication light is green. When the light is out, do not load racks or load trays onto the analyser.

3. Sample tracking: Use the Sample Tracking window to monitor the progress of sample processing. From the System Overview screen, choose Sample Tracking to open the Sample Tracking window. Obtain more detailed information on the result of a specific sample by selecting the sample from the rack information area on the right side and choosing Show Result. The Test Review window opens.

3.6 Extract Results

1. View patient results: All samples can be viewed from the Data Review screen. Choose Workplace and then Data Review to open the Data Review screen, which is used to perform tasks related to reviewing routine and QC results. Choose Search to open the Sample Search window to search for a specific sample in the database.
2. Print a Result Report: Select the required results by selecting Workplace and then Data Review before printing or viewing this report. Select a single sample, a range of samples, or nonconsecutive samples to be printed from the sample selection list on the left side of the screen. Choose Print, and then select Workplace to open the Workplace Print screen. Choose Result Report from the Workplace Items list. Choose Print to print the report or import to upload to USB.
3. Review results: Review results as they become available using the printout or on the Data Review screen. Use the Test Review window to check results in more detail. Repeat any questionable results, or those with an incomplete status, as necessary.
4. Perform daily maintenance (*see* **Note 30**).

3.7 Switching Off the Analyser

1. Switch off the analyser: Set the operation switch to off (*see* **Note 31**). The analyser goes into Sleep mode and the Sleep window opens (*see* **Note 32**).
2. Prevent evaporation of the system reagents: After switching off the analyser, close the lids on the PC and CC bottles to prevent evaporation of their contents.
3. Final power off checks: If the analyser will remain switched off for longer than 7 days, it is important to prepare the system properly and to perform the correct shutdown maintenance. Failure to observe these recommendations may result in damage to the measuring cell. To complete final power off checks, check individual parts of the instrument.

If the analyser is to be switched off at the circuit breaker, move any reagent packs from the analyser to the refrigerator as temperature control to the reagent rotor will be off. Make sure that the reagent pack lids are tightly closed.

4 Notes

1. The Roche **Cobas® e** 411 analyser is a commercially available immunoassay platform which uses electrochemiluminescence (ECL) immunoassay, based on the streptavidin-biotin technology to generate results, utilising a sandwich immunoassay principle [25]. Samples entered undergo testing for both sFlt1 and PlGF concurrently, and the platform calculates results for each of these biomarkers as well as the sFlt1/PlGF ratio. ECL is a highly sensitive luminescence detection system [26] that amplifies required signals and reduces unrequired signals, allowing high sensitivity and broad dynamic measuring ranges [25]. The system consists of an analyser and a control unit. The analyser performs all functions required for fully automated sample and assay processing and consists of the sample/reagent area, the consumables area, the measuring area, and the operation switch. The control unit consists of a touchscreen monitor, software keyboard, data storage, external printer, and service and host interfaces (Fig. 1) [25].

   The control unit controls the analyser through the user software [25]. When a sample is ready for measurement, an AssayCup is transferred to the aspiration station. The sipper probe aspirates the reaction mixture containing sample and reagents into the measuring cell and also aspirates ProCell (PC), a buffer solution for generating electrochemical signals, and CleanCell (CC), a solution for cleaning the measuring cell. The sipper rinse station externally washes the sipper probe with system water between measurements. The reaction mixture then undergoes the first incubation at 37.0 °C ± 0.3 °C [25]. During the first incubation, a biotinylated monoclonal antibody specific for either sFlt1 or PlGF and a monoclonal antibody specific for either sFlt1 or PlGF, labeled with a ruthenium complex, react to form a sandwich complex [25]. During the second incubation, strong bonding between streptavidin and biotin affixes the antigen/antibody complex to a magnetic microbead [25].

   A magnetic field is applied, and the paramagnetic beads bind to the surface of the measuring cell. PC solution is introduced to separate the bound immunoassay complexes from the free remaining particles to provide tripropylamine (TPA), which is essential for the ECL reaction [25].

2. **Cobas and Elecsys are trademarks of Roche.** The Roche **Cobas® e** 411 analyser specifically requires the reagents and consumables outlined in this chapter in order to function.

3. Reagent kits have been assembled into a single ready-for-use unit that cannot be separated. The reagent pack and reagent rotor are keyed to ensure reagents are placed on the analyser correctly (Fig. 6).

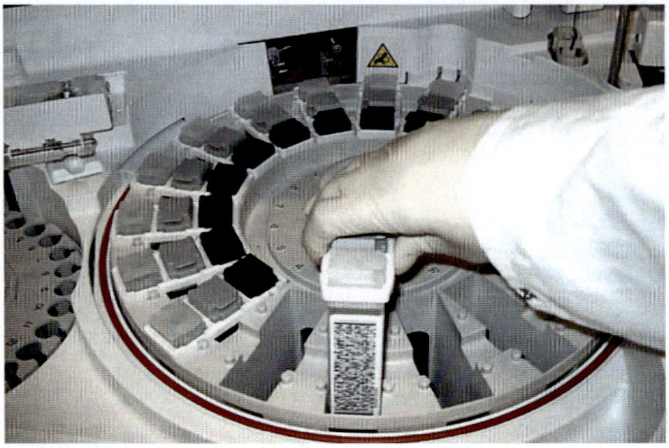

Fig. 6 Reagent rotor [25]

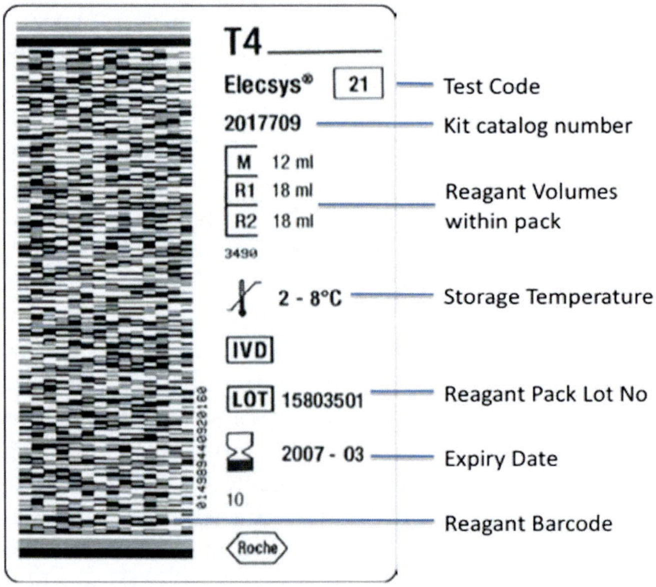

Fig. 7 Calibrator kit barcode card in PDF417 format [25]

4. For both PlGF and sFlt1 calibration kits, the exact lot-specific calibrator values are encoded in the barcode as well as printed on the enclosed calibrator barcode sheet. Each time a calibration is performed, it must be ensured that the calibration is accepted before proceeding further.
5. Each calibrator kit comes with a barcode card in PDF417 format, to be used with the corresponding calibrators (Fig. 7). Information encoded in the calibrator barcode cards includes test number, calibrator lot number, lot identifier to calibrator

barcode labels, what calibrators are to be used and their number of determinations, target or assigned values, and expiration date. Roche Diagnostics GmbH produces a factory master calibration for each calibration lot. The results are encoded into the corresponding reagent barcode. Scan the new barcode card when you use a new lot.

6. The exact lot-specific QC target values and ranges are encoded in the barcodes as well as printed on the value sheet located in the platform Operator Manual. These target values and ranges have been determined and evaluated by Roche. Results must be within the specified ranges. In the event that deviations beyond the range limits are observed, all test steps must be checked and samples should not be run. Each laboratory should establish corrective measures to be taken if values fall outside the defined limits.
7. ProCell (PC) facilitates the assay by conditioning the electrodes, transporting assay reactant mixture, and washing the streptavidin-coated microparticles and signal generation.
8. CleanCell (CC) facilitates the assay by cleansing the tubing system and measuring cell after every measurement and conditioning the electrodes.
9. PC and CC are stored on the analyser, temperature controlled at 28.0 °C ± 2.0 °C. The keyed shape of the reagent compartment ensures that the reagent bottles can only be placed in the proper position.
10. We used Hitachi cups to place samples through the analyser. If using other tubes, particularly long narrow tubes, ensure correct upright vertical position on the rack; otherwise the sample/reagent probe may attempt to sample outside the tube, causing errors and incorrect results.
11. This was a research study using stored, frozen, samples for analysis, each manually labelled with a study ID.
12. If you plan to import results data to USB stick, place in USB drive at rear of analyser prior to switching it on. When the analyser is first switched on, the system performs initialisation to reset mechanisms to their home positions. The log-on screen is displayed throughout initialisation, and then the analyser will enter Standby mode.
13. If any alarms have been issued, an audible warning will sound once the analyser is switched on and the alarm button will display red or yellow. Sound can be switched off to silence alarms at the log-on screen. Select each alarm to view the description. The remedy for each alarm will be displayed in the lower half of the screen. Correct any alarm conditions, close the alarm screen, and continue with log-on procedure.

14. The System Overview screen has a central role (Fig. 4), displaying an overview of the whole system at any time. This screen shows the status of each reagent, the details of the reagents loaded, and details of the inventory. You can open the System Overview screen from any screen by touching the double System Overview icon in the top left corner of the screen. Inventory Area displays the amount of system reagents, AssayCups, AssayTips, and solid waste on the analyser by means of seven bar charts.
15. Store reagent kits upright to ensure complete availability of the microparticles during automatic mixing prior to use. Prior to loading onto the reagent rotor, open lids on each compartment of reagent pack to exclude significant spillage of microparticles into the underside of the lid, which may compromise results obtained. Store at 2–8 °C. Do not freeze.
16. A transparent sipper shield is fitted to the pipetting area, which contains the PC and CC. The sipper shield must be opened to access the system reagent bottles. It is opened and closed by applying pressure to the white metal area at the top to release or engage the latch. The sipper shield should not be opened during operation or programmed maintenance, or the analyser will stop processing, and an alarm will be issued. Hence, you cannot exchange PC and CC during a run, or the run is aborted.
17. Place the PC and CC bottles on the analyser at least 1 h before use. Open the lids of all PC and CC bottles on board prior to starting operation or programmed maintenance functions. If the analyser stands idle for more than 3 h, the bottles should be closed to avoid evaporation effect.
18. Remove the empty PC and CC bottles, indicated in the inventory area on the System Overview screen, and replace them with a set of full bottles. Ensure that each bottle is firmly in place in the correct position with the correct orientation. Place PC only in the left-hand position of each bottle set and CC in the right-hand position (Fig. 8). Always replace PC and CC bottles as sets. If you remove and replace a full (100% volume) bottle from one of the system reagent compartment positions containing a photosensor, the analyser assumes that you have loaded a new bottle set, even if the bottle has been on the analyser for several hours or days. The analyser consequently waits 15 min for temperature equilibration, as is normal for a new bottle set. If you need to load two new bottle sets of PC/CC, load these new bottles as your first inventory check. By the time you are ready to operate, the system reagents should be at the correct temperature. If they are not, you will receive PC/CC reagent temperature alarms. The bottles on the right (Set 1) are consumed first. If replacing the bottles on the right,

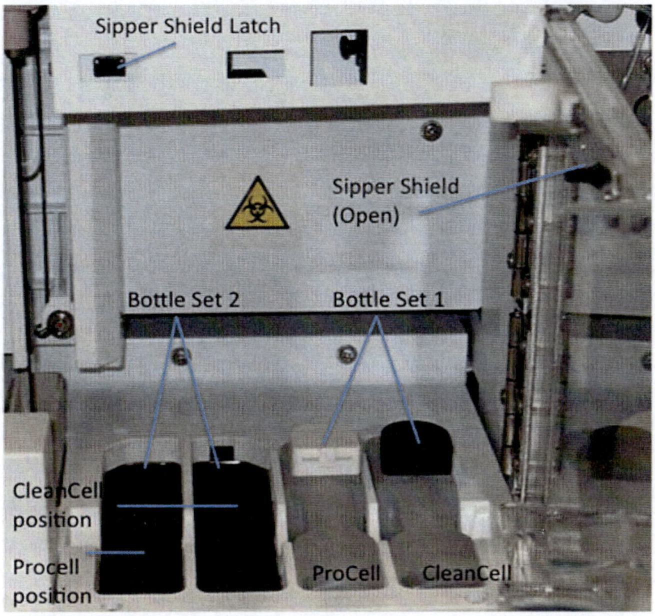

Fig. 8 Sipper shield, CleanCell, and ProCell [25]

move the bottles from the left (Set 2) to the right. Then load the new bottles in the correct positions of Set 2.

19. To load a PC bottle with a new lot number, select Reagent and choose Inventory Set. The Inventory Set window opens. Type the lot number for each PC bottle. The analyser can operate with just one bottle of PC and one bottle of CC reagent, but they must be placed together either as bottle Set 1 or as bottle Set 2.
20. Prior to sample analysis, the system water container needs to be refilled with distilled water containing SysWash.
21. Treat the waste from the waste container as potentially infectious.
22. The solid waste tray is located behind the solid waste door, beneath the AssayTip and AssayCup trays. If the tray is full, remove the Clean Liner and replace it with a new one.
23. The counter for the solid waste, which is located on the System Overview screen, automatically resets to zero (0) when the tray is removed.
24. Do not add or remove single AssayTips or AssayCups. Only load complete trays as supplied. Make sure that the trays are seated properly with the correct orientation. Trays are keyed for proper placement.
25. Calibration and quality controls should be processed prior to sample processing but can be performed at any time during

routine operation. Calibration and QC involve two steps: (1) measuring the calibrators and controls and (2) validating the results. Prepare calibrators as necessary, based on the Reagent Overview screen information updated at the last reagent scan. sFlt1 and PlGF calibrators are lyophilised and require reconstitution. Refer to the specific calibrator package insert. Prepare controls, if necessary, following the instructions on their package inserts. Perform only one calibration procedure per aliquot. Ensure the calibrators are at 20–25 °C prior to measurement.

26. Avoid foam formation in all reagents and sample types, including specimens, calibrators, and controls.
27. From the System Overview screen, select Calibration from the lowest row of buttons, and then select Status. This screen will display whether the calibration is valid by the background color displayed for the calibration. No background color indicates calibration is "available or successful"; red indicates "no calibration available or calibration failed," in which case the calibration needs to be repeated. Alternatively, a calibration Result Report is automatically printed by the analyser after each calibration, and values obtained can be checked using the Calibration Result Sheet in the Platform Operator Manual.
28. Specific calibration racks for our machine were allocated, with specified positions on these racks programmed for PlGF and sFlt1 CalSets.
29. PreciControl Multimarker can be stored at 2–8 °C for up to 72 h or frozen at −20 °C or less for up to 31 days. Ensure the controls are at 20–25 °C prior to measurement. The lyophilised control serum is stable up to the stated expiration date. Treat the reconstituted control as potentially infectious and wear eye protection and gloves to avoid eye and skin irritation. Perform only one control procedure per aliquot, and ensure controls are used within expiry date. Specific QC racks for our analyser were allocated, with specified positions on these racks programmed for PreciControl MM1 and MM2. Run controls daily in parallel with patient samples, once per reagent kit, and whenever a calibration is performed. The control intervals and limits should be adapted to each laboratory's individual requirements. In the event that deviations beyond the range limits are observed, all test steps must be checked. Each laboratory should establish corrective measures to be taken if values fall outside the defined limits.
30. Before the end of routine operation, it is important to ensure that all required maintenance is performed. Each day, the sample/reagent probe requires cleaning, and compartments should be checked for condensation. In addition to the routine daily maintenance, this could also include other scheduled maintenance, for example, weekly and monthly maintenance.

31. After routine operation is finished and you have performed all the required maintenance, you can switch off the analyser. If using a USB to back up result data, it is safe to remove the device once the analyser is switched off. Under normal circumstances, it is not necessary to shut down the analyser. Keep the circuit breaker on the right of the analyser on to maintain the temperatures in the reagent rotor and system reagent compartments.
32. In sleep mode, the analyser remains powered, and the temperatures in the reagent rotor and system reagent compartments are maintained. The monitor screen goes blank after a few minutes.

References

1. Ghulmiyyah L, Sibai B (2012) Maternal mortality from preeclampsia/eclampsia. Semin Perinatol 36(1):56–59
2. Khan KS et al (2006) WHO analysis of causes of maternal death: a systematic review. Lancet 367(9516):1066–1074
3. National Collaborating Centre for W.s. and H (2010) Children's, National Institute for Health and Clinical Excellence: guidance, in hypertension in pregnancy: the management of hypertensive disorders during pregnancy. RCOG Press Royal College of Obstetricians and Gynaecologists, London
4. WHO (2011) WHO recommendations for prevention and treatment of pre-eclampsia and eclampsia. WHO, Geneva
5. American College of Obstetricians and Gynecologists; Task Force on Hypertension in Pregnancy (2013) Hypertension in pregnancy. Report of the American College of Obstetricians and Gynecologists' Task Force on hypertension in pregnancy. Obstet Gynecol 122(5):1122–1131
6. GWHO (2011) WHO recommendations for prevention and treatment of pre-eclampsia and eclampsia. In: WHO Guidelines Approved by the Guidelines Review Committee. WHO, Geneva
7. Dekker G, Sibai B (2001) Primary, secondary, and tertiary prevention of pre-eclampsia. Lancet 357(9251):209–215
8. Levine RJ, Maynard SE, Qian C, Lim KH, England LJ, Yu KF, Schisterman EF, Thadhani R, Sachs BP, Epstein FH, Sibai BM, Sukhatme VP, Karumanchi SA (2004) Circulating angiogenic factors and the risk of preeclampsia. N Engl J Med 350:672–683
9. Redman CW, Sargent IL (2010) Immunology of pre-eclampsia. Am J Reprod Immunol 63(6):534–543
10. Maynard SE et al (2003) Excess placental soluble fms-like tyrosine kinase 1 (sFlt1) may contribute to endothelial dysfunction, hypertension, and proteinuria in preeclampsia. J Clin Invest 111(5):649–658
11. Stepan H (2009) Angiogenic factors and preeclampsia: an early marker is needed. Clin Sci (Lond) 116(3):231–232
12. Rana S et al (2012) Angiogenic factors and the risk of adverse outcomes in women with suspected preeclampsia. Circulation 125(7):911–919
13. Liu Y et al (2015) Diagnostic accuracy of the soluble Fms-like tyrosine kinase-1/placental growth factor ratio for preeclampsia: a meta-analysis based on 20 studies. Arch Gynecol Obstet 292:507
14. Zeisler H, Hund M, Verlohren S (2016) The sFlt-1:PlGF ratio in women with suspected preeclampsia. N Engl J Med 374(18):1785–1786
15. Zeisler H et al (2016) Predictive value of the sFlt-1:PlGF ratio in women with suspected preeclampsia. N Engl J Med 374(1):13–22
16. Zeisler H et al (2016) Soluble fms-like tyrosine kinase-1-to-placental growth factor ratio and time to delivery in women with suspected preeclampsia. Obstet Gynecol 128(2):261–269
17. Verlohren S et al (2012) The sFlt-1/PlGF ratio in different types of hypertensive pregnancy disorders and its prognostic potential in preeclamptic patients. Am J Obstet Gynecol 206(1):58.e1–58.e8
18. Verlohren S et al (2010) An automated method for the determination of the sFlt-1/PIGF ratio in the assessment of preeclampsia. Am J Obstet Gynecol 202(2):161.e1–161.e11
19. Engels T et al (2013) Automated measurement of sFlt1, PlGF and sFlt1/PlGF ratio in differential diagnosis of hypertensive pregnancy disorders. Hypertens Pregnancy 32(4):459–473

20. Sunderji S et al (2010) Automated assays for sVEGF R1 and PlGF as an aid in the diagnosis of preterm preeclampsia: a prospective clinical study. Am J Obstet Gynecol 202(1):40.e1–40.e7
21. Andersen LB et al (2015) Diagnosis of preeclampsia with soluble Fms-like tyrosine kinase 1/placental growth factor ratio: an inter-assay comparison. J Am Soc Hypertens 9(2):86–96
22. Benton SJ et al (2011) Angiogenic factors as diagnostic tests for preeclampsia: a performance comparison between two commercial immunoassays. Am J Obstet Gynecol 205(5):469.e1–469.e8
23. Lehnen H et al (2013) Prenatal Clinical Assessment of sFlt-1 (Soluble fms-like Tyrosine Kinase-1)/PlGF (Placental Growth Factor) Ratio as a Diagnostic Tool for Preeclampsia, Pregnancy-induced Hypertension, and Proteinuria. Geburtshilfe Frauenheilkd 73(5):440–445
24. Anderson UD et al (2015) First trimester prediction of preeclampsia. Curr Hypertens Rep 17(9):584
25. Cobas e 411 analyzer. Operator's manual. Version 2.1. Roche Diagnostics GmbH. Internal Data on File. See also www.cobas.com
26. Bramham K et al (2015) [42-OR]: diagnostic accuracy of placental growth factor in women with chronic kidney disease or hypertension and suspected preeclampsia: a prospective cohort study. Pregnancy Hypertens 5(1):21

Chapter 3

Assessing the Circulating Placental-Specific Anti-angiogenic Protein sFLT-1 e15a in Preeclampsia

Kirsten Palmer

Abstract

Preeclampsia is a common obstetric complication globally responsible for a significant burden of maternal and perinatal morbidity and mortality. The anti-angiogenic protein, sFLT-1, plays a central role in its pathophysiology. sFLT-1 is released from a range of tissues into the circulation, where it antagonizes the activity of vascular endothelial growth factor and placental growth factor leading to endothelial dysfunction. The resulting widespread endothelial dysfunction produces the clinical features of preeclampsia including hypertension and proteinuria. Multiple splice variants of sFLT-1 have been identified, with one, known as sFLT-1 e15a, present only in humans and higher-order primates. This sFLT-1 variant is also the main form of sFLT-1 produced by the placenta. Recent work has shown that sFLT-1 e15a is significantly elevated in the placenta and circulation of women with preeclampsia. It is also biologically active, capable of causing endothelial dysfunction and end-organ dysfunction seen in preeclampsia. Indeed, overexpression of sFLT-1 e15a in mice recapitulates the preeclamptic phenotype in pregnancy. No commercial assay currently exists to analyze sFLT-1 e15a protein levels. Here, a new ELISA method to determine circulating sFLT-1 variant levels is described.

Key words sFLT-1, Splice variant, Preeclampsia, Immunoassay, ELISA, Protein

1 Introduction

Soluble fms-like tyrosine kinase-1 (sFLT-1) plays a key role in the pathophysiology of preeclampsia. Circulating sFLT-1 serum levels are significantly increased in women with preeclampsia compared to normal pregnancy, with levels correlating with disease severity [1–3]. Elevated sFLT-1 causes the preeclamptic phenotype through antagonizing the actions of vascular endothelial growth factor (VEGF) and placental growth factor (PlGF) [4–7]. This leads to widespread endothelial dysfunction and end-organ dysfunction seen as the classic features of preeclampsia, being hypertension and proteinuria [5, 8]. Indeed, overexpression of sFLT-1 in animal models has been shown to produce a preeclamptic-like phenotype [5, 9, 10], while neutralizing its effects, either through reducing sFLT-1 levels or increasing VEGF and PlGF levels, leads to a resolution in preeclamptic features

Padma Murthi and Cathy Vaillancourt (eds.), *Preeclampsia: Methods and Protocols*, Methods in Molecular Biology, vol. 1710, https://doi.org/10.1007/978-1-4939-7498-6_3,

in animal models [10–13]. These findings have been supported in human trials using apheresis to transiently reduce circulating sFLT-1 levels [14]. These findings all support the pivotal role that sFLT-1 plays in producing the preeclamptic phenotype.

sFLT-1 results either from alternative splicing of the *FLT-1* pre-mRNA [15] or through cleavage of the ectodomain of FLT-1 [16]. During the last decade, four truncated splice variants have been identified [17–19]. Of these, three sFLT-1 variants appear to be translated into protein, two of which are upregulated in preeclamptic placenta [17]. The two variants altered in the setting of preeclampsia are sFLT-1 i13 (also known as sFLT-1, sFLT-1_v1 [17]) and sFLT-1 e15a (also known as sFLT-1_v2 [17], sFLT-1 14 [18]). These splice variants share significant sequence homology with the full-length FLT-1 receptor, differing only at their C-terminal ends (Fig. 1). Furthermore, these splice variants have significantly different tissue distributions [20], raising the potential for different physiological and pathological roles.

The sFLT-1 e15a variant has been found to be specific to humans and higher-order primates, having been inserted into the primate genome approximately 40 million years ago [19]. More importantly, it is primarily produced by the placenta, where it constitutes >80% of all placental transcripts from the *FLT-1* pre-mRNA [20]. Within the placenta, sFLT-1 e15a is mainly produced by the syncytiotrophoblast and the cytotrophoblasts, where its mRNA expression is 100-fold greater than in placental vascular smooth muscle cells, endothelial cells, and macrophages [19]. In preeclampsia, all *FLT-1* transcripts are upregulated [20]; however, sFLT-1 e15a shows the greatest increase, with mRNA levels appearing to correlate with severity of preeclampsia [21].

More recently, it has been shown that the sFLT-1 e15a variant protein is biologically active, being capable of antagonizing the actions of VEGF [22]. It is also capable of causing endothelial dysfunction, with evidence of impaired endothelial cell invasion, migration, and tubule formation [22]. With the development of a new enzyme-linked immunosorbent assay (ELISA) described here, circulating levels of sFLT-1 e15a protein can now also be assessed. sFLT-1 e15a levels have been shown to gradually rise with advancing gestation [22, 23] and are significantly elevated in women destined to develop preeclampsia, especially in those diagnosed with the early-onset form [22–24].

While many commercially available assay systems are available to analyze total sFLT-1 levels, there are no currently available reagents or assays to examine the sFLT-1 splice variant proteins. Here I describe a method for detecting the placental-specific sFLT-1 variant, sFLT-1 e15a, including antibody development and protein production for quantification and assay standards.

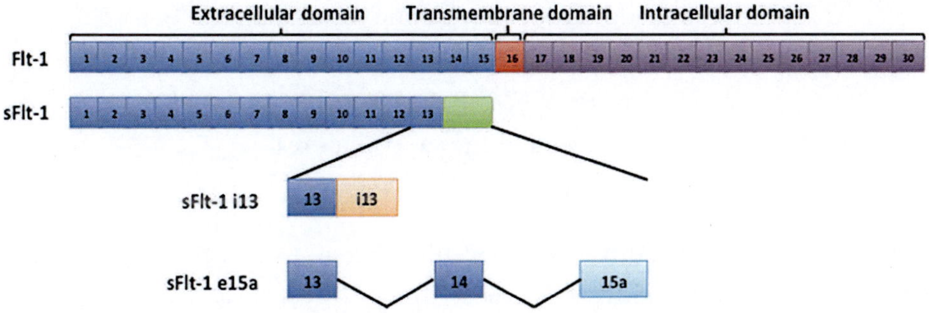

FLT-1 650 kkeitirdqeapyllrnlsdhtvaissttldchangvpepqitwfknnhkiqqepgiilgpgsstlfiervtee...

sFLT-1 i13 650 kkeitirgehcnkkavfsriskfkstrndcttqsnvkh

sFLT-1 e15a 650 kkeitirdqeapyllrnlsdhtvaissttldchangvpepqitwfknnhkiqqepelytstspssssspls[11]

Fig. 1 Schematic and amino acid sequence alignment for human FLT-1, sFLT-1 i13, and sFLT-1 e15a. Schematic demonstrating shared exons between the full-length and soluble FLT-1, as well as unique C-terminal regions. The amino acid sequence for all proteins is shown from amino acid 650, prior sequence share 100% homology between the three proteins. The unique C-terminal tails are highlighted for sFLT-1 i13 and sFLT-1 e15a (*orange*). The sFLT-1 e15a poly-serine tail continues for further 11 serine residues

2 Materials

2.1 General

1. Ultracentrifuge.
2. Orbital shaker and conical flasks.
3. Tissue culture incubator.
4. Spectrophotometer.

2.2 Plasmid Production

1. Phusion high-fidelity PCR kit, restriction enzymes, Antarctic Phosphatase, and T4 DNA ligase (New England Biolabs).
2. Real-time PCR machine.
3. Agarose, gel tank, and power pack.
4. Ultraviolet light box.
5. QIAquick gel extraction kit (Qiagen).
6. QIAquick PCR purification kit (Qiagen).
7. One Shot® TOP10 chemically competent *E. coli* (Invitrogen).
8. Agar plates.
9. LB broth.
10. QIAprep Spin Miniprep Kit (Qiagen).
11. EndoFree Plasmid Maxi Kit (Qiagen).

2.3 Protein Production

1. 293F cells.
2. FreeStyle 293 expression media (Invitrogen).

3. Antibiotic/antimycotic solution.
4. FreeStyle MAX transfection reagent (Invitrogen).
5. OptiPro SFM (Invitrogen).
6. LucraTone™ Lupin (Millipore).
7. Pluronic acid.

2.4 Protein Purification

1. Anti-FLAG M2 affinity resin (Sigma).
2. Polypropylene columns.
3. FLAG peptide (Sigma).
4. 0.1 M glycine pH 3.5.
5. Tris-buffered saline (TBS).
6. Amicon spin ultraconcentrators (Millipore).
7. Protease inhibitors.
8. Ethylenediaminetetraacetic acid (EDTA).

2.5 ELISA

1. EZ-Link-Sulfo-NHS-LC biotin (Thermo Fisher Scientific) or any appropriate biotinylation protocol.
2. Slide-A-Lyzer mini-dialysis units (Thermo Fisher Scientific) or any appropriate dialysis equipment.
3. Phosphate-buffered saline (PBS).
4. 96-well MaxiSorp immunoplates.
5. Mouse monoclonal anti-FLT-1 antibody (MAB321, R&D Systems).
6. Bovine serum albumin.
7. Streptavidin-HRP.
8. Tetramethylbenzidine (TMB).
9. 1 M H_2SO_4.

3 Methods

3.1 Polyclonal Antibody Development

1. Produce an unconjugated peptide specific to sFlt-1 e15a (KNNHKIQQEPELYTSTC). Refer to **Note 1** regarding commercial production.
2. Conjugate to keyhole limpet hemocyanin (KLH) and emulsify in incomplete Freund's adjuvant (IFA) in preparation for immunization of specific pathogen-free (SPF) rabbits.
3. Produce polyclonal antibody with a commercial company or in-house if required facilities are available (*see* **Note 1**). This involves the immunization of two rabbits over a 10-week period, obtaining serum prior to immunization and at 4, 8, and 10 weeks during the protocol. ELISA is used to assess antibody

titers and determine whether the rabbits have an adequate antibody response. Those rabbits with a good antibody response should receive an extra immunization prior to final sera collection through an exsanguination bleed.

4. Proceed to protein A purification to isolate the IgG antibody component from the sera.

3.2 sFLT-1 e15a Plasmid Production

1. Obtain a plasmid optimized for protein production. This protocol uses a pEFBOS vector (MTA from The Walter and Eliza Hall Institute of Medical Research; *see* **Note 2**).
2. Isolate sFLT-1 variant DNA from placental tissue or plasmid DNA. This protocol uses an sFlt-1 e15a pcDNA4/HisMax vector (obtained as a gift from Dr. Christie Thomas, University of Iowa).
3. Amplify sFlt-1 e15a DNA from the sFlt-1 e15a pcDNA4/HisMax vector using high-fidelity PCR using specifically designed primers. For the pEFBOS vector, an MluI restriction enzyme site is required at the 5′ and 3′ end. The primer sequences required for cloning sFLT-1 e15a and inserting the Mlu1 sites are sFlt-1 e15a forward primer 5′-TAATACGCGTAC CATGGTCAGCTACTGGGACAC-3′ and sFlt-1 e15a reverse primer 5′-TGATACGCGTTAGCTATGATGATGATGATGA TGACGA-3′.
4. Set up PCR in accordance with the recommended Phusion high-fidelity protocol.
5. Perform real-time PCR with the following cycling conditions: 98 °C for 1 min, 98 °C for 10 s, then 72 °C for 60 s for 35 cycles, and 72 °C for 10 min and then hold on 4 °C.
6. Run PCR products on a 1.2% agarose gel to isolate the DNA band.
7. Purify DNA using the QIAquick gel extraction kit in accordance with the manufacturer's instructions.
8. Prepare sFlt-1 variant DNA for pEFBOS plasmid insertion with an MluI restriction enzyme digest at 37 °C overnight. Cease reaction by heating to 65 °C for 20 min.
9. Gel purify cut DNA on a 1.2% agarose gel and extract it using the QIAquick gel extraction kit.
10. Prepare the pEFBOS vector for ligation through an MluI restriction enzyme digest at 37 °C overnight to create complementary ends.
11. Proceed immediately to dephosphorylation of the cut plasmid to prevent self-ligation through the addition of Antarctic Phosphatase and its buffer to the reaction. This reaction requires further incubation at 37 °C for 60 min, prior to heat inactivation at 65 °C for 20 min.

12. Gel purify the vector using the QIAquick PCR purification kit as per manufacturer's instructions after running on a 1.2% agarose gel.
13. Ligate cut sFlt-1 e15a DNA and pEFBOS using T4 DNA ligase with the vector in a 3:1 molar ratio at room temperature for 10 min prior to heat inactivation at 65 °C for 10 min.
14. Run ligated plasmid DNA on a 1.2% agarose prior to purification using the QIAquick PCR purification kit. This final plasmid produces a secreted sFLT-1 e15a protein with a FLAG-tag at the N-terminus.
15. Transform plasmid DNA into One Shot® TOP10 chemically competent *E. coli*, as per manufacturer's guidelines.
16. Streak cells onto ampicillin-selective agar plates and incubate overnight at 37 °C.
17. Add selected colonies to 1.5 mL LB broth (starter culture) and culture overnight at 37 °C with vigorous shaking.
18. Use 1 mL of the starter culture for DNA isolation and purification using a miniprep kit in accordance with manufacturer's instructions.
19. Elute miniprep DNA in sterile water.
20. Analyze plasmid DNA by agarose gel electrophoresis. Samples running at the correct size can be sequenced to ensure correct sFlt-1 e15a sequence and in frame orientation.
21. Expand plasmids with correct sequence through the addition of 500 μL of the transformed *E. coli* starter culture to 250 mL of LB broth. Incubate overnight at 37 °C with vigorous shaking.
22. Obtain bacterial cell pellets by centrifugation at 6000 × *g* for 15 min at 4 °C. Larger-scale plasmid isolation and purification are achieved using a Maxi Kit in accordance with manufacturer's instructions.

3.3 sFLT-1 e15a Protein Production

1. Use 293F mammalian cell system for production of FLAG-tagged sFlt-1 e15a protein (*see* **Note 3**).
2. Culture 293F cells in 8% CO_2 at 37 °C on an orbital shaker at 150 rpm.
3. The day prior to transfection, passage cells to give 0.7×10^6 cells/mL giving a cell density of $1.2–1.5 \times 10^6$ cells/mL on the day of transfection.
4. Spin cells at 375 × *g* for 5 min, remove the supernatant, and resuspend cells in fresh FreeStyle 293 expression media containing antibiotic/antimycotic solution (1:100) to give a concentration of 1×10^6 cells/mL.

5. The optimal ratio of plasmid DNA to FreeStyle MAX transfection reagent is 1:2. Dilute these two reagents separately in OptiPro SFM prior to gentle mixing and incubation at room temperature for 10 min.
6. Add the resulting DNA-lipid complexes dropwise to cells prior to returning to the 37 °C incubator.
7. Add LucraTone™ Lupin (1:40) and pluronic acid (1:100) 24 h following transfection to promote protein production and prevent cell shearing, respectively.
8. Obtain media 72 h following transfection for optimal protein yields.

3.4 sFLT-1 e15a Protein Purification

1. Purify the FLAG-tagged protein from 293F cell culture media using anti-FLAG M2 affinity resin.
2. Prepare 25 mL polypropylene columns by adding anti-FLAG M2 resin to give a resin bed of 1 mL volume.
3. Wash the resin bed with 4 × 5 mL washes in 0.1 M glycine pH 3.5.
4. Wash with 4 × 5 mL in Tris-buffered saline (TBS).
5. Spin the cell culture media at 375 × *g* for 5 min to clear all cellular material prior to the addition of NaCl to a final concentration of 0.15 M and neutralize the pH.
6. Mix the cell culture supernatant with the resin and rotate at 4 °C for 4 h to optimize binding.
7. Drain the resin-media mix through the columns to collect the resin.
8. Wash with 3 × 25 mL TBS washes.
9. Add 1 mL of TBS containing 100 μg/mL of FLAG peptide and incubate on ice for 1 h.
10. Elute the FLAG-tagged sFLT-1 e15a over five 1 mL TBS elutions.
11. Pool elutions and concentrate the protein using Amicon spin ultraconcentrators, as per the manufacturer's instructions.
12. Determine protein concentration on spectrophotometry at 280 nm.
13. Add protease inhibitors (1:100) and EDTA to a final concentration of 2 mM to inhibit protein degradation.
14. Store sFLT-1 e15a protein at 4 °C for immediate use or aliquot and freeze at −40 °C for subsequent use.

3.5 sFLT-1 e15a ELISA

1. Biotinylate sFLT-1 e15a polyclonal antibody using EZ-Link-Sulfo-NHS-LC biotin. Undertake biotinylation in accordance with manufacturer's instructions.

2. Remove excess biotin using dialysis, such as the Slide-A-Lyzer mini-dialysis units. This is performed in PBS with multiple buffer exchanges and over a period of 18–24 h.
3. Determine biotinylated antibody concentration by spectrophotometry.
4. Coat a 96-well immunoplate with 4 μg/mL of a mouse monoclonal anti-FLT-1 antibody in PBS (*see* **Note 4**).
5. Incubate plates overnight at room temperature.
6. Perform three washes in PBS Tween-20.
7. Block the wells with 1% BSA/PBS at room temperature for 1 h.
8. Perform three further washes with PBS Tween-20.
9. Add 100 μL of sample and controls to desired wells. Use a standard curve of the FLAG-tagged protein produced in Subheading 3.4 (*see* **Note 5**).
10. Incubate at room temperature for 2 h.
11. Wash three times with PBS Tween-20
12. Add the biotinylated sFLT-1 e15a polyclonal antibody at 10 μg/mL in PBS as the detection antibody.
13. Incubate for 2 h at room temperature.
14. Wash three times with PBS Tween-20.
15. Add 100 μL of streptavidin-HRP per well.
16. Incubate at room temperature for 20 min.
17. Wash three times with PBS Tween-20.
18. Add 100 μL of TMB until appropriate color change has occurred or 30 min has passed.
19. Stop the reaction by adding 50 μL of 1 M H_2SO_4.
20. Obtain results using a microplate reader at OD_{450} with an OD_{570} subtraction.

4 Notes

1. Peptide production and conjugation, as well as rabbit immunizations, are available commercially or can be produced by independent researchers if the facilities are available. This protocol used Auspep (Australia) for peptide production and Invitrogen for peptide conjugation and rabbit immunizations.
2. For sFLT-1 e15a plasmid production, any plasmid for protein production can be used. These will have a variety of required restriction enzyme sites to enable DNA insertion into the vector. This protocol describes the use of a pEFBOS vector and will need to be modified if other vector systems are used. This

vector was chosen as it produced greater protein yields than other vectors assessed.

3. sFLT-1 e15a protein production described here is for small-scale production. This process can be scaled up for large-scale protein production or commercial companies are available for large-scale custom production.
4. This protocol has been optimized using R&D Systems anti-FLT-1 monoclonal antibody, MAB321. Other anti-FLT-1 antibodies may also be suitable, however would need to be assessed prior to large-scale use.
5. Purified sFlt-1 e15a protein (FLAG-tagged protein) is used for standard curves to enable quantification of serum levels. It is recommended that control samples are run on all plates to enable inter-run comparisons, as well as assessing intraplate and interplate coefficient of variance.

Acknowledgment

I would like to acknowledge Professor Terrence Johns for his assistance with peptide design and ELISA optimization. I would also like to acknowledge Dr. Tu'uhevaha Kaitu'u-Lino for her advice with ELISA development and Dr. Sandra Nicholson for her assistance with optimizing sFLT-1 e15a protein production. This work received funding support from the Royal Australian and New Zealand College of Obstetricians and Gynaecologists Arthur Wilson Memorial scholarship and Keith Fitzmaurice Bursary, as well as the National Health and Medical Research Council (#607219).

References

1. Levine RJ, Maynard SE, Qian C, Lim K-H, England LJ, KF Y, Schisterman EF, Thadhani R, Sachs BP, Epstein FH, Sibai BM, Sukhatme VP, Karumanchi SA (2004) Circulating angiogenic factors and the risk of preeclampsia. N Engl J Med 350(7):672–683. https://doi.org/10.1056/NEJMoa031884
2. Levine RJ, Qian C, Maynard SE, KF Y, Epstein FH, Karumanchi SA (2006) Serum sFlt1 concentration during preeclampsia and mid trimester blood pressure in healthy nulliparous women. Am J Obstet Gynecol 194(4):1034–1041. https://doi.org/10.1016/j.ajog.2005.10.192
3. Shibata E, Rajakumar A, Powers RW, Larkin RW, Gilmour C, Bodnar LM, Crombleholme WR, Ness RB, Roberts JM, Hubel CA (2005) Soluble fms-like tyrosine kinase 1 is increased in preeclampsia but not in normotensive pregnancies with small-for-gestational-age neonates: relationship to circulating placental growth factor. J Clin Endocrinol Metab 90(8):4895–4903. https://doi.org/10.1210/jc.2004-1955
4. Clark DE, Smith SK, He Y, Day KA, Licence DR, Corps AN, Lammoglia R, Charnock-Jones DS (1998) A vascular endothelial growth factor antagonist is produced by the human placenta and released into the maternal circulation. Biol Reprod 59(6):1540–1548
5. Maynard S, Min J, Merchan J, Lim K, Li J, Mondal S, Libermann T, Morgan J, Sellke F, Stillman I, Epstein F, Sukhatme V, Ananth Karumanchi S (2003) Excess placental soluble fms-like tyrosine kinase 1 (sFlt-1) may contribute to endothelial dysfunction, hypertension, and proteinuria in preeclampsia. J Clin Invest 111(5):649–658
6. Christinger HW, Fuh G, de Vos AM, Wiesmann C (2004) The crystal structure of placental

growth factor in complex with domain 2 of vascular endothelial growth factor receptor-1. J Biol Chem 279(11):10382–10388. https://doi.org/10.1074/jbc.M313237200
7. Wiesmann C, Fuh G, Christinger HW, Eigenbrot C, Wells JA, de Vos AM (1997) Crystal structure at 1.7 A resolution of VEGF in complex with domain 2 of the Flt-1 receptor. Cell 91(5):695–704
8. Ahmad SAA (2004) Elevated placental soluble vascular endothelial growth factor receptor-1 inhibits angiogenesis in preeclampsia. Circ Res 95(9):884–891. https://doi.org/10.1161/01.RES.0000147365.86159.f5
9. Gilbert JS, Babcock SA, Granger JP (2007) Hypertension produced by reduced uterine perfusion in pregnant rats is associated with increased soluble fms-like tyrosine kinase-1 expression. Hypertension 50(6):1142–1147. https://doi.org/10.1161/HYPERTENSIONAHA.107.096594
10. Kumasawa K, Ikawa M, Kidoya H, Hasuwa H, Saito-Fujita T, Morioka Y, Takakura N, Kimura T, Okabe M (2011) Pravastatin induces placental growth factor (PGF) and ameliorates preeclampsia in a mouse model. Proc Natl Acad Sci U S A 108:1451. https://doi.org/10.1073/pnas.1011293108
11. Bergmann A, Ahmad S, Cudmore M, Gruber AD, Wittschen P, Lindenmaier W, Christofori G, Gross V, Gonzalves A, Grone HJ, Ahmed A, Weich HA (2010) Reduction of circulating soluble Flt-1 alleviates preeclampsia-like symptoms in a mouse model. J Cell Mol Med 14(6B):1857–1867. https://doi.org/10.1111/j.1582-4934.2009.00820.x
12. Gilbert JS, Verzwyvelt J, Colson D, Arany M, Karumanchi SA, Granger JP (2010) Recombinant vascular endothelial growth factor 121 infusion lowers blood pressure and improves renal function in rats with placentalischemia-induced hypertension. Hypertension 55(2):380–385. https://doi.org/10.1161/HYPERTENSIONAHA.109.141937
13. Li Z, Zhang Y, Ying Ma J, Kapoun AM, Shao Q, Kerr I, Lam A, O'Young G, Sannajust F, Stathis P, Schreiner G, Karumanchi SA, Protter AA, Pollitt NS (2007) Recombinant vascular endothelial growth factor 121 attenuates hypertension and improves kidney damage in a rat model of preeclampsia. Hypertension 50(4):686–692. https://doi.org/10.1161/HYPERTENSIONAHA.107.092098
14. Thadhani R, Hagmann H, Schaarschmidt W, Roth B, Cingoez T, Karumanchi SA, Wenger J, Lucchesi KJ, Tamez H, Lindner T, Fridman A, Thome U, Kribs A, Danner M, Hamacher S, Mallmann P, Stepan H, Benzing T (2016) Removal of soluble Fms-like tyrosine kinase-1 by dextran sulfate apheresis in preeclampsia. J Am Soc Nephrol 27(3):903–913. https://doi.org/10.1681/ASN.2015020157
15. He Y, Smith SK, Day KA, Clark DE, Licence DR, Charnock-Jones DS (1999) Alternative splicing of vascular endothelial growth factor (VEGF)-R1 (FLT-1) pre-mRNA is important for the regulation of VEGF activity. Mol Endocrinol 13(4):537–545. https://doi.org/10.1210/mend.13.4.0265
16. Rahimi N, Golde TE, Meyer RD (2009) Identification of ligand-induced proteolytic cleavage and ectodomain shedding of VEGFR-1/FLT1 in leukemic cancer cells. Cancer Res 69(6):2607–2614. https://doi.org/10.1158/0008-5472.CAN-08-2905
17. Heydarian M, McCaffrey T, Florea L, Yang Z, Ross MM, Zhou W, Maynard SE (2009) Novel splice variants of sFlt1 are upregulated in preeclampsia. Placenta 30(3):250–255. https://doi.org/10.1016/j.placenta.2008.12.010
18. Sela S, Itin A, Natanson-Yaron S, Greenfield C, Goldman-Wohl D, Yagel S, Keshet E (2008) A novel human-specific soluble vascular endothelial growth factor receptor 1: cell type-specific splicing and implications to vascular endothelial growth factor homeostasis and preeclampsia. Circ Res 102(12):1566–1574. https://doi.org/10.1161/circresaha.108.171504
19. Thomas CP, Andrews JI, Raikwar NS, Kelley EA, Herse F, Dechend R, Golos TG, Liu KZ (2009) A recently evolved novel trophoblast-enriched secreted form of fms-like tyrosine kinase-1 variant is up-regulated in hypoxia and preeclampsia. J Clin Endocrinol Metab 94(7):2524–2530. https://doi.org/10.1210/jc.2009-0017
20. Jebbink J, Keijser R, Veenboer G, van der Post J, Ris-Stalpers C, Afink G (2011) Expression of placental FLT1 transcript variants relates to both gestational hypertensive disease and fetal growth. Hypertension 58(1):70–76. https://doi.org/10.1161/HYPERTENSIONAHA.110.164079
21. Whitehead CL, Palmer KR, Nilsson U, Gao Y, Saglam B, Lappas M, Tong S (2011) Placental expression of a novel primate-specific splice variant of sFlt-1 is upregulated in pregnancies complicated by severe early onset preeclampsia. BJOG 118(10):1268–1271. https://doi.org/10.1111/j.1471-0528.2011.02962.x
22. Palmer KR, Kaitu'u-Lino TJ, Hastie R, Hannan NJ, Ye L, Binder N, Cannon P, Tuohey L, Johns TG, Shub A, Tong S (2015) Placental-specific sFLT-1 e15a protein is increased in

preeclampsia, antagonizes vascular endothelial growth factor signaling, and has antiangiogenic activity. Hypertension 66(6):1251–1259. https://doi.org/10.1161/HYPERTENSIONAHA.115.05883

23. Souders CA, Maynard SE, Yan J, Wang Y, Boatright NK, Sedan J, Balyozian D, Cheslock PS, Molrine DC, Simas TA (2015) Circulating levels of sFlt1 splice variants as predictive markers for the development of preeclampsia. Int J Mol Sci 16(6):12436–12453. https://doi.org/10.3390/ijms160612436

24. Palmer KR, Kaitu'u-Lino TJ, Cannon P, Tuohey L, De Silva MS, Varas-Godoy M, Acuna S, Galaz J, Tong S, Illanes SE (2017) Maternal plasma concentrations of the placental specific sFLT-1 variant, sFLT-1 e15a, in fetal growth restriction and preeclampsia. J Matern Fetal Neonatal Med 30:635–639. https://doi.org/10.1080/14767058.2016.1182975

Chapter 4

Role of Activin A in the Pathogenesis of Endothelial Cell Dysfunction in Preeclampsia

Sebastian R. Hobson, Rebecca Lim, Joanne C. Mockler, Seshini Gurusinghe, and Euan M. Wallace

Abstract

This chapter describes the methodologies which may be used in evaluating in vitro endothelial cell dysfunction in preeclampsia.

Key words Preeclampsia, Endothelial function, Activin A, Follistatin, Endothelin, ICAM-1, VCAM-1

1 Introduction

Preeclampsia is a serious multisystem disorder unique to human pregnancy that remains a major cause of maternal and fetal morbidity and mortality worldwide [1]. While typically presenting as new-onset hypertension, insights into the pathogenesis of the disease have revealed that preeclampsia is much more than simply high blood pressure [2]. In essence, the clinical features of preeclampsia are thought to be due to widespread maternal endothelial dysfunction arising from impaired placentation leading to placental dysfunction and the excessive release of anti-angiogenic factors and pro-inflammatory cytokines [3, 4]. In particular, the anti-angiogenic factors sFlt-1 and soluble endoglin (sEng) have received much interest as likely candidates underlying the maternal endothelial dysfunction [5–9]. These insights have offered the prospects of new therapeutic approaches to the care of women with preeclampsia [10].

One anti-angiogenic factor that has attracted less attention as a possible contributor to the pathogenesis of preeclampsia is activin A. Activin is a member of the TGFβ superfamily that is secreted by the placenta across pregnancy with maximum levels at term [11–13]. Irrespective of gestation, circulating levels of activin A in women

Padma Murthi and Cathy Vaillancourt (eds.), *Preeclampsia: Methods and Protocols*, Methods in Molecular Biology, vol. 1710, https://doi.org/10.1007/978-1-4939-7498-6_4, © Springer Science+Business Media LLC 2018

with established preeclampsia are manyfold higher than those in women with a healthy pregnancy [14, 15], secondary to increased placental production [16]. Excessive placental oxidative stress is thought to underlie the increased placental production of activin A [17]. In regard to pathogenesis of preeclampsia, maternal serum levels of activin A are also elevated in early pregnancy in women who subsequently develop preeclampsia, months before the onset of clinical symptoms [18, 19] and significantly earlier than the rise in levels of sFlt-1 and sEng [6]. Indeed, activin A has long been known to impair endothelial cell function [20], and recently it has been shown that the endothelial dysfunction induced by pre-eclamptic serum is due, at least in part, to induction of oxidative stress by activin A [21]. These endothelial effects of activin A appear quite separate from any effects of sFlt and sEng [22].

Accordingly, in this current study, we wished to examine whether activin A had any other effects on endothelial function, specifically exploring changes in endothelin-1 (ET-1) and cell adhesion molecule expression. Activated or injured endothelial cells produce vasoactive substances and lose their ability to maintain vascular integrity [23]. The sensitivity of maternal preeclamptic endothelium to angiotensin II [24] coupled with an increase in ET-1 [25] culminates in the hypertensive aspect of the disease. End-organ dysfunction results from increasing maternal vascular permeability and edema brought about through increased expression of adhesion molecules on the activated endothelial surface [26]. The expression of cell adhesion molecules, such as intracellular adhesion molecule-1 (ICAM-1) and vascular adhesion molecule-1 (VCAM-1), and the vasoconstrictor ET-1 are considered reliable markers for impaired endothelial cell function [27, 28].

2 Materials

2.1 Equipment

1. Venepuncture equipment.
2. 5 mL clot-activator separator Vacutainer tubes.
3. Shaking water bath.
4. Water-jacketed CO_2 incubator.
5. Chamber slides.
6. Laboratory microscope and cell counting slide/chamber.
7. Real-time qPCR machine with associated computer hardware and software requirements.
8. Microplate assay reader with associated computer hardware and software requirements.
9. Gel doc analyzer.

2.2 Solutions

Concentrated stock solutions of cell culture reagents are reconstituted according to manufacturer's instructions if applicable, aliquoted into appropriate volumes and stored at −20 °C. Thawed reagents should be held at 4 °C or on ice during experiments.

1. Hank's balanced salt solution (HBSS).
2. M199 media with phenol red (containing Hank's salts, 25 mM HEPES buffer, and L-glutamine).
3. M199 media without phenol red (containing Earle's salts, L-glutamine, and 2200 mg/L sodium bicarbonate).
4. Fetal bovine serum (FBS) and newborn calf serum (NCS) (heat inactivated at 56 °C for 60 min in a shaking water bath).
5. Antibiotic-antimycotic solution (containing 10,000 units penicillin, 10,000 μg streptomycin, and 25 μg amphotericin B/mL utilizing penicillin G (sodium salt), streptomycin sulfate, and amphotericin B as antimycotic in 0.85% saline).
6. Dulbecco's phosphate buffered saline (DPBS, without calcium chloride and magnesium chloride).
7. RIPA buffer (containing 50 mM tris-hydrochloric acid, pH 8.0 with 150 mM sodium chloride, 1% octylphenoxypolyethoxyethanol, 0.5% sodium deoxycholate, and 1% sodium dodecyl sulfate).
8. Type-B gelatin (dissolved in distilled water to a final concentration of 0.2%).
9. High-resolution DNA-grade agarose.
10. Electrophoresis (TBE) buffer (1 L of 5× stock solution): 54 g of Tris base, 27.5 g of boric acid, 20 mL of 0.5 M EDTA, and adjust pH to 8.3 by HCl (*see* **Note 1**).

2.3 Reagents

1. TrypLE Express (stable trypsin replacement enzyme).
2. Human recombinant epidermal growth factor (EGF).
3. Human recombinant fibroblast growth factor (FGF).
4. 200 mM L-glutamine.
5. Random primers.
6. Moloney murine leukemia virus (MMLV) reverse transcriptase.
7. Recombinant noncompetitive pancreatic-type ribonuclease inhibitor.
8. Dithiothreitol (DTT).
9. Deoxyribonucleotide triphosphate (dNTP).
10. Reverse transcriptase.
11. Dimethyl sulfoxide (DMSO).
12. Gel electrophoresis loading dye.

13. Type-II collagenase (dissolved in HBSS to a final concentration of 0.1%).
14. Recombinant human activin A (reconstituted in M199 media).
15. Recombinant mouse follistatin 288 (reconstituted in M199 media).
16. DNA master mix plus SYBR green I dye.
17. 1 kb DNA ladder.
18. QIAquick gel extraction kit (Qiagen).

3 Methods

3.1 Human Tissues

3.1.1 Serum

Maternal blood is collected for serum extraction from the antecubital vein of subjects with a singleton pregnancy in the absence of labor. Samples are obtained from ~20 women with established preeclampsia and from ~20 gestational age-matched normal healthy pregnant women with a singleton pregnancy. Gestational ages range from 24 to 39 weeks. Serum from the preeclamptic subjects should be taken within 72 h of their diagnosis. A total of 10–15 mL of blood is collected into 5 mL serum clot-activator separator Vacutainer tubes. Samples should be left to sit at room temperature for 30–60 min before centrifuge at 1100 × *g* for 20 min also at room temperature. Serum is then withdrawn and transferred into 2 mL cell freezing tubes and stored at −20 °C until needed.

Two gestational age-matched serum pools can then be established; one comprising normal pregnant and the other comprising preeclamptic serum. From each individual patient's serum store, 5 mL is withdrawn and added to a central pool and stored at −20 °C, until required for the serum studies.

3.1.2 Umbilical Cords

Umbilical cords for human umbilical vein endothelial cell (HUVEC) isolation are obtained from healthy subjects with a singleton pregnancy undergoing elective caesarean section for either breech presentation or previous caesarean section at term (37–40 weeks gestation). Umbilical cords are collected ($n = 15$) in M199 media containing 2 mM glutamine and antibiotic-antimycotic solution (*see* **Note 2**).

3.2 HUVEC Isolation and Culture

All aspects of cell isolation and culture should be performed under sterile conditions in a class II biological safety cabinet. Incubations are carried out at 37 °C, 20% O_2, and 5% CO_2 in a water-jacketed CO_2 incubator under sterile conditions. HUVEC isolation can be performed according to an established method with minor alterations [29].

1. Harvested umbilical cords are prepared for endothelial cell isolation in warm HBSS. The cords are cleaned and blood gently

manually expressed out from each end. Areas of cord damaged by surgical clamping should be excised, and the remaining cord cut into 20 cm sections. Sections are then placed in a clean HBSS bath and a cannula with an attached three-way valve inserted into the umbilical vein at each end and secured tightly with a surgical silk.

2. The cord is then carefully flushed with warm HBSS via the cannula to remove remaining blood and debris. One three-way valve is closed, and the other end of the umbilical vein transfused with approximately 10 mL of warm 0.1% type-II collagenase solution. The second three-way valve is then closed and the cord section incubated at 37 °C for 10 min in a warm DPBS bath.
3. Following incubation, the section of cord should be removed and massaged along its entire length to detach remaining endothelial cells from the vein. The three-way valves are then opened with alternating syringe suction applied to each end to draw out the cell suspension.
4. The resulting cell suspension is placed into a 50 mL centrifuge tube containing 10 mL NCS to inactivate the collagenase and then centrifuged at 300 × *g* for 5 min. The supernatant is discarded and the cell pellet washed twice by resuspension in 20 mL M199 (containing 2 mM glutamine and antibiotic-antimycotic solution) and repeated centrifugation.
5. The isolated HUVECs are resuspended in M199 complete medium containing 20% heat-inactivated FBS, epidermal and fibroblast growth factors (10 ng/mL each), 2 mM glutamine, and antibiotic-antimycotic solution for counting on a hemocytometer.
6. HUVECs are then seeded at an appropriate density into tissue culture plastic ware previously coated with 0.2% gelatin for 2 h or more (Table 1).
7. The media is then changed every 48 h until the HUVECs reach confluence (Figs. 1 and 2 showing incomplete and complete confluence, respectively).
8. Once confluent, HUVECs are passaged and either transferred into a larger flask for further growth or seeded into wells/chambers for experimental use at passage 2 or 3.
9. When passaging, exhausted media and dead cells are aspirated, and healthy adherent HUVECs are washed twice with DPBS. TrypLE Express is then added to completely cover the HUVEC monolayer, and cells are incubated at 37 °C for 5 min (refer to Table 1 for TrypLE Express volumes). The flask is then firmly tapped several times to dislodge cells, and the resulting cell suspension is transferred to a 50 mL centrifuge

Table 1
Cell seeding densities and media volumes for different culture conditions

Receptacle type	Cell count	Media volume	TrypLE Express volume
Chamber slides	1×10^4	400 μL	–
96 well plate	1×10^4	200 μL	–
24 well plate	5×10^4	1 mL	–
6 well plate	2×10^5	2 mL	–
T25 flask	2×10^5	5 mL	4 mL
T75 flask	5×10^5–1×10^6	12 mL	8 mL
T175 flask	1×10^6–2×10^6	28 mL	18 mL

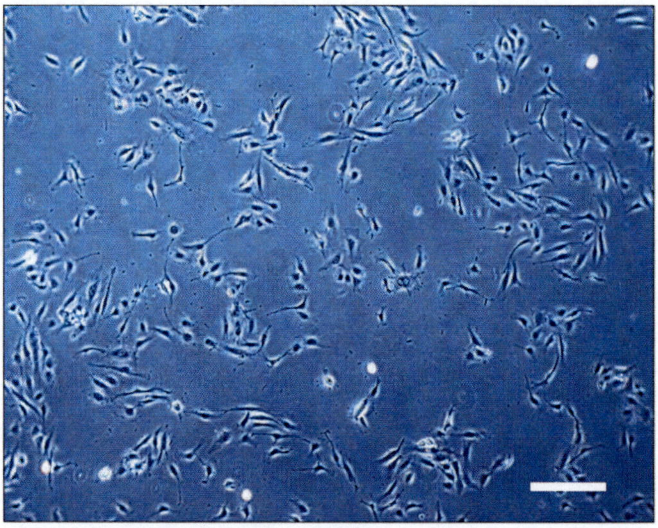

Fig. 1 Photograph of HUVECs after 2-day culture showing incomplete confluence at 50-times magnification (scale bar represents 300 μm)

tube containing an equal volume of NCS to inactivate the TrypLE Express.

10. The suspension is then centrifuged at $300 \times g$ for 5 min and supernatant discarded. The cell pellet is washed twice by resuspending the cell pellet with 20 mL M199 with phenol-red collection media (containing 2 mM glutamine and antibiotic-antimycotic solution) and repeated centrifugation (*see* **Note 3**).
11. Passaged HUVECs can be transferred into a freezing solution comprising 90% FBS and 10% DMSO at 2×10^6 cells per mL.

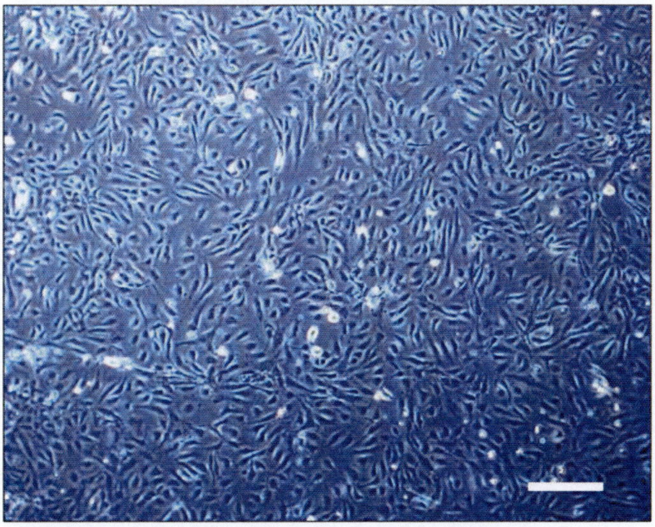

Fig. 2 Photograph of HUVECs after 6-day culture showing complete confluence at 50-times magnification (scale bar represents 300 μm)

This cell suspension is immediately aliquoted into 2 mL cryovials for rate controlled freezing and eventual transfer into liquid nitrogen for long-term cryopreservation.

12. When required, frozen ampoules are removed from storage and immediately placed in a 37 °C water bath to thaw rapidly. The ampoule is swabbed with ethanol and contents transferred into 10 mL of cold M199 complete media. Cells can then be transferred into an appropriate receptacle as described above.
13. Immediately prior to any treatment, the set volume of treatment solution to be administered should be withdrawn from the culture in order to maintain identical final culture media volumes between treatment groups.

3.3 Effects of Treatments on Endothelial Cell Function

1. All treatments should be carried out using confluent HUVECs cultured in 6- and 96-well plates.
2. At the time of treatment, cells are washed with DPBS and cultured with their respective treatments (Fig. 3).
3. Cellular viability should be quantified at the end of each experiment using an MTT assay as per manufacturer's instructions.

3.4 Quantitative Measurement of mRNA

1. Total cell-associated RNA is isolated from HUVECs cultured in 96-well plates using cell-to-signal lysis buffer.
2. Culture supernatant is removed and discarded and cells then washed twice with 100 μL DPBS before the addition of 100 μL of lysis buffer and incubation at room temperature for 2 min.

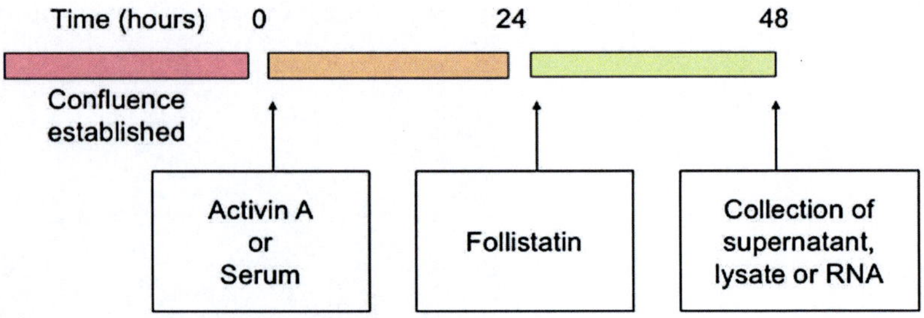

Fig. 3 Diagram showing the time line of treatment and cell product collection throughout the study experiments

RNA solution is then collected and stored at −80 °C until required.

3. Reverse transcriptase reaction is achieved by adding 12 μL of total RNA sample to a microfuge tube along with a 15 μL volume comprising 12.7 μL sterile distilled H_2O, 0.3 μL random primer, and 2 μL 10 mM dNTP.
4. Samples are then run in a PCR machine at 65 °C for 5 min. Following, a second volume of 13 μL comprising 8 μL first strand buffer, 2 μL DTT, 2 μL recombinant noncompetitive pancreatic-type ribonuclease inhibitor and 1 μL MMLV reverse transcriptase is added to each sample tube.
5. These are then run in the PCR machine to achieve reverse transcription at 25 °C for 5 min, 50 °C for 60 min, and 70 °C for 15 min and then cooled to handling temperature.
6. Real-time quantitative polymerase chain reaction (RT-qPCR) can then be achieved by adding 5 μL of sample cDNA from the reverse transcriptase reaction to 10 μL sterile distilled H_2O, 0.5 μL of both the forward and reverse primer of interest (Table 2) and 4 μL SYBR Green I, in a sterile microfuge tube.
7. Normalization of results is achieved through the amplification of 2 μL of cDNA to detect 18S mRNA in conjunction with the mRNA of interest.
8. Samples are placed in the real-time qPCR machine and held at 95 °C for 10 min for initial denaturation.
9. This is followed by a cycling profile unique to each gene of interest (Table 3), with 18s run at every profile for comparison and eventual quantification of results using the $2^{-\Delta\Delta C_T}$ method as described previously [30].
10. To confirm that the products of RT-qPCR are specifically the products of interest, gel electrophoresis and sequencing should be performed on representative PCR products. Prepare an

Table 2
Forward (F) and reverse (R) primers used for endothelin-1 (ET), intercellular adhesion molecule-1 (ICAM), vascular cell adhesion molecule-1 (VCAM), and 18s

mRNA of interest	Forward and reverse primer sequences
ET	F: 5′-GAG AAA CCC ACT CCC AGT CC-3′ R: 5′-GAT GTC CAG GTG GCA GAA GT-3′
ICAM	F: 5′ CTG CAG ACA GTG ACC ATC 3′ R: 5′ GTC CAG TTT CCC GGA CAA 3′
VCAM	F: 5′ TGG ACC CCG GAT TGC TGC 3′ R: 5′ AAA ACT CAC AGG GCT CAG GGT C 3′
18s	F: 5′ CGG CTA CCA CAT CCA AGG AA 3′ R: 5′ GCT GGA ATT ACC GCG GCT 3′

Table 3
Real-time qPCR machine profiles used in the analysis of endothelin-1 (ET), intercellular adhesion molecule-1 (ICAM), and vascular cell adhesion molecule-1 (VCAM) mRNA

mRNA of interest	Profile	Cycles
ET	94 °C for 15 s, 60 °C for 30 s	40
ICAM	95 °C for 15 s, 60 °C for 10 s, 72 °C for 15 s	45
VCAM	95 °C for 15 s, 60 °C for 5 s, 72 °C for 10 s	40

agarose gel (1.7%) containing ethidium bromide (1 μL/50 mL) using TBE buffer.

11. Each 20 μL sample is then combined with 2.5 μL of loading dye and loaded onto the gel (*see* **Note 4**).
12. Gels undergo electrophoresis at 100 V in the TBE buffer solution for 1.5–2.5 h and are photographed on a gel doc analyzer.
13. Product bands are then excised from the gel and purified using a QIAquick gel extraction kit. The excised gel samples should be processed according to the provided protocol with buffers and incubated at 50 °C for 10 min, dissolving the gel.
14. Reagents can then be added to the gel solution and centrifuged in a QIAquick column before being washed through with further buffer.

Table 4
Products of the sequencing process confirmed through the BLAST nucleotide-nucleotide database

Product	Base-pair length
Endothelin-1	104
Intercellular adhesion molecule-1	168
Vascular cell adhesion molecule-1	319

15. The remaining DNA product is then eluted in 10 mM tris-chloride and centrifuged to create the final product solution for sequencing.
16. Sequencing is then performed by local methods using 10 μg of purified DNA product along with 10 μL of 5 μM forward primer for a single product.
17. Retrieved sequences are then entered into the BLAST nucleotide-nucleotide database to confirm products (Table 4).

3.5 Assays

1. Secreted protein is isolated from HUVECs cultures in 6-well plates through the collection of culture supernatant and stored at −20 °C for quantitative ET-1 protein measurement by enzyme-linked immunosorbent assay (ELISA).
2. Cell-associated protein should be isolated through cell lysis with RIPA buffer. Following removal of supernatant, cells are washed twice with 1000 μL DPBS and 220 μL RIPA buffer added before incubation at 4 °C for 5 min.
3. Cell lysate is then scraped from the wells, collected and stored at −80 °C until analyzed for quantitative ICAM-1 and VCAM-1 protein measurement.
4. All ELISAs should be read on a single microplate assay reader and an assessment of inter- and intra-assay variability be made.

3.5.1 Activin A ELISA

Total activin A protein in subject serum can be quantified using a commercial two-site ELISA, according to manufacturer's instructions.

1. Briefly, the assay plates are pre-coated with an antibody against a peptide of the βA-subunit of activin.
2. Standards and samples are diluted in provided calibrator diluent.
3. 100 μL of each sample is placed into each well along with 100 μL of assay diluent and the plates then covered and incubated at room temperature for 3 h.
4. Each well is then washed with 400 μL of wash buffer and 50 μL of the secondary antibody diluted 1:1200 added.

5. After 2 h incubation and further washing, 50 μL of streptavidin diluted 1:300 in assay buffer is added to each well for 1 h.
6. The bound alkaline phosphatase should then be quantified by means of a commercially available enzyme immunoassay amplification kit and absorbency read on a microplate reader at 490 and 620 nm.
7. The intra- and inter-assay variability (%) and sensitivity (pg/mL) should be reported.

3.5.2 Follistatin Radioimmunoassay

Total follistatin protein in subject serum can be quantified using a discontinuous radioimmunoassay as described previously [31]. The intra- and inter-assay variability (%) and sensitivity (pg/mL) should be reported.

3.5.3 Endothelin-1 ELISA

A commercial human ET-1 ELISA kit can be used to quantitate the levels of ET-1 protein in culture supernatant and serum according to manufacturer's instructions. Briefly, the reagents, working standards, controls, and samples are prepared according to the manufacturer's protocol. Serum can usually be analyzed neat and culture supernatant diluted 1:15 in the provided assay buffer.

1. 100 μL of prepared sample, standards (0–100 pg/mL), and controls are added to their respective wells in duplicate.
2. The plate is then sealed and incubated at 37 °C for 1 h before the well contents are discarded and each well washed with 400 μL of wash buffer for a total of seven washes.
3. Labelled antibody (100 μL) is then added to each well, except the blank, and the plate sealed and incubated at 37 °C for 30 min before the well contents are discarded and each well washed with 400 μL of wash buffer nine times.
4. Substrate solution (100 μL) is then added to each well and the plate incubated for 30 min at room temperature in the dark.
5. Each well then requires blocking with 100 μL of stop solution and the plate read at optical densities of 450 and 590 nm using an optical microplate reader.
6. The intra- and inter-assay variability (%) and sensitivity (pg/mL) should be reported.

3.5.4 Intracellular Adhesion Molecule-1 ELISA

A commercial human soluble ICAM-1 (CD54) immunoassay kit can be used to quantitate the levels of ICAM-1 in cell lysate and/or serum. Reagents, working standards, controls, and samples should be prepared according to the manufacturer's protocol. Lysate can be assayed neat and serum diluted 1:5 using the provided sample diluent.

1. Diluted conjugate (100 μL) is added to each well followed by 100 μL of sample, standards (0–49.55 ng/mL), or controls, each in duplicate.

2. The plate is then sealed and incubated at room temperature for 1.5 h before the well contents are discarded and each well washed with 300 μL of wash buffer for a total of six washes.
3. Immediately, 100 μL of prepared substrate should be added to each well and the plate sealed and incubated at room temperature for 3 min.
4. After this incubation, 100 μL of stop solution is added to each well and the plate read at 450 and 650 nm using the microplate reader.
5. The intra- and inter-assay variability (%) and sensitivity (pg/mL) should be reported.

3.5.5 Vascular Cell Adhesion Molecule-1 ELISA

A commercial human soluble VCAM-1 (CD54) ELISA kit can be used to quantitate the levels of VCAM-1 in culture supernatant, cell lysate, and/or serum. Reagents, working standards, and samples should be prepared according to the manufacturer's protocol, with culture supernatant, cell lysate, and serum assayed neat.

1. Diluted conjugate (100 μL) is added to each well followed by 100 μL of sample or standards (0–200 ng/mL) in duplicate.
2. The plate is then sealed and incubated at room temperature for 1.5 h before the well contents are discarded and each well washed with 400 μL of wash buffer for a total of four washes.
3. Immediately, 100 μL of prepared substrate solution should be added to each well and the plate sealed and incubated at room temperature for 20 min in the dark.
4. After incubation, 50 μL of stop solution is added to each well and the plate read at 450 and 570 nm using the microplate reader.
5. The intra- and inter-assay variability (%) and sensitivity (pg/mL) should be reported.

4 Notes

1. TBE can be diluted to 1× prior to use in electrophoresis, and 0.5× is acceptable as well. Higher concentrations will result in poor results due to excessive heat generation.
2. Cords should be processed for HUVEC isolation (Subheading 3.2) as soon as possible after collection as this yields higher cell numbers; otherwise they may be stored at 4 °C overnight.
3. The same protocol for HUVEC culture can then be used to transfer the cells to an appropriate receptacle.
4. A 1 kb DNA ladder is used to ascertain PCR product size.

References

1. Lyall F, Greer IA (1994) Pre-eclampsia: a multifaceted vascular disorder of pregnancy. J Hypertens 12(12):1339–1345
2. Roberts JM, Redman CW (1993) Pre-eclampsia: more than pregnancy-induced hypertension. Lancet 341(8858):1447–1451
3. Redman CW, Sargent IL (2005) Latest advances in understanding preeclampsia. Science 308(5728):1592–1594
4. Roberts JM, Hubel CA (2009) The two stage model of preeclampsia: variations on the theme. Placenta 30(Suppl A):S32–S37
5. Maynard SE, Min JY, Merchan J, Lim KH, Li J, Mondal S, Libermann TA, Morgan JP, Sellke FW, Stillman IE, Epstein FH, Sukhatme VP, Karumanchi SA (2003) Excess placental soluble fms-like tyrosine kinase 1 (sFlt1) may contribute to endothelial dysfunction, hypertension, and proteinuria in preeclampsia. J Clin Invest 111(5):649–658
6. Levine RJ, Maynard SE, Qian C, Lim KH, England LJ, Yu KF, Schisterman EF, Thadhani R, Sachs BP, Epstein FH, Sibai BM, Sukhatme VP, Karumanchi SA (2004) Circulating angiogenic factors and the risk of preeclampsia. N Engl J Med 350(7):672–683
7. Levine RJ, Lam C, Qian C, Yu KF, Maynard SE, Sachs BP, Sibai BM, Epstein FH, Romero R, Thadhani R, Karumanchi SA (2006) Soluble endoglin and other circulating antiangiogenic factors in preeclampsia. N Engl J Med 355(10):992–1005
8. Venkatesha S, Toporsian M, Lam C, Hanai J, Mammoto T, Kim YM, Bdolah Y, Lim KH, Yuan HT, Libermann TA, Stillman IE, Roberts D, D'Amore PA, Epstein FH, Sellke FW, Romero R, Sukhatme VP, Letarte M, Karumanchi SA (2006) Soluble endoglin contributes to the pathogenesis of preeclampsia. Nat Med 12(6):642–649
9. Steinberg G, Khankin EV, Karumanchi SA (2009) Angiogenic factors and preeclampsia. Thromb Res 123(Suppl 2):S93–S99
10. Fenton C, Hobson SR, Wallace EM, Lim R (2014) Future therapies for pre-eclampsia: beyond treading water. Aust N Z J Obstet Gynaecol 54:3
11. Petraglia F (1997) Inhibin, activin and follistatin in the human placenta--a new family of regulatory proteins. Placenta 18(1):3–8
12. Fowler PA, Evans LW, Groome NP, Templeton A, Knight PG (1998) A longitudinal study of maternal serum inhibin-A, inhibin-B, activin-A, activin-AB, pro-alphaC and follistatin during pregnancy. Hum Reprod 13(12):3530–3536
13. Schneider-Kolsky M, D'Antona D, Evans LW, Taylor N, O'Connor A, Groome NP, de Kretser D, Wallace EM (2000) Maternal serum total activin A and follistatin in pregnancy and parturition. BJOG 107(8):995–1000
14. Muttukrishna S, Knight PG, Groome NP, Redman CW, Ledger WL (1997) Activin A and inhibin A as possible endocrine markers for pre-eclampsia. Lancet 349(9061):1285–1288
15. Schneider-Kolsky M, Manuelpillai U, Gargett C, Wallace EM (2001) Activin betaA-subunit and activin receptors in human myometrium at term and during labour. BJOG 108(8): 869–874
16. Manuelpillai U, Schneider-Kolsky M, Dole A, Wallace EM (2001) Activin A and activin receptors in gestational tissue from preeclamptic pregnancies. J Endocrinol 171(1):57–64
17. Mandang S, Manuelpillai U, Wallace EM (2007) Oxidative stress increases placental and endothelial cell activin A secretion. J Endocrinol 192(3):485–493
18. Muttukrishna S, North RA, Morris J, Schellenberg JC, Taylor RS, Asselin J, Ledger W, Groome N, Redman CW (2000) Serum inhibin A and activin A are elevated prior to the onset of pre-eclampsia. Hum Reprod 15(7): 1640–1645
19. Schneider-Kolsky ME, Manuelpillai U, Waldron K, Dole A, Wallace EM (2002) The distribution of activin and activin receptors in gestational tissues across human pregnancy and during labour. Placenta 23(4):294–302
20. McCarthy SA, Bicknell R (1993) Inhibition of vascular endothelial cell growth by activin-A. J Biol Chem 268(31):23066–23071
21. Lim R, Acharya R, Delpachitra P, Hobson S, Sobey CG, Drummond GR, Wallace EM (2015) Activin and NADPH-oxidase in preeclampsia: insights from in vitro and murine studies. Am J Obstet Gynecol 212:86.e1
22. Gurusinghe S, Wallace EM, Lim R (2014) The relationship between Activin A and anti-angiogenic factors in the development of pre-eclampsia. Pregnancy Hypertens 4(1):3–6
23. Deanfield JE, Halcox JP, Rabelink TJ (2007) Endothelial function and dysfunction: testing and clinical relevance. Circulation 115(10): 1285–1295
24. Signore C, Mills JL, Qian C, Yu K, Lam C, Epstein FH, Karumanchi SA, Levine RJ (2006) Circulating angiogenic factors and placental abruption. Obstet Gynecol 108(2):338–344
25. Nova A, Sibai BM, Barton JR, Mercer BM, Mitchell MD (1991) Maternal plasma level of

endothelin is increased in preeclampsia. Am J Obstet Gynecol 165(3):724–727

26. Wang Y, Gu Y, Granger DN, Roberts JM, Alexander JS (2002) Endothelial junctional protein redistribution and increased monolayer permeability in human umbilical vein endothelial cells isolated during preeclampsia. Am J Obstet Gynecol 186(2):214–220
27. Blann AD, Taberner DA (1995) A reliable marker of endothelial cell dysfunction: does it exist? Br J Haematol 90(2):244–248
28. Lerman A, Holmes DR Jr, Bell MR, Garratt KN, Nishimura RA, Burnett JC Jr (1995) Endothelin in coronary endothelial dysfunction and early atherosclerosis in humans. Circulation 92(9):2426–2431
29. Jaffe EA, Nachman RL, Becker CG, Minick CR (1973) Culture of human endothelial cells derived from umbilical veins. Identification by morphologic and immunologic criteria. J Clin Invest 52(11):2745–2756
30. Livak KJ, Schmittgen TD (2001) Analysis of relative gene expression data using real-time quantitative PCR and the 2(-Delta Delta C(T)) Method. Methods 25(4):402–408

31 O'Connor AE, McFarlane JR, Hayward S, Yohkaichiya T, Groome NP, de Kretser DM (1999) Serum activin A and follistatin concentrations during human pregnancy: a cross-sectional and longitudinal study. Hum Reprod 14(3):827–832

Chapter 5

Genetic Approaches in Preeclampsia

Hannah E.J. Yong, Padma Murthi, Shaun P. Brennecke, and Eric K. Moses

Abstract

Preeclampsia (PE) is a serious hypertensive disorder that affects up to 8% of all pregnancies annually. An established risk factor for PE is family history, clearly demonstrating an underlying genetic component to the disorder. To date, numerous genetic studies, using both the candidate gene and genome-wide approach, have been undertaken to tease out the genetic basis of PE and understand its origins. Such studies have identified some promising candidate genes such as STOX1 and ACVR2A. Nevertheless, researchers face ongoing challenges of replicating these genetic associations in different populations and performing the functional validation of identified genetic variants to determine their causality in the disorder. This chapter will review the genetic approaches used in the study of PE, discuss their limitations and possible confounders, and describe current strategies.

Key words Preeclampsia, Genetic approaches, Genome-wide association, Linkage analysis, Transcriptome profiling, Candidate gene, STOX1, ACVR2A

1 Introduction

1.1 Preeclampsia

Preeclampsia (PE) is a leading cause of perinatal mortality and morbidity worldwide. An estimated 2–8% of all pregnancies are complicated with PE [1]. The International Society for the Study of Hypertension in Pregnancy defines de novo PE as new-onset gestational hypertension accompanied by one or more of the following features: proteinuria, maternal organ dysfunction, and uteroplacental dysfunction (Table 1) [2]. Women with preexisting hypertension are diagnosed with superimposed PE, when they develop one or more of the additional features [2]. The severity of PE is often classified by the gestation at disease onset, significant elevation of blood pressures, and involvement of multiple organs, which have worse perinatal outcomes [3–5]. The combination of hemolysis, elevated liver enzymes, and low platelet counts in a pregnant woman is termed the HELLP syndrome, which is a severe variant of PE [6].

Padma Murthi and Cathy Vaillancourt (eds.), *Preeclampsia: Methods and Protocols*, Methods in Molecular Biology, vol. 1710, https://doi.org/10.1007/978-1-4939-7498-6_5,

Table 1
Clinical characteristics for the diagnosis of preeclampsia

Features	Definition
Hypertension	• Systolic ≥140 mmHg or diastolic ≥90 mmHg after 20 weeks' gestation
Accompanied by one or more of the following:	
Proteinuria	• ≥300 mg of protein in 24 h urine collection or spot urine protein/creatinine ratio ≥30 mg/mmol or '2+' on dipstick testing (equivalent to ≥1 g/L)
Other maternal organ dysfunction	• Renal insufficiency (creatinine ≥90 μmol/L; 1.02 mg/dl) • Liver involvement (elevated transaminases—at least twice upper limit of normal ± upper right quadrant or epigastric abdominal pain) • Neurological complications (examples include eclampsia, altered mental status, blindness, stroke, hyperreflexia accompanied by clonus, severe headaches accompanied by hyperreflexia, persistent visual scotomata) • Hematological complications (thrombocytopenia—platelet count below 150,000/dl, disseminated intravascular coagulation, hemolysis)
Uteroplacental dysfunction	• Fetal growth restriction (failure to achieve full growth potential in utero) • Abnormal Doppler ultrasound findings

Adapted from the International Society for the Study of Hypertension in Pregnancy Statement [2]

1.2 Genetic Basis of PE

The complex pathophysiology of PE suggests that some women are inherently predisposed to suffering from PE (Fig. 1). Having a family history of PE significantly increases an individual woman's risk of PE by between 24% and 163% [7]. The risk for developing PE is inheritable, when the genetic code is passed from one generation to the next. Familial clustering of PE was reported in the literature as early as the 1870s [8]. The familial form of PE is associated with a more severe phenotype [9], which demonstrates a strong genetic basis for PE.

Population studies of families reveal clear transmission of PE across generations. A Norwegian study using a national birth registry showed that being born of a preeclamptic pregnancy increased the risk of a woman having PE herself by 2.2-fold, while a man increased the risk of PE in his partner by 1.5-fold [9]. Even sisters born of a normotensive pregnancy, who had siblings affected with PE, had a twofold increased risk of developing PE themselves [9]. Another population study performed in Canada identified a similar increased risk for PE of 2.6-fold in primiparous sisters of

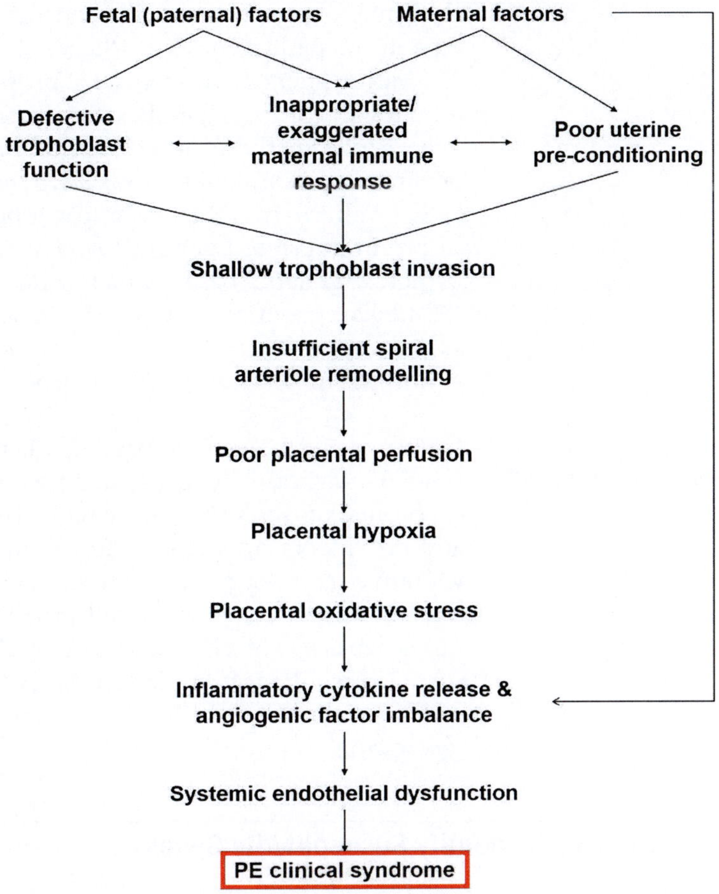

Fig. 1 Pathophysiology of preeclampsia

preeclamptic women, compared with primiparous women in the general population [10]. In a separate case-control study, mothers of preeclamptic women had a greater than threefold incidence of PE compared with mothers-in-law, who had a baseline rate similar to mothers of controls [11].

Twin studies, which are commonly used to understand disease heritability, were also performed to increase understanding of PE genetics. While some twins show concordance for the disorder [12], multiple studies performed in various populations demonstrated generally poor concordance between twin sisters [13]. These findings support some fetal (paternal) genotype and environmental contributions in the development of PE.

Heritability estimates of PE range from 31% to 54% [14–16]. Almost half of the familial aggregation of PE is estimated to be due to maternal genetic factors, with the environment and fetal (paternal) factors accounting for the remainder [17]. These data collectively suggest a greater contribution of the maternal genotype in the pathogenesis of PE.

Various genetic models were proposed to explain the mode of inheritance for PE in families. Suggested models include a recessive gene active in the mother or a dominant gene with incomplete penetrance assuming a classical Mendelian mode of inheritance [18] or alternatives such as mitochondrial genes [19] and parent-of-origin imprinted genes [20]. The current view is that PE has a complex genetic basis, which cannot be explained by simple Mendelian genetics alone [21]. PE susceptibility is thus regarded as a complex interplay between the maternal and fetal (paternal) genotypes in addition to the environment [22].

1.3 Rationale Behind Study of Genetics in PE

Determining the genetic basis of PE has three significant implications. Firstly, casual gene(s) identified can be used to develop clinical biomarker tests to identify high-risk women through screening and provide an opportunity to improve patient outcomes by preventative treatment and closer surveillance. Secondly, understanding how these genes work will provide new insights into the still unknown cause of PE. Lastly, potential novel treatments may eventuate from enhanced understanding of the PE pathogenesis, which will alleviate the risk of PE and minimize its impact on future generations.

2 Approaches to Identify Susceptibility Genes

As PE can only develop in pregnant females, susceptibility cannot be directly determined from males or females who never become pregnant. The susceptibility of a male, particularly if the gene acts solely in the female during pregnancy, can only be inferred if he has a daughter who becomes pregnant. However, this may be confounded by the maternal contribution, as both parents contribute equally to the fetal genome. Additionally, as PE is usually observed in the first pregnancies [23], only one child can be genetically tested for the fetal (paternal) contribution. Therefore, the vast majority of genetic studies have focused on identifying maternal PE susceptibility genes in women affected with PE. The candidate gene and the genome-wide study approaches are widely used to identify maternal PE susceptibility genes.

2.1 Candidate Gene Studies

Candidate gene studies determine if one or more genetic variants of a candidate gene are associated with the disease of interest. Such studies are performed in large cohorts of affected and unaffected individuals. The selection of a candidate gene is often based on the contemporary understanding of the disease pathophysiology. Genes may be selected based on signalling or biochemical pathways. For example, in studying alcoholism, plausible choices would be to focus on genes involved in addiction or alcohol metabolism such as neurotransmitters or enzymes, respectively [24]. Based on the cumulative knowledge of the PE pathophysiology, the candidate gene approach has predominantly examined genes in endothelial function, hemodynamics, immune response, lipid metabolism, oxidative stress, and thrombophilia [25]. Most of the early candidate gene studies were focused on just nine genes: *AGT*, *ACE*, *AGTR1*, *AGTR2*, *F2*, *F5*, *MTHFR*, *NOS3*, and *TNF* [21].

2.1.1 Endothelial Function and Hemodynamics

With the abnormal blood pressure regulation observed in PE, numerous studies have investigated candidate genes involved in blood pressure regulation [22]. Much of the focus is on the renin-angiotensin system (RAS). The activation of this system leads to vasoconstriction, plasma volume expansion, activation of the sympathetic nervous system, and increased blood pressures (Fig. 2). Several genetic variants of the multiple genes involved in the RAS pathway—*ACE*, *AGT*, and *AGTR1*—are positively associated with PE in meta-analyses and systemic reviews, although they are not always reproducible in different populations [26, 27].

Another gene that can regulate blood pressure is *NOS3*, which codes for endothelial nitric oxide synthase (eNOS) that synthesizes

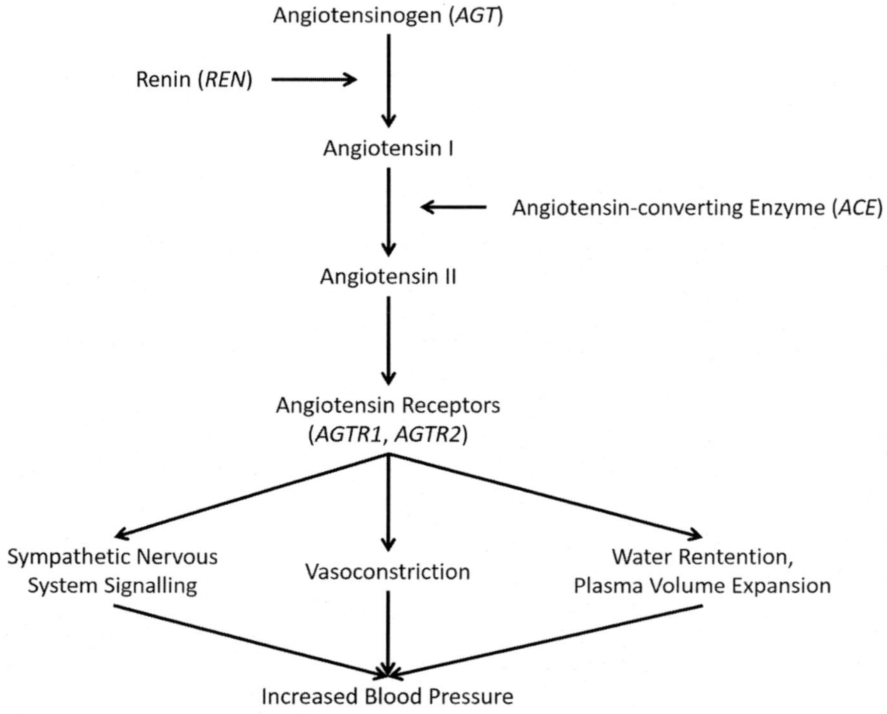

Fig. 2 Renin-angiotensin system in blood pressure regulation. Activation of the RAS pathway leads to increased blood pressure through multiple mechanisms

nitric oxide in endothelial cells for vasodilation. A recent meta-analysis demonstrated that two commonly studied *NOS3* polymorphisms—4b/a and −786 T>C—which correlate with lower nitric oxide serum levels, were associated with a greater risk of PE, particularly in the European population [28]. In contrast, the *NOS3* Glu298Asp polymorphism shows no overall difference between control or preeclamptic women, although individual studies have previously demonstrated significant associations with PE [29]. Therefore, the linkage between PE and eNOS remains to be further investigated.

2.1.2 Immune Response

As PE is thought to partly arise due to immune maladaptation, studies have also examined genes involved in the immune response. The human leukocyte class C, E, and G (HLA-C, HLA-E, and HLA-G) antigens are a unique repertoire of histocompatibility antigens expressed on extravillous trophoblast cells, which are ligands for maternal uterine killer cell receptors (KIR). The interaction between the fetal antigens and maternal immune cells allows immune tolerance to be established for normal placentation to occur. The pairing of the maternal KIR-AA haplotype and the fetal HLA-C2 haplotype is associated with the greatest risk of PE among the different possible combinations [30]. This association was recently reproduced in Chinese Han [31] and sub-Saharan [32] populations. Nevertheless, PE develops in women with other haplotype combinations as well, suggesting that further studies are required to dissect out the role of maternal-fetal histoincompatibility in the pathogenesis of the disorder.

Pro-inflammatory cytokines such as tumor necrosis factor α (TNFα) and interleukin 6 (IL6), which are involved in the exaggerated inflammatory response in PE, circulate at increased concentrations in the blood of preeclamptic women [33, 34]. Meta-analyses of past studies demonstrated null genetic associations of *TNF* and *IL6* variants with PE [34, 35]. However, a more recent study in a large cohort of more than 1000 women suggests that *TNF* is associated with PE in Americans with European ancestry [36], while another study shows that the G308A allele increases the odds of PE and its severity [37]. Therefore, the genetic links of these inflammatory cytokines with PE remain unclear.

2.1.3 Lipid Metabolism and Oxidative Stress

Dyslipidemia, as a result of oxidative stress, can also be damaging to the endothelium and may contribute to the vascular endothelial dysfunction in PE. As such, genes involved in regulating lipid metabolism such as *APOE* and *LPL*, which code for apolipoprotein E and lipoprotein lipase, respectively, are alternative candidate genes for PE [25]. While recent genetic and animal model studies suggest a role for *APOE* in PE [38, 39], meta-analyses of past studies so far have not supported this [26, 27]. Nevertheless, study sizes for *APOE* were relatively smaller compared with similar studies conducted for other genes, and the role of APOE in PE remains to be resolved. In contrast, meta-analyses support *LPL* as a potential candidate gene [26]. A study showed that the interaction between the maternal and fetal *LPL* genotypes could alter maternal lipid profiles and disease severity in PE [40].

Oxidative stress is another key feature of PE. Reactive oxygen species (ROS), which are damaging to the vascular endothelium, circulate at increased concentrations in the blood of preeclamptic women [41]. Additionally, antioxidants that can attenuate the activity of ROS are present at significantly lower concentrations in PE, demonstrating an imbalance of factors [42]. Therefore, genetic studies examining genes involved in the oxidative stress pathway (e.g., *EPHX*, *GST*, *NOX1*, *SOD2*) were performed [22, 25]. While some individual studies demonstrate positive associations of these genes with PE, most studies and systemic reviews show negative associations overall [22, 26, 27, 35, 43].

2.1.4 Thrombophilia

Blood coagulation is abnormal in preeclamptic women, particularly in those with the HELLP syndrome, where they develop thrombocytopenia. As such, numerous studies have examined the association of multiple thrombophilia genes with PE [22]. Several genetic variants of three widely studied thrombophilic factors, prothrombin (*F2*), factor V Leiden (*F5*), and methylenetetrahydrofolate reductase (*MTHFR*), show consistent associations with PE in multiple meta-analyses, although a few do show contradictory results [26, 27, 35, 44, 45]. Nevertheless, more individual studies actually show null associations of these genes, compared to those that do [25].

2.2 Genome-Wide Linkage and Association Studies

While the majority of genetic studies for PE have focused on using the candidate gene approach, several groups have undertaken the genome-wide approach, of which there are two aspects. One is referred to as linkage mapping, while the other an association study. Genome-wide linkage mapping or positional cloning studies are performed using family pedigrees to ascertain, without bias, any genetic loci that are associated with the condition. The entire genome is first scanned in a process termed “chromosome walking” to identify and localize disease susceptibility loci to specific chromosomal regions. These regions are then subjected to further genetic investigation to identify plausible candidate genes. Alternatively, genome-wide association studies can be performed in large cohorts of unrelated cases and controls to identify novel genetic loci through large-scale single nucleotide polymorphism (SNP) analyses.

To date, genome-wide studies have been conducted in Australia and New Zealand [46–48], Finland [49], Iceland [50], the Netherlands [51], Norway [52], the United Kingdom [53], and the USA [54]. Details of the genetic studies are available in Table 2.

Table 2
Genome-wide linkage and association studies performed in the study of preeclampsia

Population	Study type	Sample size	Study authors
American	Association	293 unrelated individuals	Zhao et al. (2012) [54]
Australian	Linkage	15 families	Harrison et al. (1997) [46]
Australian	Linkage	26 families	Guo et al. (1999) [55]
Australian/New Zealand	Linkage	34 families	Moses et al. (2000) [48]
Australian/New Zealand	Linkage	34 families	Fitzpatrick et al. (2004) [56]
Australian/New Zealand	Linkage	34 families	Moses et al. (2006) [57]
Australian/New Zealand	Linkage	34 families	Johnson et al. (2007) [14]
Australian/New Zealand	Linkage	34 families	Johnson et al. (2009) [58]
Australian/New Zealand	Linkage	74 families	Fitzpatrick et al. (2009) [59]
Australian/New Zealand	Linkage	74 families	Fenstad et al. (2010) [60]
Australian	Association	1078 unrelated individuals	Johnson et al. (2012) [47]
Australian/New Zealand	Linkage and association	74 families and 1095 unrelated individuals	Johnson et al. (2013) [61]
British	Linkage	35 families	Hayward et al. (1992) [53]
Dutch	Linkage	67 families	Lachmeijer et al. (2001) [51]
Dutch	Linkage	24 families	Oudejans et al. (2004) [62]
Dutch	Linkage	24 families	van Djik et al. (2005) [63]
Finnish	Linkage	15 families	Laivuori et al. (2003) [49]
Finnish	Association	248 unrelated individuals	Laasanen et al. (2003) [64]
Finnish	Linkage	15 families	Majander et al. (2013) [65]
Finnish	Association	2052 unrelated individuals in main study + additional 6118 unrelated individuals available from population database	Kaartokallio et al. (2016) [66]
Icelandic/Scottish	Linkage	50 families	Arngrimsson et al. (1997) [67]
Icelandic	Linkage	124 families	Arngrimsson et al. (1999) [50]
Norwegian	Association	3537 unrelated individuals	Johnson et al. (2009) [58]
Norwegian	Association	3537 unrelated individuals	Roten et al. (2009) [68]
Norwegian	Association	2291 unrelated individuals	Fenstad et al. (2010) [60]
Australia/New Zealand, Dutch, Finnish, Icelandic	Linkage	Meta-analysis of 159 families	Zintzaras et al. (2006) [69]

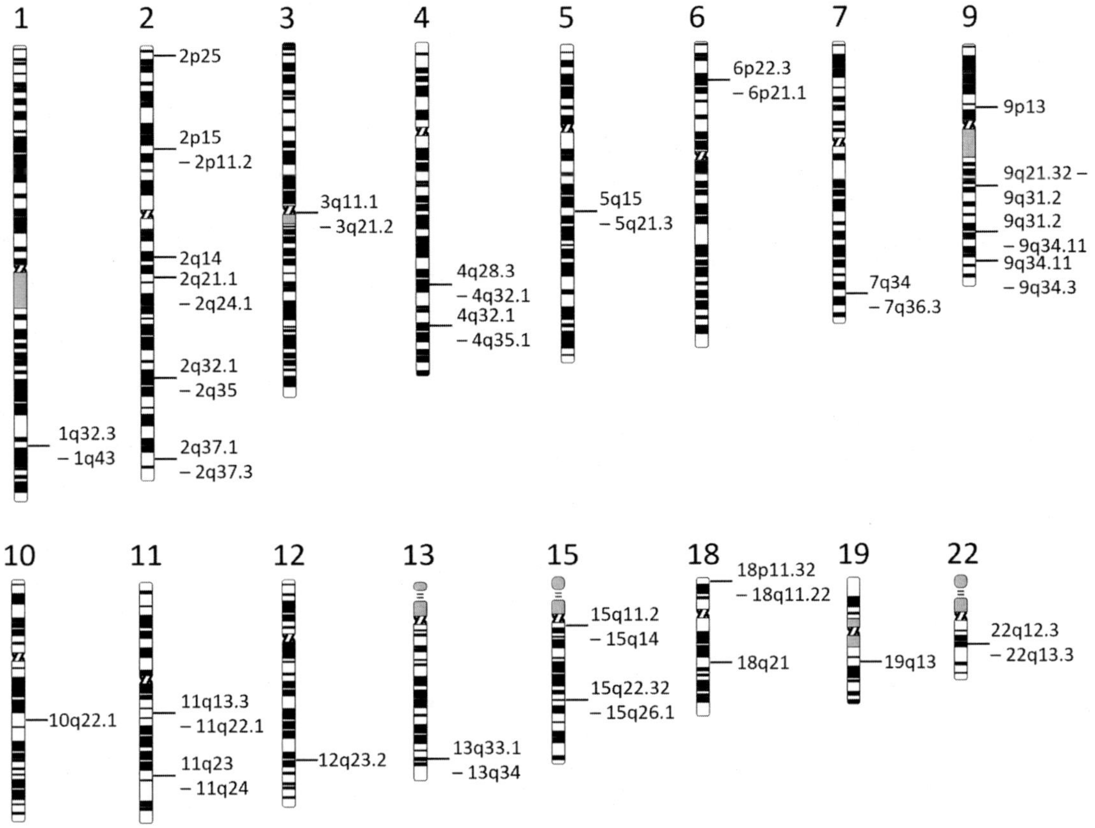

Fig. 3 Susceptibility loci and their chromosomal localizations identified through the genome-wide study approach. All loci contain regions for maternal susceptibility, with the exception of the fetal 18q21 susceptibility locus. Modified from Adler [70]

A summary of the susceptibility loci identified thus far and their chromosomal locations is presented in Fig. 3.

The earliest reported PE genome-wide linkage study tested 43 loci on 21 chromosomes and found nonsignificant and inconclusive associations of PE with either chromosomes 1, 3, 9, or 18 in the United Kingdom [53]. In contrast, a subsequent study in the Australian/New Zealand population demonstrated possible linkage with PE on 4q [46]. A potential linkage at the 7q36 locus was also demonstrated in the Australian/New Zealand and Icelandic population linkage analyses [55, 67]. The lack of replication between these early studies as explained by Harrison et al. [46] is possibly due to the use of different genetic models of inheritance when analyzing the linkage data and definitions of PE.

With the advancement of genetic sequencing, particularly with the success of the Human Genome Project, successive genetic studies for PE were of a higher density and demonstrated more conclusive genetic linkages. Using multiple family pedigrees, the

Icelandic group reported the first significant susceptibility locus for PE at 2p13 [50]. Further evidence for a susceptibility locus on chromosome 2 was supported by a subsequent genome-wide scan in 34 affected families from the Australian/New Zealand population; the identified region of linkage was designated as the PREG1 locus [48]. A subsequent reanalysis of the original Australian/New Zealand scan, using an alternative variance component-based linkage approach, showed novel susceptibility loci on chromosomes 5q and 13q [14]. The association of PE with chromosome 2 was replicated in a Finnish study of 15 affected families, which found a peak at the 2p25 locus [49]. The Finnish group also demonstrated significant linkage with the 9p13 locus [49]. A follow-up Finnish study found novel linkage of PE with chromosome 18q for the fetal genotype [65]. An additional case-control analysis in the Finnish population demonstrated a nominal association at the 2p13 locus [64]. The Dutch analyses on 67 affected families showed suggestive linkage of PE with chromosomes 10q and 22q [51]. A subset analysis of HELLP families showed distinct linkage of the HELLP syndrome on chromosome 12q, which suggests that PE and the HELLP syndrome may have different genetic origins. A meta-analysis of these multiple population genome scans confirmed linkage with seven of the loci and revealed an additional six novel loci [69]. Later association studies were expanded to genotype multiple SNPs in large cohorts of unrelated preeclamptic cases and controls. These studies show further associations with the 2q14 locus in an Australian/New Zealand cohort [47] and the 19q31.31 locus in a cohort from the state of Iowa in the USA [54]. The association of PE with the 2q14 locus was recently replicated in the Chinese Han population [71].

Fine mapping of the PREG1 locus identified in the Australian/New Zealand families revealed the presence of two loci on both arms of chromosome 2 [56]. SNP analyses of two candidate genes—*TACR1* and *TCF7L1*—in the 2p region achieved genome-wide significance [56]. The quantitative bioinformatics analysis of differential expression and SNP association of the 2q locus prioritized *ACVR2A* as a candidate PE susceptibility gene [57]. In this study, multiple *ACVR2A* SNPs showed preliminary associations with PE, and a greater than tenfold differential expression of *ACVR2A* in preeclamptic decidua compared with controls was observed [57]. While a subsequent study in an extended family cohort in the Australian/New Zealand population [59] and an independent Finnish study did not replicate the SNP findings [72], significant associations of *ACVR2A* SNPs were demonstrated in a large independent Norwegian population cohort of unrelated preeclamptic cases and controls [68]. Additionally, the significant association of *ACVR2A* with PE was recently replicated in the Brazilian and Turkish populations, particularly in women who developed severe early-onset PE before 34 weeks' gestation [73,

74]. Further genetic dissection of the 2q22 locus showed an overlap between PE and cardiovascular disease, underscoring a shared genetic mechanism for both conditions [61], which remains to be further investigated.

Resolution of the quantitative trait loci on chromosomes 5q and 13q revealed several positional candidate genes, *CRHBP*, *ERAP1*, *LNPEP*, *COL4A1*, and *COL4A2*, for further genetic and functional investigation [14]. Subsequent analysis of the 5q quantitative trait locus demonstrated significant associations of several *ERAP2* SNPs with PE in the Australian/New Zealand familial cohort and a large independent Norwegian cohort of unrelated preeclamptic cases and controls [58]. Fetal *ERAP2* was also associated with PE in an African-American population [75]. Additional analysis of the 13q susceptibility locus in the Australian/New Zealand and Norwegian cohorts identified *TNFSF13B* as a promising candidate gene [60]. Three rare genetic variants of *TNFSF13B* showed nominal associations with PE in the Australian/New Zealand familial cohort but not in the Norwegian replication cohort [60]. One of these variants results in altered transcription factor binding, which may have implications in the development of PE and remains to be further investigated [60].

Using a sib-pair linkage analysis, Dutch researchers confirmed a significant association of PE with the 10q22.1 locus [62]. Maternal allele transmission was demonstrated by haplotype analysis [62], showing for the first time that a parent-of-origin effect exists in PE. This suggested that paternally derived alleles were imprinted, leaving only the maternal copy to be expressed that results in PE. Hence, to test for imprinting effects, the Dutch group examined gene expression in androgenetic placentas, where all genes are derived solely from the father. Two gene clusters near *CTNNA3* and *KCNMA1* were downregulated in these androgenetic placentas, which corresponded with the chromosomal regions identified in affected sisters, providing evidence for epigenetics in the pathogenesis of PE [62]. Further refinement of this susceptibility locus at 10q22.1 showed that missense mutations in the *STOX1* gene were identical in affected sisters [63].

3 Confounders and Limitations

The genetic study of PE has largely been hampered by a lack of reproducibility and conflicting results, when trying to replicate genetic associations in multiple populations. There are several possible reasons for this. Firstly, a major issue for the candidate gene approach is that etiology of PE remains unknown and the knowledge of its pathophysiology is incomplete, thus significantly impacting the selection of candidate genes for analysis. Nevertheless, the use of the genome-wide approach has partially helped to improve this selection process and allowed the identification of novel candidate genes such as *STOX1* and *ACVR2A*. Another issue is that populations will have different genetic backgrounds and likely have a diverse range of causal gene variants, thus lowering study reproducibility of a single causal gene variant. Yet another confounder is that most of the earlier studies were inadequately powered with small sample sizes, which results in more false positives. Effect sizes of causal gene variants are also likely to be small, further reducing the ability of past studies, which are designed to identify larger effect sizes, to detect them. Hence, even the large-scale GOPEC consortium analyses of over 500 preeclamptic women and their families failed to identify any casual gene variants [76]. While the use of meta-analyses may improve statistical power by combining past studies, they are reliant on the quality of the original studies. For example, the use of varying definitions of PE in each study can confound the results [77]. Therefore, no universally accepted single causative gene has yet been identified. Nevertheless, given the complexity of PE, it is most likely a variety of genes with small effect size from multiple functional pathways rather than a single gene or gene family with a large effect size, which cumulatively confers susceptibility of PE to an individual woman. Extremely large sample sizes will thus be required to properly determine the genetic contributions to PE, and only a worldwide collaborative effort with well-defined samples will achieve this [78]. Encouragingly, efforts are currently underway to establish new PE cohorts [79], standardize collection methods and definitions used in the field, and promote international collaborative networks through the Global Pregnancy Collaboration (CoLab) initiative [80].

4 What's Next?

4.1 Expression and Functional Analyses of Identified Candidate Genes

As the genetic association of a gene variant with PE does not equate to a casual role in the development of PE, expression and functional analyses should be performed to examine causal involvement of identified genes. The two most closely studied candidate genes identified from the genome-wide approach are *STOX1* and *ACVR2A*.

STOX1, which was first identified as a candidate gene in the Dutch population [63], codes for a winged helix transcription factor and is involved in the trophoblast differentiation pathway. The high-risk *STOX1* allele Y153H results in decreased trophoblast invasion, which is commonly observed in PE [81]. This was the first report of a high-risk genotype with a functional consequence that directly contributes to the development of PE. The genetic association for *STOX1* was however not reproducible in two independent replication studies performed in the Finnish and Norwegian populations [82, 83]. Nevertheless, the Norwegian study found that expression of the *STOX1* paralogue, *STOX2*, was significantly decreased in the preeclamptic decidua and that the transcriptional alterations in the preeclamptic decidua were consistent with that observed when *STOX1* was overexpressed in choriocarcinoma cells [82]. Choriocarcinoma cells overexpressing *STOX1* also effectively reproduced the transcriptional changes seen in the preeclamptic placenta [84]. Transgenic mice overexpressing human *STOX1* also show a preeclamptic phenotype [85] and have similar cardiovascular alterations compared with that seen in preeclamptic women [86]. A possible mechanism for this is that *STOX1* overexpression alters free radical production and mitochondrial function, which impacts the vasodilator availability of nitric oxide and switches the equilibrium to favor increased blood pressure [87]. Hence, functional investigation of the role of *STOX1* in PE is ongoing.

Genetic variants of *ACVR2A*, which codes for the main activin A binding type II receptor, are associated with PE in multiple populations worldwide [57, 59, 68, 73, 74]. Activin A and its related receptors belong to the transforming growth factor β-family [88], and are ubiquitously expressed throughout the body, where they mediate numerous cellular functions such as proliferation, differentiation, and apoptosis [89]. The PE-associated rs1424954 variant results in decreased *ACVR2A* mRNA expression [90]. An earlier study in our laboratory showed significantly decreased *ACVR2A* receptor mRNA expression in preeclamptic *decidua basalis* tissues at the maternal-fetal interface [57]. A similar reduction was observed by Manuelpillai et al. [91] in the chorio-decidua obtained from preeclamptic women. Mimicking decreased *ACVR2A* expression in decidualized stromal cells resulted in lowered mRNA expression of the decidualization marker, prolactin, and abnormal regulation of trophoblast adhesion, proliferation, migration, and invasion in vitro [92]. Additionally, decreasing *ACVR2A* expression could increase permeability and inhibit proliferation of vascular endothelial cells [93]. Collectively, these studies support a potential role for decreased *ACVR2A* expression in the development of PE.

4.2 Integrative Approaches

Nevertheless, a major limitation of current functional studies is that knowledge gained is often confined to the role of individual genes in individual cell types. In a complex disorder like PE, with over a hundred genes described as having genetic associations with PE [78], interactions between many genes in multiple cell types are likely to be involved and thereby contribute to the common development of PE. To identify novel interactions and possible functions of susceptibility genes, and prioritize efforts for future functional studies, we previously pursued a novel integrative bioinformatics approach based on transcriptome profiling [94]. Having demonstrated significantly altered preeclamptic expression of several maternal susceptibility genes, *ACVR1*, *ACVR1C*, *ACVR2A*, *COL4A1*, *COL4A2*, *ERAP1*, *ERAP2*, *INHA*, *INHBB*, and *LNPEP*, which were identified through the genome-wide approach [57, 95], the bioinformatics study was focused on this set of genes [94]. Through this integrative approach, we were able to show novel interactive links between ACVR2A, AGT, and ERAP1, which would not have been apparent through traditional study approaches. Additionally, an unbiased and unexpected functional role of the structural collagen gene, *COL4A1*, on blood pressure regulation was identified. We subsequently showed that arresten, the anti-angiogenic cleavage product derived from COL4A1 [96], was significantly increased in the maternal circulation before the clinical onset of PE and associated with clinical severity in the third trimester [97], providing supporting evidence for a causal role in the development of PE rather than a consequence of subsequent PE dysfunction.

The advancement of gene technologies presents an exciting future ahead for the genetic study of PE. Although a recent study using the latest exome sequencing with over 8000 samples failed to find any significant genetic variants for PE [66], it merely underscores how critical sample size is in determining the genetic architecture of PE. Ongoing studies in our laboratory are utilizing a combined approach of comparing the genome, transcriptome, and methylome profiles in PE. Thus, the ability to rapidly determine genome sequences and related transcriptome and methylation profiles will undoubtedly enhance genetic studies in PE.

5 Conclusion

In summary, resolving the genetic basis of PE will require further studies with large-scale international collaborative efforts. Using an integrated approach incorporating various platforms to interrogate genes at the genome, transcriptome and functional levels may provide novel insights into the causes of PE.

References

1. Duley L (2009) The global impact of pre-eclampsia and eclampsia. Semin Perinatol 33(3):130–137. https://doi.org/10.1053/j.semperi.2009.02.010
2. Tranquilli AL, Dekker G, Magee L, Roberts J, Sibai BM, Steyn W, Zeeman GG, Brown MA (2014) The classification, diagnosis and management of the hypertensive disorders of pregnancy: a revised statement from the ISSHP. Pregnancy Hypertens 4(2):97–104. https://doi.org/10.1016/j.preghy.2014.02.001
3. Murphy DJ, Stirrat GM (2000) Mortality and morbidity associated with early-onset preeclampsia. Hypertens Pregnancy 19(2):221–231
4. Sibai B, Dekker G, Kupferminc M (2005) Preeclampsia. Lancet 365(9461):785–799. https://doi.org/10.1016/S0140-6736(05)17987-2
5. Tranquilli AL, Brown MA, Zeeman GG, Dekker G, Sibai BM (2013) The definition of severe and early-onset preeclampsia. Statements from the International Society for the Study of

hypertension in pregnancy (ISSHP). Pregnancy Hypertens 3(1):44–47. https://doi.org/10.1016/j.preghy.2012.11.001

6. Lowe SA, Brown MA, Dekker GA, Gatt S, McLintock CK, McMahon LP, Mangos G, Moore MP, Muller P, Paech M, Walters B (2009) Guidelines for the management of hypertensive disorders of pregnancy 2008. Aust N Z J Obstet Gynaecol 49(3):242–246. https://doi.org/10.1111/j.1479-828X.2009.01003.x
7. Boyd HA, Tahir H, Wohlfahrt J, Melbye M (2013) Associations of personal and family preeclampsia history with the risk of early-, intermediate- and late-onset preeclampsia. Am J Epidemiol 178(11):1611–1619. https://doi.org/10.1093/aje/kwt189
8. Chesley LC, Annitto JE, Cosgrove RA (1968) The familial factor in toxemia of pregnancy. Obstet Gynecol 32(3):303–311
9. Skjaerven R, Vatten LJ, Wilcox AJ, Ronning T, Irgens LM, Lie RT (2005) Recurrence of preeclampsia across generations: exploring fetal and maternal genetic components in a population based cohort. BMJ 331(7521):877. https://doi.org/10.1136/bmj.38555.462685.8F
10. Dawson LM, Parfrey PS, Hefferton D, Dicks EL, Cooper MJ, Young D, Marsden PA (2002) Familial risk of preeclampsia in Newfoundland: a population-based study. J Am Soc Nephrol 13(7):1901–1906
11. Sutherland A, Cooper DW, Howie PW, Liston WA, MacGillivray I (1981) The incidence of severe preeclampsia amongst mothers and mothers-in-law of preeclamptics and controls. Br J Obstet Gynaecol 88(8):785–791
12. O'Shaughnessy KM, Ferraro F, Fu B, Downing S, Morris NH (2000) Identification of monozygotic twins that are concordant for preeclampsia. Am J Obstet Gynecol 182(5):1156–1157
13. Treloar SA, Cooper DW, Brennecke SP, Grehan MM, Martin NG (2001) An Australian twin study of the genetic basis of preeclampsia and eclampsia. Am J Obstet Gynecol 184(3):374–381. https://doi.org/10.1067/mob.2001.109400
14. Johnson MP, Fitzpatrick E, Dyer TD, Jowett JB, Brennecke SP, Blangero J, Moses EK (2007) Identification of two novel quantitative trait loci for preeclampsia susceptibility on chromosomes 5q and 13q using a variance components-based linkage approach. Mol Hum Reprod 13(1):61–67. https://doi.org/10.1093/molehr/gal095
15. Nilsson E, Salonen Ros H, Cnattingius S, Lichtenstein P (2004) The importance of genetic and environmental effects for preeclampsia and gestational hypertension: a family study. BJOG 111(3):200–206
16. Salonen Ros H, Lichtenstein P, Lipworth L, Cnattingius S (2000) Genetic effects on the liability of developing preeclampsia and gestational hypertension. Am J Med Genet 91(4):256–260. https://doi.org/10.1002/(SICI)1096-8628(20000410)91:4<256::AID-AJMG3>3.0.CO;2-T
17. Cnattingius S, Reilly M, Pawitan Y, Lichtenstein P (2004) Maternal and fetal genetic factors account for most of familial aggregation of preeclampsia: a population-based Swedish cohort study. Am J Med Genet A 130A(4):365–371. https://doi.org/10.1002/ajmg.a.30257
18. Arngrimsson R, Bjornsson S, Geirsson RT, Bjornsson H, Walker JJ, Snaedal G (1990) Genetic and familial predisposition to eclampsia and preeclampsia in a defined population. Br J Obstet Gynaecol 97(9):762–769
19. Torbergsen T, Oian P, Mathiesen E, Borud O (1989) Preeclampsia – a mitochondrial disease? Acta Obstet Gynecol Scand 68(2):145–148
20. Graves JA (1998) Genomic imprinting, development and disease – is preeclampsia caused by a maternally imprinted gene? Reprod Fertil Dev 10(1):23–29
21. Chappell S, Morgan L (2006) Searching for genetic clues to the causes of preeclampsia. Clin Sci (Lond) 110(4):443–458. https://doi.org/10.1042/CS20050323
22. Mutze S, Rudnik-Schoneborn S, Zerres K, Rath W (2008) Genes and the preeclampsia syndrome. J Perinat Med 36(1):38–58. https://doi.org/10.1515/JPM.2008.004
23. Luo ZC, An N, Xu HR, Larante A, Audibert F, Fraser WD (2007) The effects and mechanisms of primiparity on the risk of preeclampsia: a systematic review. Paediatr Perinat Epidemiol 21(Suppl 1):36–45. https://doi.org/10.1111/j.1365-3016.2007.00836.x
24. Kwon JM, Goate AM (2000) The candidate gene approach. Alcohol Res Health 24(3):164
25. Williams PJ, Broughton Pipkin F (2011) The genetics of preeclampsia and other hypertensive disorders of pregnancy. Best Pract Res Clin Obstet Gynaecol 25(4):405–417. https://doi.org/10.1016/j.bpobgyn.2011.02.007
26. Buurma AJ, Turner RJ, Driessen JH, Mooyaart AL, Schoones JW, Bruijn JA, Bloemenkamp KW, Dekkers OM, Baelde HJ (2013) Genetic variants in preeclampsia: a meta-analysis. Hum Reprod Update 19(3):289–303. https://doi.org/10.1093/humupd/dms060
27. Staines-Urias E, Paez MC, Doyle P, Dudbridge F, Serrano NC, Ioannidis JP, Keating BJ,

Hingorani AD, Casas JP (2012) Genetic association studies in preeclampsia: systematic meta-analyses and field synopsis. Int J Epidemiol 41(6):1764–1775. https://doi.org/10.1093/ije/dys162

28. Dai B, Liu T, Zhang B, Zhang X, Wang Z (2013) The polymorphism for endothelial nitric oxide synthase gene, the level of nitric oxide and the risk for preeclampsia: a meta-analysis. Gene 519(1):187–193. https://doi.org/10.1016/j.gene.2013.01.004
29. Yu CK, Casas JP, Savvidou MD, Sahemey MK, Nicolaides KH, Hingorani AD (2006) Endothelial nitric oxide synthase gene polymorphism (Glu298Asp) and development of preeclampsia: a case-control study and a meta-analysis. BMC Pregnancy Childbirth 6:7. https://doi.org/10.1186/1471-2393-6-7
30. Hiby SE, Walker JJ, O'Shaughnessy KM, Redman CW, Carrington M, Trowsdale J, Moffett A (2004) Combinations of maternal KIR and fetal HLA-C genes influence the risk of preeclampsia and reproductive success. J Exp Med 200(8):957–965. https://doi.org/10.1084/jem.20041214
31. Yu H, Pan N, Shen Y, Jin S, Zhai J, Qiao D, Shen Y, Miao F, Wang L, He Y, Ren M, Zhang J (2014) Interaction of parental KIR and fetal HLA-C genotypes with the risk of preeclampsia. Hypertens Pregnancy 33(4):402–411. https://doi.org/10.3109/10641955.2014.920026
32. Nakimuli A, Chazara O, Hiby SE, Farrell L, Tukwasibwe S, Jayaraman J, Traherne JA, Trowsdale J, Colucci F, Lougee E, Vaughan RW, Elliott AM, Byamugisha J, Kaleebu P, Mirembe F, Nemat-Gorgani N, Parham P, Norman PJ, Moffett A (2015) A KIR B centromeric region present in Africans but not Europeans protects pregnant women from preeclampsia. Proc Natl Acad Sci U S A 112(3):845–850. https://doi.org/10.1073/pnas.1413453112
33. Lau SY, Guild SJ, Barrett CJ, Chen Q, McCowan L, Jordan V, Chamley LW (2013) Tumor necrosis factor-alpha, interleukin-6, and interleukin-10 levels are altered in preeclampsia: a systematic review and meta-analysis. Am J Reprod Immunol 70(5):412–427. https://doi.org/10.1111/aji.12138
34. Xie C, Yao MZ, Liu JB, Xiong LK (2011) A meta-analysis of tumor necrosis factor-alpha, interleukin-6, and interleukin-10 in preeclampsia. Cytokine 56(3):550–559. https://doi.org/10.1016/j.cyto.2011.09.021
35. Fong FM, Sahemey MK, Hamedi G, Eyitayo R, Yates D, Kuan V, Thangaratinam S, Walton RT (2014) Maternal genotype and severe preeclampsia: a HuGE review. Am J Epidemiol 180(4):335–345. https://doi.org/10.1093/aje/kwu151
36. Harmon QE, Engel SM, Wu MC, Moran TM, Luo J, Stuebe AM, Avery CL, Olshan AF (2014) Polymorphisms in inflammatory genes are associated with term small for gestational age and preeclampsia. Am J Reprod Immunol 71(5):472–484. https://doi.org/10.1111/aji.12241
37. Zubor P, Dokus K, Zigo I, Skerenova M, Pullmann R, Danko J (2014) TNF alpha G308A gene polymorphism has an impact on renal function, microvascular permeability, organ involvement and severity of preeclampsia. Gynecol Obstet Investig 78(3):150–161. https://doi.org/10.1159/000364865
38. Mao L, Zhou Q, Zhou S, Wilbur RR, Li X (2013) Roles of apolipoprotein E (ApoE) and inducible nitric oxide synthase (iNOS) in inflammation and apoptosis in preeclampsia pathogenesis and progression. PLoS One 8(3):e58168. https://doi.org/10.1371/journal.pone.0058168
39. Procopciuc LM, Caracostea G, Zaharie G, Stamatian F (2015) Newborn APOE genotype influences maternal lipid profile and the severity of high-risk pregnancy – preeclampsia. Interaction with maternal genotypes as a modulating risk factor in preeclampsia. Hypertens Pregnancy:1–13. https://doi.org/10.3109/10641955.2015.1009541
40. Procopciuc LM, Zaharie G, Caracostea G, Stamatian F (2014) Newborn LpL (Ser447Stop, Asn291Ser) genotypes and the interaction with maternal genotypes influence the risk for different types of preeclampsia: modulating effect on lipid profile and pregnancy outcome. Gynecol Endocrinol 30(3):221–225. https://doi.org/10.3109/09513590.2013.871512
41. Matsubara K, Higaki T, Matsubara Y, Nawa A (2015) Nitric oxide and reactive oxygen species in the pathogenesis of preeclampsia. Int J Mol Sci 16(3):4600–4614. https://doi.org/10.3390/ijms16034600
42. Gupta S, Aziz N, Sekhon L, Agarwal R, Mansour G, Li J, Agarwal A (2009) Lipid peroxidation and antioxidant status in preeclampsia: a systematic review. Obstet Gynecol Surv 64(11):750–759. https://doi.org/10.1097/OGX.0b013e3181bea0ac
43. Mistry HD, Gill CA, Kurlak LO, Seed PT, Hesketh JE, Meplan C, Schomburg L, Chappell LC, Morgan L, Poston L, SCOPE Consortium (2015) Association between maternal micronutrient status, oxidative stress, and common genetic variants in antioxidant

enzymes at 15 weeks gestation in nulliparous women who subsequently develop preeclampsia. Free Radic Biol Med 78:147–155. https://doi.org/10.1016/j.freeradbiomed.2014.10.580

44. Wang X, Bai T, Liu S, Pan H, Wang B (2014) Association between thrombophilia gene polymorphisms and preeclampsia: a meta-analysis. PLoS One 9(6):e100789. https://doi.org/10.1371/journal.pone.0100789
45. Wang XM, Wu HY, Qiu XJ (2013) Methylenetetrahydrofolate reductase (MTHFR) gene C677T polymorphism and risk of preeclampsia: an updated meta-analysis based on 51 studies. Arch Med Res 44(3):159–168. https://doi.org/10.1016/j.arcmed.2013.01.011
46. Harrison GA, Humphrey KE, Jones N, Badenhop R, Guo G, Elakis G, Kaye JA, Turner RJ, Grehan M, Wilton AN, Brennecke SP, Cooper DW (1997) A genomewide linkage study of preeclampsia/eclampsia reveals evidence for a candidate region on 4q. Am J Hum Genet 60(5):1158–1167
47. Johnson MP, Brennecke SP, East CE, Goring HH, Kent JW Jr, Dyer TD, Said JM, Roten LT, Iversen AC, Abraham LJ, Heinonen S, Kajantie E, Kere J, Kivinen K, Pouta A, Laivuori H, Austgulen R, Blangero J, Moses EK (2012) Genome-wide association scan identifies a risk locus for preeclampsia on 2q14, near the inhibin, beta B gene. PLoS One 7(3):e33666. https://doi.org/10.1371/journal.pone.0033666
48. Moses EK, Lade JA, Guo G, Wilton AN, Grehan M, Freed K, Borg A, Terwilliger JD, North R, Cooper DW, Brennecke SP (2000) A genome scan in families from Australia and New Zealand confirms the presence of a maternal susceptibility locus for preeclampsia, on chromosome 2. Am J Hum Genet 67(6):1581–1585. https://doi.org/10.1086/316888
49. Laivuori H, Lahermo P, Ollikainen V, Widen E, Haiva-Mallinen L, Sundstrom H, Laitinen T, Kaaja R, Ylikorkala O, Kere J (2003) Susceptibility loci for preeclampsia on chromosomes 2p25 and 9p13 in Finnish families. Am J Hum Genet 72(1):168–177. https://doi.org/10.1086/345311
50. Arngrimsson R, Siguroardottir S, Frigge ML, Bjarnadottir RI, Jonsson T, Stefansson H, Baldursdottir A, Einarsdottir AS, Palsson B, Snorradottir S, Lachmeijer AM, Nicolae D, Kong A, Bragason BT, Gulcher JR, Geirsson RT, Stefansson K (1999) A genome-wide scan reveals a maternal susceptibility locus for preeclampsia on chromosome 2p13. Hum Mol Genet 8(9):1799–1805
51. Lachmeijer AM, Arngrimsson R, Bastiaans EJ, Frigge ML, Pals G, Sigurdardottir S, Stefansson H, Palsson B, Nicolae D, Kong A, Aarnoudse JG, Gulcher JR, Dekker GA, ten Kate LP, Stefansson K (2001) A genome-wide scan for preeclampsia in the Netherlands. Eur J Hum Genet 9(10):758–764. https://doi.org/10.1038/sj.ejhg.5200706
52. Roten LT, Johnson MP, Thompsen LC, Gundersen AS, Solberg P, Tollaksen K, Lyslo I, Tappert C, Odland ML, Strand KM, Fenstad MH, Drablos F, Skorpen F, Moses EK, Austgulen R, Bjorge L (2013) OP006. A preeclampsia genome-wide linkage scan in Norwegian families. Pregnancy Hypertens 3(2):64. https://doi.org/10.1016/j.preghy.2013.04.022
53. Hayward C, Livingstone J, Holloway S, Liston WA, Brock DJ (1992) An exclusion map for preeclampsia: assuming autosomal recessive inheritance. Am J Hum Genet 50(4):749–757
54. Zhao L, Triche EW, Walsh KM, Bracken MB, Saftlas AF, Hoh J, Dewan AT (2012) Genome-wide association study identifies a maternal copy-number deletion in PSG11 enriched among preeclampsia patients. BMC Pregnancy Childbirth 12:61. https://doi.org/10.1186/1471-2393-12-61
55. Guo G, Lade JA, Wilton AN, Moses EK, Grehan M, Fu Y, Qiu H, Cooper DW, Brennecke SP (1999) Genetic susceptibility to preeclampsia and chromosome 7q36. Hum Genet 105(6):641–647
56. Fitzpatrick E, Goring HH, Liu H, Borg A, Forrest S, Cooper DW, Brennecke SP, Moses EK (2004) Fine mapping and SNP analysis of positional candidates at the preeclampsia susceptibility locus (PREG1) on chromosome 2. Hum Biol 76(6):849–862
57. Moses EK, Fitzpatrick E, Freed KA, Dyer TD, Forrest S, Elliott K, Johnson MP, Blangero J, Brennecke SP (2006) Objective prioritization of positional candidate genes at a quantitative trait locus for preeclampsia on 2q22. Mol Hum Reprod 12(8):505–512. https://doi.org/10.1093/molehr/gal056
58. Johnson MP, Roten LT, Dyer TD, East CE, Forsmo S, Blangero J, Brennecke SP, Austgulen R, Moses EK (2009) The ERAP2 gene is associated with preeclampsia in Australian and Norwegian populations. Hum Genet 126(5):655–666. https://doi.org/10.1007/s00439-009-0714-x
59. Fitzpatrick E, Johnson MP, Dyer TD, Forrest S, Elliott K, Blangero J, Brennecke SP, Moses EK (2009) Genetic association of the activin A receptor gene (ACVR2A) and preeclampsia. Mol Hum Reprod 15(3):195–204. https://doi.org/10.1093/molehr/gap001

60. Fenstad MH, Johnson MP, Roten LT, Aas PA, Forsmo S, Klepper K, East CE, Abraham LJ, Blangero J, Brennecke SP, Austgulen R, Moses EK (2010) Genetic and molecular functional characterization of variants within TNFSF13B, a positional candidate preeclampsia susceptibility gene on 13q. PLoS One 5(9). https://doi.org/10.1371/journal.pone.0012993
61. Johnson MP, Brennecke SP, East CE, Dyer TD, Roten LT, Proffitt JM, Melton PE, Fenstad MH, Aalto-Viljakainen T, Makikallio K, Heinonen S, Kajantie E, Kere J, Laivuori H, Austgulen R, Blangero J, Moses EK (2013) Genetic dissection of the preeclampsia susceptibility locus on chromosome 2q22 reveals shared novel risk factors for cardiovascular disease. Mol Hum Reprod 19(7):423–437. https://doi.org/10.1093/molehr/gat011
62. Oudejans CB, Mulders J, Lachmeijer AM, van Dijk M, Konst AA, Westerman BA, van Wijk IJ, Leegwater PA, Kato HD, Matsuda T, Wake N, Dekker GA, Pals G, ten Kate LP, Blankenstein MA (2004) The parent-of-origin effect of 10q22 in preeclamptic females coincides with two regions clustered for genes with down-regulated expression in androgenetic placentas. Mol Hum Reprod 10(8):589–598. https://doi.org/10.1093/molehr/gah080
63. van Dijk M, Mulders J, Poutsma A, Konst AA, Lachmeijer AM, Dekker GA, Blankenstein MA, Oudejans CB (2005) Maternal segregation of the Dutch preeclampsia locus at 10q22 with a new member of the winged helix gene family. Nat Genet 37(5):514–519. https://doi.org/10.1038/ng1541
64. Laasanen J, Hiltunen M, Romppanen EL, Punnonen K, Mannermaa A, Heinonen S (2003) Microsatellite marker association at chromosome region 2p13 in Finnish patients with preeclampsia and obstetric cholestasis suggests a common risk locus. Eur J Hum Genet 11(3):232–236. https://doi.org/10.1038/sj.ejhg.5200951
65. Majander KK, Villa PM, Kivinen K, Kere J, Laivuori H (2013) A follow-up linkage study of Finnish preeclampsia families identifies a new fetal susceptibility locus on chromosome 18. Eur J Hum Genet 21(9):1024–1026. https://doi.org/10.1038/ejhg.2013.6
66. Kaartokallio T, Wang J, Heinonen S, Kajantie E, Kivinen K, Pouta A, Gerdhem P, Jiao H, Kere J, Laivuori H (2016) Exome sequencing in pooled DNA samples to identify maternal preeclampsia risk variants. Sci Rep 6:29085. https://doi.org/10.1038/srep29085
67. Arngrimsson R, Hayward C, Nadaud S, Baldursdottir A, Walker JJ, Liston WA, Bjarnadottir RI, Brock DJ, Geirsson RT, Connor JM, Soubrier F (1997) Evidence for a familial pregnancy-induced hypertension locus in the eNOS-gene region. Am J Hum Genet 61(2):354–362. https://doi.org/10.1086/514843
68. Roten LT, Johnson MP, Forsmo S, Fitzpatrick E, Dyer TD, Brennecke SP, Blangero J, Moses EK, Austgulen R (2009) Association between the candidate susceptibility gene ACVR2A on chromosome 2q22 and preeclampsia in a large Norwegian population-based study (the HUNT study). Eur J Hum Genet 17(2):250–257. https://doi.org/10.1038/ejhg.2008.158
69. Zintzaras E, Kitsios G, Harrison GA, Laivuori H, Kivinen K, Kere J, Messinis I, Stefanidis I, Ioannidis JP (2006) Heterogeneity-based genome search meta-analysis for preeclampsia. Hum Genet 120(3):360–370. https://doi.org/10.1007/s00439-006-0214-1
70. Adler D (1994) Idiogram album. http://www.pathology.washington.edu/research/cytopages/idiograms/human/. Accessed 2015
71. Wang Q, Wang G, Guo C, Cao X, An L, Du M, Qiu Y, Yang Y, Wang Y, Wang S, Wang X, Ma X (2015) Single nucleotide polymorphisms near the inhibin beta B gene on 2q14 are associated with preeclampsia in Han Chinese women. Eur J Obstet Gynecol Reprod Biol 193:127–131. https://doi.org/10.1016/j.ejogrb.2015.04.001
72. Lokki AI, Klemetti MM, Heino S, Hiltunen L, Heinonen S, Laivuori H (2011) Association of the rs1424954 polymorphism of the ACVR2A gene with the risk of preeclampsia is not replicated in a Finnish study population. BMC Res Notes 4:545. https://doi.org/10.1186/1756-0500-4-545
73. Ferreira LC, Gomes CE, Araujo AC, Bezerra PF, Duggal P, Jeronimo SM (2015) Association between ACVR2A and early-onset preeclampsia: replication study in a Northeastern Brazilian population. Placenta 36(2):186–190. https://doi.org/10.1016/j.placenta.2014.11.007
74. Zeybek B, Celik HA, Aydin HH, Askar N (2013) Polymorphisms in the activin A receptor type 2A gene affect the onset time and severity of preeclampsia in the Turkish population. J Perinat Med 41(4):389–399. https://doi.org/10.1515/jpm-2012-0187
75. Hill LD, Hilliard DD, York TP, Srinivas S, Kusanovic JP, Gomez R, Elovitz MA, Romero R, Strauss JF III (2011) Fetal ERAP2 variation is associated with preeclampsia in African Americans in a case-control study. BMC Med Genet 12:64. https://doi.org/10.1186/1471-2350-12-64

76. GOPEC Consortium (2005) Disentangling fetal and maternal susceptibility for preeclampsia: a British multicenter candidate-gene study. Am J Hum Genet 77(1):127–131. https://doi.org/10.1086/431245
77. Williams PJ, Morgan L (2012) The role of genetics in preeclampsia and potential pharmacogenomic interventions. Pharmgenomics Pers Med 5:37–51. https://doi.org/10.2147/PGPM.S23141
78. Jebbink J, Wolters A, Fernando F, Afink G, van der Post J, Ris-Stalpers C (2012) Molecular genetics of preeclampsia and HELLP syndrome - a review. Biochim Biophys Acta 1822(12):1960–1969. https://doi.org/10.1016/j.bbadis.2012.08.004
79. Roten LT, Thomsen LC, Gundersen AS, Fenstad MH, Odland ML, Strand KM, Solberg P, Tappert C, Araya E, Baerheim G, Lyslo I, Tollaksen K, Bjorge L, Austgulen R (2015) The Norwegian preeclampsia family cohort study: a new resource for investigating genetic aspects and heritability of preeclampsia and related phenotypes. BMC Pregnancy Childbirth 15:319. https://doi.org/10.1186/s12884-015-0754-2
80. Myatt L, Redman CW, Staff AC, Hansson S, Wilson ML, Laivuori H, Poston L, Roberts JM, Global Pregnancy C (2014) Strategy for standardization of preeclampsia research study design. Hypertension 63(6):1293–1301. https://doi.org/10.1161/HYPERTENSIONAHA.113.02664
81. van Dijk M, van Bezu J, van Abel D, Dunk C, Blankenstein MA, Oudejans CB, Lye SJ (2010) The STOX1 genotype associated with preeclampsia leads to a reduction of trophoblast invasion by alpha-T-catenin upregulation. Hum Mol Genet 19(13):2658–2667. https://doi.org/10.1093/hmg/ddq152
82. Fenstad MH, Johnson MP, Loset M, Mundal SB, Roten LT, Eide IP, Bjorge L, Sande RK, Johansson AK, Dyer TD, Forsmo S, Blangero J, Moses EK, Austgulen R (2010) STOX2 but not STOX1 is differentially expressed in decidua from preeclamptic women: data from the second Nord-Trondelag health study. Mol Hum Reprod 16(12):960–968. https://doi.org/10.1093/molehr/gaq064
83. Kivinen K, Peterson H, Hiltunen L, Laivuori H, Heino S, Tiala I, Knuutila S, Rasi V, Kere J (2007) Evaluation of STOX1 as a preeclampsia candidate gene in a population-wide sample. Eur J Hum Genet 15(4):494–497. https://doi.org/10.1038/sj.ejhg.5201788
84. Rigourd V, Chauvet C, Chelbi ST, Rebourcet R, Mondon F, Letourneur F, Mignot TM, Barbaux S, Vaiman D (2008) STOX1 overexpression in choriocarcinoma cells mimics transcriptional alterations observed in preeclamptic placentas. PLoS One 3(12):e3905. https://doi.org/10.1371/journal.pone.0003905
85. Doridot L, Passet B, Mehats C, Rigourd V, Barbaux S, Ducat A, Mondon F, Vilotte M, Castille J, Breuiller-Fouche M, Daniel N, le Provost F, Bauchet AL, Baudrie V, Hertig A, Buffat C, Simeoni U, Germain G, Vilotte JL, Vaiman D (2013) Preeclampsia-like symptoms induced in mice by fetoplacental expression of STOX1 are reversed by aspirin treatment. Hypertension 61(3):662–668. https://doi.org/10.1161/HYPERTENSIONAHA.111.202994
86. Ducat A, Doridot L, Calicchio R, Mehats C, Vilotte JL, Castille J, Barbaux S, Couderc B, Jacques S, Letourneur F, Buffat C, Le Grand F, Laissue P, Miralles F, Vaiman D (2016) Endothelial cell dysfunction and cardiac hypertrophy in the STOX1 model of preeclampsia. Sci Rep 6:19196. https://doi.org/10.1038/srep19196
87. Doridot L, Chatre L, Ducat A, Vilotte JL, Lombes A, Mehats C, Barbaux S, Calicchio R, Ricchetti M, Vaiman D (2014) Nitroso-redox balance and mitochondrial homeostasis are regulated by STOX1, a preeclampsia-associated gene. Antioxid Redox Signal 21(6):819–834. https://doi.org/10.1089/ars.2013.5661
88. Pangas SA, Woodruff TK (2000) Activin signal transduction pathways. Trends Endocrinol Metab 11(8):309–314
89. Harrison CA, Gray PC, Vale WW, Robertson DM (2005) Antagonists of activin signaling: mechanisms and potential biological applications. Trends Endocrinol Metab 16(2):73–78. https://doi.org/10.1016/j.tem.2005.01.003
90. Thulluru HK, Michel OJ, Oudejans CB, van Dijk M (2015) ACVR2A promoter polymorphism rs1424954 in the Activin-A signaling pathway in trophoblasts. Placenta 36(4):345–349. https://doi.org/10.1016/j.placenta.2015.01.010
91. Manuelpillai U, Schneider-Kolsky M, Dole A, Wallace EM (2001) Activin A and activin receptors in gestational tissue from preeclamptic pregnancies. J Endocrinol 171(1):57–64
92. Yong HE, Murthi P, Kalionis B, Brennecke SP, Keogh RJ (2015) Altered activin receptor ACVR2A expression in preeclampsia contributes to abnormal placentation. Placenta 36(9):A3. https://doi.org/10.1016/j.placenta.2015.07.194
93. Brennecke SP, Yong HE, Murthi P, Kalionis B, Cartwright JE, Keogh RJ (2016) 52 altered ACVR2A expression modifies the response of vascular endothelial cells to normotensive and

preeclamptic activin a concentrations: endothelial dysfunction, anti-angiogenic factors. Pregnancy Hypertens 6(3):161. https://doi.org/10.1016/j.preghy.2016.08.053

94. Yong HE, Melton PE, Johnson MP, Freed KA, Kalionis B, Murthi P, Brennecke SP, Keogh RJ, Moses EK (2015) Genome-wide transcriptome directed pathway analysis of maternal preeclampsia susceptibility genes. PLoS One 10(5):e0128230. https://doi.org/10.1371/journal.pone.0128230
95. Yong HE, Murthi P, Borg A, Kalionis B, Moses EK, Brennecke SP, Keogh RJ (2014) Increased decidual mRNA expression levels of candidate maternal preeclampsia susceptibility genes are associated with clinical severity. Placenta 35(2):117–124. https://doi.org/10.1016/j.placenta.2013.11.008
96. Colorado PC, Torre A, Kamphaus G, Maeshima Y, Hopfer H, Takahashi K, Volk R, Zamborsky ED, Herman S, Sarkar PK, Ericksen MB, Dhanabal M, Simons M, Post M, Kufe DW, Weichselbaum RR, Sukhatme VP, Kalluri R (2000) Anti-angiogenic cues from vascular basement membrane collagen. Cancer Res 60(9):2520–2526
97. Yong HE, Murthi P, Wong MH, Kalionis B, Brennecke SP, Keogh RJ (2015) Anti-angiogenic collagen fragment arresten is increased from 16 weeks' gestation in preeclamptic plasma. Placenta 36(11):1300–1309. https://doi.org/10.1016/j.placenta.2015.08.013

Chapter 6

Epigenetics and Preeclampsia: Programming of Future Outcomes

Alberto Borges Peixoto, Liliam Cristine Rolo, Luciano Marcondes Machado Nardozza, and Edward Araujo Júnior

Abstract

Pregnancy is known to induce rapid, progressive, and substantial changes to the cardiovascular system, ultimately facilitating successful pregnancy outcomes. Women who develop hypertensive disorders during pregnancy are considered to have "failed" the cardiovascular stress test of pregnancy and likely represent a subpopulation with inadequate cardiovascular accommodation. Preeclampsia is a serious complication with a myriad of manifestations in both mother and offspring. This pregnancy syndrome is a polygenic disease and has now been linked to a greater incidence of cardiovascular disease. Moreover, offsprings born to preeclamptic mothers exhibit an elevated risk of cardiovascular disease, stroke, and mental disorders during adulthood. This suggests that preeclampsia not only exposes the mother and the fetus to complications during pregnancy but also programs chronic diseases during adulthood in the offspring. The etiology of preeclampsia remains unknown, with various theories being suggested to explain its origin. It is primarily thought to be associated with poor placentation and entails excessive maternal inflammation and endothelial dysfunction. It is well established now that the maternal immune system and the placenta are involved in a highly choreographed cross talk that underlies adequate spiral artery remodeling required for uteroplacental perfusion and free flow of nutrients to the fetus. Although it is not clear whether immunological alterations occur early during pregnancy, studies have proposed that dysregulated systemic and placental immunity contribute to impaired angiogenesis and the onset of preeclampsia. Recently emerged strong evidence suggests a potential link among epigenetics, microRNAs (miRNAs), and pregnancy complications. This chapter will focus on important aspects of epigenetics, immunological aspects, and cardiovascular and vascular remodeling of preeclampsia.

Key words Preeclampsia, Epigenetic, Remodeling, Immunology, Cardiovascular system

1 Introduction

Preeclampsia (PE) is a pregnancy-associated syndrome, characterized by hypertension and proteinuria, affecting 2–8% of the population worldwide [1]. It remains a major obstetric concern owing to the associated high prevalence of maternal and fetal mortality and morbidity. Although the etiology is not well characterized, several pathophysiological mechanisms combined have proven to

Padma Murthi and Cathy Vaillancourt (eds.), *Preeclampsia: Methods and Protocols*, Methods in Molecular Biology, vol. 1710, https://doi.org/10.1007/978-1-4939-7498-6_6, © Springer Science+Business Media LLC 2018

be involved in at least the clinical course of PE. Antiangiogenic imbalance, excessive inflammation, hypoxia, and/or autoantibodies targeting the renin-angiotensin system form the harsh intrauterine environment during PE [2, 3]. All these factors may interact with the genome of the mother and the fetus in terms of gene expression modulation, ultimately affecting the expressed phenotype.

The placenta is extremely important for intrauterine fetal development and growth. Deregulation of placentation can lead to adverse outcomes for both mother and fetus, including gestational trophoblastic disease, fetal growth restriction, and PE [4]. Early gamete alterations (of epigenetic origin) may be adequate to induce placental defects [5]. The clinical complications of PE may originate from defective trophoblast invasion and aberrant placental formation, resulting in placental insufficiency due to inadequate remodeling of the maternal vasculature during early pregnancy [6, 7]. Two concepts are mostly accepted: hypertension results either from defects in fetal or placental tissues itself or from a maladapted maternal response to pregnancy. Most genetic studies on PE have focused on maternal susceptibility and have tried to identify genetic aberrations in the mother/fetus [8].

There is evidence that environmental factors can cause epigenetic marks in the DNA and proteins that may be associated with increased susceptibility to several diseases, including PE [9, 10].

2 Epigenetics and Preeclampsia

Epigenetics is the study of heritable changes in gene function that occur without a change in the DNA sequence. These modifications typically turn genes on or off, allowing or preventing the gene from being used to make a protein [11].

Exposure to different environmental stimuli (ethanol, oxygen tension, and assisted reproduction technologies), particularly during critical windows of development, results in the formation of adaptive epigenetic marks as part of the adaptive stress response [12]. The epigenetic marking system includes changes in DNA methylation, histone modifications, and noncoding RNA (ncRNA) expression. These are usually established early during development and act as regulators of developmental, tissue, and sex-specific gene expression [13]. These may be heritable if they occur in the gametes and can have phenotypic consequences in the next generation [14].

Although the precise mechanism is still unknown, epigenetic features within the placenta have been implicated in the pathogenesis of PE [15].

DNA methylation is a unique form of gene regulation because it involves direct covalent modification within the genome and can provide long-term stability in a heritable transgenerational manner [16]. Methylation of vital regulatory sites such as gene promoters or enhancers is mostly connected to gene repression, resulting in downregulation of gene expression [17].

DNA methylation analysis of cord blood cells is a valuable target when studying early epigenetic consequences of PE on the fetus. Several studies have analyzed DNA methylation of genes involved in fetal growth and development that are also highly sensitive to environmental perturbations. Hypomethylation has been observed in the promoter region of 11b-hydroxysteroid dehydrogenase type 2 (HSD11B2) in cord blood samples from neonates exposed to PE [18]. In addition, decreased methylation was reported for insulin-like growth factor 2 (IGF2) in differentially methylated regions, important for gene regulation of imprinted genes [19]. In contrast, in preeclamptic placentas, HSD11B2 and IGF2, gene expression levels are decreased [20, 21]. Therefore, there is a discrepancy between the reported hypomethylated status and the observed downregulated activity of these genes in other studies. It is tempting to speculate that this is a compensatory change in methylation to ensure favorable offspring functioning, but on the other hand, it can be an atypical decrease in gene expression that can lead to metabolic maladaptation.

A recent study used a genome-wide methylation analysis wherein neonatal cord blood DNA from mothers diagnosed with early-onset PE showed promoter hypo- or hyper-methylation for different gene subsets. Prominent DNA modifications were primarily discovered in genes involved in lipid metabolism and inflammation, indicating that early epigenetic disruptions can be identified in preeclamptic children [22]. Taken together, these findings support an effect of PE on the methylation status of cord blood in neonates, but it is unclear whether this is a protective or maladaptive effect. Although this does not prove any causal relationship with long-term health effects, it can be used as an initial proof of concept to conduct new cohort studies [23].

There are no data concerning histone modifications and/or ncRNAs in offsprings from preeclamptic mothers [23]. Communication between DNA methylation and chromatin modifiers or promoter regions of ncRNAs has been established [24, 25], and abnormal methylation, either solely or via other epigenetic marks, can be an important mediator of fetal metabolism. It was clarified that these molecules are implicated in several diseases, and successful revelation of their role in developmental programming can lead to possible biological biomarkers or targets for therapy [23].

3 Preeclampsia: Vascular Remodeling

There is evidence in available literature that implicates PE as a cardiovascular risk factor, predictive of subsequent cardiovascular disease and death [26, 27]. Women with history of PE are at a threefold greater risk of developing hypertension and a twofold greater risk of ischemic heart disease and stroke [26, 27].

PE has been classified according to time of disease onset into early- and late-onset PE; these two modalities of PE have distinct clinical forms with specific pathophysiological features. Early-onset PE is commonly associated with placental insufficiency, intrauterine growth restriction, and adverse maternal and perinatal outcomes [28, 29]. Conversely, late-onset PE is associated with minor placental involvement and milder clinical disease [28, 29]. Intrinsic placental factors are more frequently altered in early-onset PE [28, 29], whereas late-onset PE is usually associated with predisposing maternal factors [30].

Recent findings have suggested that early-onset PE has impaired myocardial relaxation and left ventricular (LV) diastolic dysfunction [31], lipid profile alterations, such as increased cholesterol concentrations, and a trend toward insulin resistance [32]. On the other hand, late-onset PE is characterized by changes in maternal metabolism [33, 34], as well as cardiovascular and endothelial functions [28]. Structural and functional changes in the vasculature are considered independent risk factors for long-term cardiovascular events [35, 36]. Structural remodeling of the vasculature can be evaluated by measurement of the carotid intima-media thickness (IMT) [37] and lumen diameters, while vascular function can be assessed by arterial stiffness indices such as pulse wave velocity, augmentation index, carotid artery distensibility (CD), and circumferential wall stress (CWS) [38]. Moreover, inferior vena cava (IVC) compliance is reflective of the venous responsiveness to hemodynamic changes [39].

Stergiotou et al. [40] evaluated 100 cases of PE subdivided into 50 early- and 50 late-onset cases according to gestational age at onset and 100 controls paired by maternal age and gestational age at ultrasound examination with cases; the results revealed that compared to normotensive pregnancies, early-onset PE was characterized by increased carotid IMT, lumen diameters, and arterial stiffness but with no significant changes in IVC collapsibility. On the other hand, compared to early-onset PE, late-onset PE was characterized by more prominent carotid IMT but less pronounced changes in lumen diameter and arterial stiffness. Furthermore, a significant decrease of IVC collapsibility was observed in late-onset PE.

Yuan et al. [36] prospectively evaluated 22 women with late-onset PE who had not received any antihypertensive treatment before admission and 28 normotensive pregnant women. The authors reported that 18 months after parturition, internal diameter, pressure, and wall tension of the carotid artery remained greater in women with late-onset PE.

The release of factors from an underperfused placenta in early-onset PE [28, 29] may cause vascular dysfunction and elevated blood pressure. Enlarged IMT could possibly represent an adaptive response to preserve the arterial wall stress [41]. Moreover, disturbances in endothelial function and high blood pressure may affect arterial elasticity and consequently enhance stiffness [42]. Lumen diameters in early-onset PE are significantly increased owing to complex interactions among parameters such as cardiac output, blood volume, heart rate, and vessel diameter. IVC collapsibility can be assessed to evaluate venous functioning in PE. Venous distensibility differs in distinct vascular beds [43]. In any case, the ninefold increase in cardiovascular mortality [44] in early-onset PE could possibly be attributed to the cardiovascular changes observed in such patients [45].

Women with late-onset PE have increased mean carotid IMT possibly because of an earlier vascular impairment and maternal predisposition [40]. Arterial stiffness is increased in late-onset PE but to a lesser extent when compared with early-onset PE [40]. A study postulated the hypothesis that timely arterial hypertrophy could favor a "structural" increase in compliance by decreasing the relative amount of connective tissue [46]. Decreased collapsibility index in late-onset PE, suggesting reduced venous reserve capacity, is in favor of the concept of maternal preexisting vascular maladaptation. Regarding arterial diameters, less prominent increase in carotid diameters in late-onset PE is concordant with milder changes in cardiac output as compared to early-onset PE [47]. In this context, the development of less prominent vascular disorders in late-onset PE, when compared with early-onset PE, could support the concept of a milder (twofold) increase in the risk of cardiovascular disease.

4 Preeclampsia: Immunological Findings

PE is a polygenic and potentially fatal pregnancy disorder and a leading cause of maternal and neonatal morbidity and mortality worldwide. To date, the only effective treatment for controlling maternal manifestations associated with PE is delivery, rising preterm birth in cases of severity [48].

The placenta is a heterogeneous tissue with a chimeric pattern of gene expression and DNA methylation; consequently, differences in methylation across different sites, and at different depths, within the same placenta have been identified in several studies [49]. It is believed that PE occurs because of an imbalance between angiogenic and antiangiogenic factors resulting in defective placentation. The dysregulation in gene and protein expression within key biological pathways that control angiogenesis has been implicated in the development of PE, although the specific etiology remains unknown [50].

According to certain studies, the exaggerated systemic inflammatory response in PE is a result of oxidative stress, increased release of microparticles, autoantibodies, misfolded and aggregated proteins, and nuclear and mitochondrial damage-associated molecular patterns (DAMPS) that impart both local and systemic adverse effects, leading to poor trophoblast invasion and vascular growth, endothelial dysfunction, and excessive inflammation [48].

Recently, studies have revealed that both immunological tolerance and immunocompetent cells are important contributors to normal placentation or spiral artery remodeling by extravillous trophoblasts, which establish adequate flow of nutrients to the fetus. Perhaps, a systemic inflammatory response involving leukocytes and endothelium is an important trigger for development of the maternal syndrome of PE. Therefore, a majority of publications have indicated the role of natural killer (NK) and regulatory T cells in the development of this pregnancy pathology because of "poor placentation" [48, 51].

It is known that NK cells correspond to 70% of all mononuclear cells present at the maternal–fetal interface during the first trimester. NK cells are also present in the peripheral blood, but there are remarkable differences between both cell groups. A majority of peripheral blood NK cells are CD56−CD16+ with high cytotoxicity. On the other hand, 90% of decidual NK (dNK) cells are CD56+CD16− [Bulmer]. dNK cells suffer an increase and persist around the trophoblast cells, but they have a tendency to progressively decline from midgestation, almost disappearing at term [52]. However, during normal placentation, dNK cells are not cytotoxic but are responsible for promoting trophoblast invasion and spiral artery remodeling during early normal pregnancy by secretion of chemokines (IL-8 and interferon-inducible protein-10) and various angiogenic factors (e.g., vascular endothelial growth factor C [VEGFC], placental growth factor [PLGF], and angiopoietin 2). The production of cytokine and angiogenic factors by dNK cells during early pregnancy is commanded by the interactions of NK cell-specific receptors and their specific ligands [48].

Second of some studies, whether levels of HLA-interacting receptors are reduced on populations of dNK cells, it could represent implications for interactions of dNK with trophoblast, causing a defective invasion and poor spiral artery remodeling, increasing the risk of development of pregnancy disorders as PE [53–55]. Therefore, the inhibition of dNK cell regulatory activation should be considered in context of accompanying inflammation.

Several reports have concluded that patients with PE exhibit decreased Treg expansion in peripheral blood and decidua, suggesting an association between the failure of pregnancy-compatible regulatory T cell transformation and the pathogenesis of PE. Thus, it is believed that overwhelming transgenic gene expression overrides the control of hypertension and other factors. Accordingly, if regulatory T cells are not hormonally propagated to be recruited to the endometrium, these may not counter all pathological features of PE [48].

5 Preeclampsia: Cardiovascular Remodeling

Diverse hemodynamic patterns could be present depending on the severity of PE, use of medication, and presence of comorbidities. A substantial increase in sympathetic vasoconstrictor activity occurs, reflecting a significant burden on the heart, causing changes in cardiac structure and functions [56]. In fact, certain studies have revealed that women who had complications of PE can present persistence of cardiac adjustments even after delivery and are also more likely to develop systemic hypertension and die at an early age from cardiovascular disease [57].

Approximately 50% of women affected by preterm PE (classification according to severity in relation to the need for iatrogenic delivery before 37 weeks) could manifest mild to moderate isolated LV chamber diastolic dysfunction with preserved ejection fraction and 20% with biventricular chamber longitudinal systolic dysfunction and severe LV hypertrophy. LV remodeling/hypertrophy in PE is characteristically asymmetrical, predominantly involving the basal anteroseptum [56]. Moreover, severe and preterm PE have a greater association with impaired myocardial contractility, biventricular chamber systolic dysfunction, and severe hypertrophy, representing potential markers of early subendocardial damage [56].

Cardiac changes because of acute PE could persist during initial years after delivery; in addition, LV hypertrophy and a prehypertension state could persist at 1 year after delivery, particularly in preterm PE (60%). Over half of preterm women with PE have asymptomatic LV cardiac dysfunction or hypertrophy after delivery, and 40% develop essential hypertension within 1–2 years after pregnancy [56, 58].

Women who had PE previously could be at a sevenfold higher risk of recurrence compared with normal pregnant women [57, 59]. Although women who experience PE recurrence exhibited lower LV mass index and stroke volume, their cardiac adaptation patterns in subsequent pregnancies did not differ considerably from those observed in women without any PE recurrence [59].

Although there is no definitive evidence to prove that PE causes permanent myocardial damage or that such women had previous cardiovascular deficits, the development of PE represents an opportunity to identify women at a high risk of long-term cardiovascular disease before other conventional cardiovascular disease [56]. Table 1 summarizes the characteristics between PE and time of disease onset.

Table 1
Characteristics between preeclampsia and time of disease onset

	PE	Early-onset PE	Late-onset PE
Clinical symptoms at onset	>20 weeks	<34 weeks	>34 weeks
Risk of adverse outcomes	Depending on severity and time of onset	High	Negligible
Association with IUGR	Depending on severity and time of onset	Yes	No
Familial component	Depending on time of onset	Yes	No
Placental morphology	Depending on time of onset	Abnormal	Normal
Etiology	Depending on time of onset	Placental	Maternal
Immunological findings	– Decreased level of angiogenic factors (VEGF, PLGF e IL10) – Increased levels of antiangiogenic factors (IL 6, IL17, and TNF alpha)		
Cardiovascular remodeling	– Mild to moderate isolated LV chamber diastolic dysfunction with preserved ejection fraction – Biventricular chamber longitudinal systolic dysfunction – Severe asymmetrical LV hypertrophy – Impaired myocardial contractility and biventricular chamber systolic dysfunction		
Epigenetics	– Hypomethylation in the promoter region of the 11b-hydroxysteroid dehydrogenase type 2 (HSD11B2) in neonates – Decreased methylation of insulin-like growth factor 2 (IGF2) in neonates		
Vascular remodeling		– Increased carotid IMT, lumen diameter, and arterial stiffness, no significant changes in IVC collapsibility	– More prominent carotid IMT but by less pronounced changes in lumen diameter and arterial stiffness, significant decrease in IVC collapsibility

PE preeclampsia, *IUGR* intrauterine growth restriction, *VEGF* vascular endothelial growth factor, *PLGF* placental growth factor, *IL10* interleukin 10, *IL 6* interleukin 6, *IL 17* interleukin 17, *TNF alpha* tumor necrosis factor alpha, *IGF2* insulin-like growth factor 2, *IVC* inferior vena cava, *IMT* intima-media thickness

6 Conclusion

PE is a pregnancy-specific syndrome with unknown etiology. Various theories have been postulated to explain the etiologies of early- and late-onset PE. Considering the cumulative amount of evidence, it is reasonable to suggest that PE constrains the cardio-metabolic health of both mother and offspring. The understanding regarding epigenetics and PE is still in the early phases, but it is certainly an attractive and promising field of study.

References

1. Duley L (2009) The global impact of pre-eclampsia and eclampsia. Semin Perinatol 33: 130–137
2. Laresgoiti-Servitje E, Gomez-Lopez N (2012) The pathophysiology of preeclampsia involves altered levels of angiogenic factors promoted by hypoxia and autoantibody-mediated mechanisms. Biol Reprod 87:36–36
3. Redman CW, Sargent IL (2010) Immunology of pre-eclampsia. Am J Reprod Immunol 63:534–543
4. Silasi M, Cohen B, Karumanchi SA, Rana S (2010) Abnormal placentation, angiogenic factors, and the pathogenesis of preeclampsia. Obstet Gynecol Clin N Am 37:239–253
5. Wang JX, Knottnerus AM, Schuit G, Norman RJ, Chan A, Dekker GA (2002) Surgically obtained sperm, and risk of gestational hypertension and pre-eclampsia. Lancet 359:673–674
6. Goldman-Wohl DS, Yagel S (2007) Examination of distinct fetal and maternal molecular pathways suggests a mechanism for the development of preeclampsia. J Reprod Immunol 76:54–60
7. Chaddha V, Viero S, Huppertz B, Kingdom J (2004) Developmental biology of the placenta and the origins of placental insufficiency. Semin Fetal Neonatal Med 9:357–369
8. Duckitt K, Harrington D (2005) Risk factors for pre-eclampsia at antenatal booking: systematic review of controlled studies. BMJ 330:565
9. Bell CG, Beck S (2010) The epigenomic interface between genome and environment in common complex diseases. Brief Funct Genomics 9:477–485
10. Robins JC, Marsit CJ, Padbury JF, Sharma SS (2011) Endocrine disruptors, environmental oxygen, epigenetics and pregnancy. Front Biosci (Elite Ed) 3:690–700
11. Choudhury M, Friedman JE (2012) Epigenetics and microRNAs in preeclampsia. Clin Exp Hypertens 34:334–341
12. Jiménez-Chillarón JC, Díaz R, Martínez D, Pentinat T, Ramón-Krauel M, Ribó S, Plösch T (2012) The role of nutrition on epigenetic modifications and their implications on health. Biochimie 94:2242–2263
13. Cantone I, Fisher AG (2013) Epigenetic programming and reprogramming during development. Nat Struct Mol Biol 20:282–289
14. Waterland RA, Jirtle RL (2004) Early nutrition, epigenetic changes at transposons and imprinted genes, and enhanced susceptibility to adult chronic diseases. Nutrition 20:63–68
15. Nelissen EC, van Montfoort AP, Dumoulin JC, Evers JL (2011) Epigenetics and the placenta. Hum Reprod Update 17:397–417
16. Orozco LD, Rubbi L, Martin LJ, Fang F, Hormozdiari F, Che N, Smith AD, Lusis AJ, Pellegrini M (2014) Intergenerational genomic DNA methylation patterns in mouse hybrid strains. Genome Biol 15:R68
17. Nissenbaum J, Bar-Nur O, Ben-David E, Benvenisty N (2013) Global indiscriminate methylation in cell-specific gene promoters following reprogramming into human induced pluripotent stem cells. Stem Cell Rep 1:509–517
18. Hu W, Weng X, Dong M, Liu Y, Li W, Huang H (2014) Alteration in methylation level at 11b-hydroxysteroid dehydrogenase type 2 gene promoter in infants born to preeclamptic women. BMC Genet 15:96
19. He J, Zhang A, Fang M, Fang R, Ge J, Jiang Y, Zhang H, Han C, Ye X, Yu D, Huang H, Liu Y et al (2013) Methylation levels at IGF2 and GNAS DMRs in infants born to preeclamptic pregnancies. BMC Genomics 14:472
20. Aufdenblatten M, Baumann M, Raio L, Dick B, Frey BM, Schneider H, Surbek D, Hocher B, Mohaupt MG (2009) Prematurity is related to high placental cortisol in preeclampsia. Pediatr Res 65:198–202
21. Bourque DK, Avila L, Peñaherrera M, von Dadelszen P, Robinson WP (2010) Decreased

placental methylation at the H19/IGF2 imprinting control region is associated with normotensive intrauterine growth restriction but not preeclampsia. Placenta 31:197–202
22. Ching T, Ha J, Song M-A, Tiirikainen M, Molnar J, Berry MJ, Towner D, Garmire LX (2015) Genome-scale hypomethylation in the cord blood DNAs associated with early onset preeclampsia. Clin Epigenetics 7:21
23. Stojanovska V, Scherjon SA, Plösch T (2016) Preeclampsia as modulator of offspring health. Biol Reprod 94:53
24. Reddington JP, Perricone SM, Nestor CE, Reichmann J, Youngson NA, Suzuki M, Reinhardt D, Dunican DS, Prendergast JG, Mjoseng H, Ramsahoye BH, Whitelaw E et al (2013) Redistribution of H3K27me3 upon DNA hypomethylation results in de-repression of Polycomb target genes. Genome Biol 14:R25
25. Li Y, Zhang Y, Li S, Lu J, Chen J, Wang Y, Li Y, Xu J, Li X (2015) Genome-wide DNA methylome analysis reveals novel epigenetically dysregulated non-coding RNAs in human-breast cancer. Sci Rep 5:8790
26. Bellamy L, Casas JP, Hingorani AD, Williams DJ (2007) Pre-eclampsia and risk of cardiovascular disease and cancer in later life: systematic review and meta-analysis. BMJ 335:974–977
27. McDonald SD, Malinowski A, Zhou Q, Yusuf S, Devereaux PJ (2008) Cardiovascular sequelae of preeclampsia/eclampsia: a systematic review and meta-analyses. Am Heart J 156:918–930
28. Crispi F, Domínguez C, Llurba E, Martín-Gallán P, Cabero L, Gratacós E (2006) Placental angiogenic growth factors and uterine artery Doppler findings for characterization of different subsets in preeclampsia and in isolated intra-uterine growth restriction. Am J Obstet Gynecol 195:201–207
29. Crispi F, Llurba E, Domínguez C, Martín-Gallán P, Cabero L, Gratacós E (2008) Predictive value of angiogenic factors and uterine artery Doppler for early versus late-onset pre-eclampsia and intrauterine growth restriction. Ultrasound Obstet Gynecol 31:303–309
30. Huppertz B (2008) Placental origins of preeclampsia: challenging the current hypothesis. Hypertension 51:970–975
31. Melchiorre K, Sutherland GR, Liberati M, Thilaganathan B (2012) Maternal cardiovascular impairment in pregnancies complicated by severe fetal growth restriction. Hypertension 60:437–443
32. Manten GT, Sikkema MJ, Voorbij HA, Visser GH, Bruinse HW, Franx A (2007) Risk factors for cardiovascular disease in women with a history of pregnancy complicated by preeclampsia or intrauterine growth restriction. Hypertens Pregnancy 26:39–50
33. Caruso A, Paradisi G, Ferrazzani S, Lucchese A, Moretti S, Fulghesu AM (1998) Effect of maternal carbohydrate metabolism on fetal growth. Obstet Gynecol 92:8–12
34. Hermes W, Tamsma JT, Grootendorst DC, Franx A, van der Post J, van Pampus MG, Bloemenkamp KW, Porath M, Mol BW, de Groot CJ (2013) Cardiovascular risk estimation in women with a history of hypertensive pregnancy disorders at term: a longitudinal follow-up study. BMC Pregnancy Childbirth 13:126
35. Goynumer G, Yucel N, Adali E, Tan T, Baskent E, Karadag C (2013) Vascular risk in women with a history of severe preeclampsia. J Clin Ultrasound 41:145–150
36. Yuan LJ, Xue D, Duan YY, Cao TS, Yang HG, Zhou N (2013) Carotid intima media thickness and arterial stiffness in pre-eclampsia by analysis with a radiofrequency ultrasound technique. Ultrasound Obstet Gynecol 42: 644–652
37. Stein JH, Korcarz CE, Hurst RT, Lonn E, Kendall CB, Mohler ER, Najjar SS, Rembold CM, Post WS, American Society of Echocardiography Carotid Intima-Media Thickness Task Force (2008) Use of carotid ultrasound to identify subclinical vascular disease and evaluate cardiovascular disease risk: a consensus statement from the American Society of Echocardiography Carotid Intima-Media Thickness Task Force. Endorsed by the Society for Vascular Medicine. J Am Soc Echocardiogr 21:93–111
38. Laurent S, Boutouyrie P (2007) Recent advances in arterial stiffness and wave reflection in human hypertension. Hypertension 49: 1202–1206
39. Dipti A, Soucy Z, Surana A, Chandra S (2012) Role of inferior vena cava diameter in assessment of volume status: a metaanalysis. Am J Emerg Med 30:1414–1419
40. Stergiotou I, Crispi F, Valenzuela-Alcaraz B, Bijnens B, Gratacos E (2013) Patterns of maternal vascular remodeling and responsiveness in early versus late-onset preeclampsia. Am J Obstet Gynecol 209:558.e1–558.e14
41. Bots ML, Hofman A, Grobbee DE (1997) Increased common carotid intima-media thickness: adaptive response or a reflection of atherosclerosis? Findings from the Rotterdam study. Stroke 28:2442–2447
42. Tihtonen KM, Kööbi T, Uotila JT (2006) Arterial stiffness in preeclamptic and chronic

hypertensive pregnancies. Eur J Obstet Gynecol Reprod Biol 128:180–186

43. Gyselaers W (2008) Hemodynamics of the maternal venous compartment: a new area to explore in obstetric ultrasound imaging. Ultrasound Obstet Gynecol 32:716–717
44. Mongraw-Chaffin ML, Cirillo PM, Cohn BA (2010) Preeclampsia and cardiovascular disease death: prospective evidence from the child health and development studies cohort. Hypertension 56:166–171
45. Yinon Y, Kingdom JC, Odutayo A, Moineddin R, Drewlo S, Lai V, Cherney DZ, Hladunewich MA (2010) Vascular dysfunction in women with a history of preeclampsia and intrauterine growth restriction: insights into future vascular risk. Circulation 122:1846–1853
46. Laurent S, Girerd X, Mourad JJ et al (1994) Elastic modulus of the radial artery wall material is not increased in patients with essential hypertension. Arterioscler Thromb 14: 1223–1231
47. Melchiorre K, Sutherland GR, Baltabaeva A, Liberati M, Thilaganathan B (2011) Maternal cardiac dysfunction and remodeling in women with preeclampsia at term. Hypertension 57:85–93
48. Cheng SB, Sharma S (2016) Preeclampsia and health risks later in life: an immunological link. Seminars in immunopathology. Semin Immunopathol 48:669–708
49. Novakovic B, Saffery R (2012) The ever growing complexity of placental epigenetics – role in adverse pregnancy outcomes and fetal programming. Placenta 33:959–970
50. Martin E, Ray PD, Smeester L, Grace MR, Boggess K, Fry RC (2015) Epigenetics and preeclampsia: defining functional epimutations in the preeclamptic placenta related to the TGF-β pathway. PLoS One 10(10):1–14
51. Chazara O, Xiong S, Moffett A (2011) Maternal KIR and fetal HLA-C: a fine balance. J Leukoc Biol 90:703–716
52. King A (2000) Uterine leukocytes and decidualization. Hum Reprod Update 6:28–36
53. Nevers T, Kalkunte S, Sharma S (2011) Uterine regulatory T cells, IL-10 and hypertension. Am J Reprod Immunol 66 Suppl 1:88–92
54. Norris W, Nevers T, Sharma S, Kalkunte S (2011) Review: HCG, preeclampsia and regulatory T cells. Placenta 32 Suppl 2:S182–S185
55. Sargent IL, Borzychowski AM, Redman CW (2006) NK cells and human pregnancy – an inflammatory view. Trends Immunol 27: 399–404
56. Melchiorre K, Sharma R, Thilaganathan B (2014) Cardiovascular implications in preeclampsia: an overview. Circulation 130: 703–714
57. Valensise H, Lo Presti D, Gagliardi G, Tiralongo GM, Pisani I, Novelli GP, Vasapollo B (2016) Persistent maternal cardiac dysfunction after preeclampsia identifies patients at risk for recurrent preeclampsia. Hypertension 67:748–753
58. Ghossein-Doha C, Peeters L, Van Heijster S, Van Kuijk S, Spaan J, Delhaas T, Spaanderman M (2013) Hypertension after preeclampsia is preceded by changes in cardiac structure and function. Hypertension 62:382–390
59. Ghossein-Doha C, Spaanderman ME, Al Doulah R, Van Kuijk SM, Peeters LL (2016) Maternal cardiac adaptation to subsequent pregnancy in formerly pre-eclamptic women according to recurrence of pre-eclampsia. Ultrasound Obstet Gynecol 47:96–103

Chapter 7

Inflammatory and Immune System Markers

Kelly J. McKelvey, Gaayathri Ariyakumar, and Sharon A. McCracken

Abstract

Since preeclampsia was first described by Hippocrates in 400 BC, the theory of its causation has shifted from toxins to a current theory that incorporates both vascular and immunological causation. Poor placentation whether it is genetically predisposed or due to low expression of defective HLA-G on fetal trophoblasts is believed to be the initial insult. Oxidative stress from placental ischemia/hypoxia leads to an overload of trophoblast debris by stimulating apoptosis or necrosis. Partial failure of the maternal immune system to tolerate the paternal alloantigens activates maternal immune cells to secrete cytokines whose pleiotropic functions lead to dysfunction of the maternal vascular and placental endothelium, blood coagulation, and fibrinolytic system. This chapter describes some of the key methodologies (flow cytometry, ELISAs, and multiplex immunoassays) for the identification and quantification of inflammation and immune system markers in the study of preeclampsia pathogenesis, as well as diagnostic and therapeutic development. The methodologies may be utilized for a variety of tissue sources in the study of preeclampsia: maternal peripheral blood, umbilical cord blood, intervillous blood, decidua, chorionic villous, amnion and chorion membranes, and cell culture supernatant.

Key words Flow cytometry, Antibodies, Fluorochrome-conjugated, Cytokine, Chemokine, Autoantibody, Enzyme, Multiplex

1 Introduction

Immunological assays are powerful tools used in the field of pregnancy complications and have increased our understanding of preeclampsia diagnosis, prognosis, and therapeutic development in the last 30 years. Advances in technology of the instruments, software, and reagents have now made it possible to simultaneously measure 20–40 antigen in a single heterogeneous sample [1]. Preeclampsia is associated with placental insult and chronic immune activation [2–4] with changes in cytokines, chemokines, blood coagulation factors, and apoptotic markers (summarized in Table 1). The most commonly utilized assays to detect and quantify inflammatory and immune system markers are flow cytometry (FACS), enzyme-linked immunosorbent assays (ELISAs), and multiplex immunoassays.

Padma Murthi and Cathy Vaillancourt (eds.), *Preeclampsia: Methods and Protocols*, Methods in Molecular Biology, vol. 1710, https://doi.org/10.1007/978-1-4939-7498-6_7, © Springer Science+Business Media LLC 2018

Table 1
Inflammation and immune cell markers in preeclampsia. This table summarizes the inflammatory and immune system markers reported to change in biological samples from women with preeclampsia. It is not an exhaustive list of all research but indicates that a wide range of markers are perturbed

	Antigen	PE vs normal (↑, ↓)	References
Immune cells			
T-lymphocyte	CD3	↓ Decidua	[5]
Th1	CXCR3, CCR5, Tbet, IFNγ	↑ PBMC	[6]
Th2	CRTH2, CCR4, CCR3, CCR8, GATA3, IL-4	↓ PBMC	[6]
Th17	CCR6, CCR4, RORγt, IL-17	↓ Decidua	[5]
Treg	CD25, CTLA-4, FOXP3, TGFβ	↓ PBMC	[4, 7]
		↓ Decidua	[7]
B-lymphocyte	CD19		
Monocytes	CD11b, CD64, CD14	↑ PBMC	[8]
Macrophage	CD68		
Granulocytes	CD62L, soluble L-selectin	↓ PBMC	[8]
NK cells	CD16, CD56, and CD57	↓ Decidua	[9]
		↑ Decidua	[5, 10]
Cytotoxic T-lymphocyte	CD8	↑ PBMC	[11]
		↓ Decidua	[9]
		↑ Decidua	[10]
αβ-T cell	TCRαβ	↓ Decidua	[9]
Myeloid DC	CD1c, CD123^{hi}	↑ Decidua	[12]
	Immature:CD209, CCR6		
	Mature: CD83		
Lymphoid DC	CD11c, CD123^{lo}		
	BDCA-2/CD303	↑ PB	[13]
Cytokines/chemokines			
CCL2		↑ Decidua	[12]
CCL4		↑ Decidua	[12]
CCL7/MCP3		↑ Decidua	[12]
CCL20/LARC/MIP3A		↑ Decidua	[12]
CXCL16		↑ Plasma	[14]
Soluble E-selectin		↑ Serum/plasma	[15, 16]
Soluble ICAM1		↑ Serum/plasma	[15, 16]
IFNγ		↑ Serum	[17]
		↓ PBMC	[18]
		↑ Decidual lymphocytes	[5]
IL-1β		↑ Serum	[19]
		↑ Monocytes	[20]
IL-2		↑ Serum	[17, 21]
		↓ PBMC	[18]
Soluble IL-2R		↑ Serum	[19]
Soluble IL-4R		↑ Serum	[22]
IL-6		↑ Serum	[19, 22–25]
		↑ Monocytes	[20]
		↓ Decidual lymphocytes	[5]

(continued)

Table 1 (continued)

Antigen	PE vs normal (↑, ↓)	References
IL-8	↑ Serum	[19, 22, 26]
	↑ Monocytes	[20]
IL-10	↑ Serum	[25]
	↓ PBMC	[18]
	↓ Decidual lymphocytes	[5]
IL-12	↓ Decidual lymphocytes	[5]
MCP1	↑ Plasma	[14]
Pentraxin	↑ Plasma	[14]
TGFβ1	↑ Serum	[25]
TNFα	↑ Serum	[17, 19, 23, 24, 26, 27]
	↑ Amniotic fluid	[27]
Soluble TNFR	↑ Serum/plasma	[14, 25]
Soluble VCAM1	↑ Serum/plasma	[14–16, 28–30]
Autoantibodies		
AT_1-AA	↑ Serum	[31–34]
Anti-oxLDL	↑ Serum	[35]
Anticardiolipin	↑ Serum	[36–38]
Anti-phosphatidylserine	↑ Serum	[38]
Total IgA	↑ Serum	[36]
Total IgG	↑ Serum	[36]
	↑ Placental villous	[38]
Total IgM	↑ Serum	[36]
Clotting and complement		
C3	↑ Serum	[36]
C4	↑ Serum	[36]
Factor V Leiden	↑ Serum	[39]
Protein C	↑ Serum	[39]
vWF	↑ Plasma	[26]

FACS employs highly focused lasers to directly detect properties of cells (e.g., size and granularity), or indirectly, by attaching fluorochrome-conjugated antibodies to the antigen of interest. The sample antigen(s) are injected into a stream of fluid, where they are focused at a point of measurement. Here, the fluorochromes are illuminated by the laser, and the collected light energy is detected (i.e., the scattered light and fluorescence). The combination of lasers and bandpass filters present on the flow cytometer determines the fluorochromes available for detection and the number of antigen that can be simultaneously measured (Table 2). As FACS requires the passing of cells through a fluid stream, it restricts analysis to single cell suspensions.

Table 2
Example optical configuration of flow cytometric instruments with commonly used fluorochromes

Instrument	Laser	Bandpass filters[a]	Mirror	Fluorochromes[b]
BD FACSCalibur™	488	525/50	505LP	Alexa Fluor® 488 FITC
		582/15	550LP	PE
		710/50	640LP	PE-Cy5 PerCP-Cy5.5 PerCP[c]
	635	661/16	N/A	APC Alexa Fluor® 647
BD LSRFortessa™	405	450/40	N/A	Brilliant Violet™ 421 Alexa Fluor® 405 BD Horizon™ V450[c] Pacific Blue™[c]
		525/50	475LP	Brilliant Violet™ 480 BD Horizon™ V500 Amcyan
		610/20	600LP	Brilliant Violet™ 605
		710/50	690LP	Brilliant Violet™ 711
		780/60	750LP	Brilliant Violet™ 786
	488	530/30	505LP	Alexa Fluor® 488 FITC
		585/15	550LP	PE
		610/20	600LP	PE-CF594 PE-Texas Red
		710/50	690LP	PerCP-Cy5.5
	561	585/15	550LP	PE
		610/20	600LP	PE-CF594 PE-Texas Red
		670/30	635LP	PE-Cy5
		710/50	690LP	PE-Cy5.5
		780/60	750LP	PE-Cy7
	640	670/30	N/A	APC Alexa Fluor® 647
		730/45	710LP	Alexa Fluor® 700[c]
		780/60	750LP	APC-Cy7[c] APC-H7[c]

[a]Bandpass filters indicate the detection limits (e.g., 525/50 will detect fluorochrome emission between 500 nm and 550 nm).The peak fluorochrome emission should ideally sit within this range

[b]Only one fluorochrome from each box may be used as these fluorochromes share the same/similar excitation and emission spectra. Fluorochromes in the same box are listed in order of brightness from top to bottom

[c]These fluorochromes are dim. Avoid unless a multicolor panel utilizing these fluorochromes is required

In ELISA and multiplex immunoassays, the antigen is directly affixed to the microtiter plate or indirectly via a bound capture antibody. The bound antigen is then detected and amplified using a conjugated antibody or a two-step biotin-conjugated secondary and streptavidin conjugate. The conjugate varies from enzyme and fluorochromes to radioisotopes and gold which may increase assay sensitivity and specificity depending on the antigen examined [40, 41]. For example, fluorescent-based ELISAs have a ~1000-fold increase in dynamic range when compared to chromogen-based ELISAs which are limited by a 2.0–4.0 range in optical density. The range of different ELISA and multiplex immunoassay formats are summarized in Tables 3 and 4, respectively. An obvious limitation of ELISA/EIA is that only a single antigen can be detected, making FACS or multiplex immunoassays viable alternative methods when multiple antigens need to be assessed in a single sample [42, 43].

Table 3
Formats and detection strategies of ELISA/EIA

Formats	Capture	Detection
Direct	Adsorb to microtiter plate	Conjugated primary antibody
Indirect	Adsorb to microtiter plate	Primary antibody bound by conjugated secondary antibody[a]
Sandwich	Primary antibody affixed to microtiter plate	Conjugated secondary antibody[a]
Competitive[b]	Adsorb to microtiter plate	Conjugated primary antibody
ELIspot	Primary antibody affixed to a PVDF membrane microtiter plate	Conjugated secondary antibody[a]
Cell-based	Cells cultured on microtiter plate	Primary antibody bound by conjugated secondary antibody[a]
Detection strategies	*Antibody conjugation*	*Substrate*
Chromogenic	Enzyme: alkaline phosphatase	PNPP BCIP/NBT
	Enzyme: horseradish peroxidase	ABTS OPD TMB 4CN DAB AEC
	Enzyme: β-galactosidase	OPG CPRG
Fluorescent	Fluorochrome: PE, APC, FITC, Cy	
Chemifluorescent	Enzyme: horseradish peroxidase	QuantaBlu™ QuantaRed™ Amplex red® Attophos®
	Enzyme: β-galactosidase	

(continued)

Table 3 (continued)

Formats	Capture	Detection
Chemiluminescent	Enzyme: alkaline phosphatase Enzyme: horseradish peroxidase	CSDP Luminol
Bioluminescent	Enzyme: luciferase	D-Luciferin
Autoradiography	Radioisotope: ^{125}I	
Immunogold	Metal: Gold[c]	

[a]The enzyme-conjugated secondary antibody may be substituted for a two-step biotin-conjugated antibody and streptavidin conjugate to increase sensitivity
[b]Performed in the presence of antigen competing for the primary antibody
[c]Silver precipitation can be used to amplify to immunogold signal

Table 4
Formats of multiplex immunoassays

Format	Capture	Detection	Substrate
Bead	Primary antibody affixed to bead	Fluorochrome-conjugated secondary antibody	
Flow cytometry	Bead coated with primary antibodies	Fluorochrome- conjugated secondary antibody	
Fluorescent	Spotted array of primary antibodies affixed to microtiter plate	Fluorochrome or IRDye-conjugated secondary antibody	
Chemiluminescence	Spotted array of primary antibodies affixed to microtiter plate	Secondary antibody bound by streptavidin-HRP	Luminol
Electrochemiluminescence	Primary antibodies affixed to a microtiter plate with carbon electrode[a]	$Ru(bpy)_3$-conjugated secondary antibody	DBAE[b] TPA[b]

[a]Alternatively a biotinylated primary antibody bound by a streptavidin-conjugated magnetic bead affixed to the microtiter plate upon the application of voltage
[b]Electrical current is required to catalyze the reaction

In women with preeclampsia, the above assays have been used to show that levels of anti-oxidized low-density lipoprotein (oxLDL) [35], angiotensin II type 1 receptor (AT_1-AA) [31], anti-cardiolipin [36], and endothelial and platelet microparticles [44] are increased compared to normal pregnancies and correlate with disease severity and poor neonatal outcomes [31]. Furthermore, the use of these immunoassays may aid in identification of antigen and combinations of antigen not previously considered in preeclampsia biomarker analyses. For example, assessment of maternal plasma at 16 weeks' gestation using 34-marker human cancer multiplex assays identified fibroblast growth factor basic and plasminogen activator urokinase as a potential preeclampsia predictive combination [45]. Overviews of FACS, ELISAs, and multiplex immunoassays are described in detail below.

2 Materials

All solutions should be prepared with ultrapure water (18.2 MΩ·cm at 25 °C) in endotoxin-free glassware and with reagents that are American Chemical Society (ACS) grade or above. Read the Material and Safety Data Sheets for all chemicals before use and use recommended personal protective equipment (PPE). Follow institutional guidelines for disposal of chemicals.

2.1 General Materials

1. 1% (w/v) E-Toxa-Clean® solution.
2. Endotoxin-free glassware: Fully submerge the glassware in the 1% (w/v) E-Toxa-Clean® solution and soak overnight (16 h). Rinse glassware with tap water eight times, followed by distilled water eight times, and ultrapure water eight times. Autoclave the glassware before use (*see* **Note 1**).
3. Endotoxin-free PBS (PBS-E): PBS prepared in endotoxin-free glassware.
4. 0.4% Trypan blue in PBS-E.
5. Turk's white blood cell count: 1% (w/v) Gentian violet in 1% (v/v) acetic acid.

2.2 FACS

1. FACS buffer: 0.1% (w/v) bovine serum albumin (BSA) in PBS-E (*see* **Note 2**). Store at 4 °C.
2. FACS fixation buffer: 1% (w/v) paraformaldehyde, 1% (w/v) BSA in PBS (*see* **Note 3**). PBS must be warm (60 °C) to enable the paraformaldehyde to go into solution. When dissolved, store at 4 °C for up to 1 week or freeze at −20 °C.
3. FACS permeabilization buffer: 0.1% (w/v) saponin in FACS buffer (*see* **Note 3**). Store at 4 °C.
4. Fluorochrome-conjugated antibodies. Store at 4 °C. An example multicolor panel: Surface antibodies, CD3-AF488, CD4-BV480, CD8-BV786, and CD56-BV605; intracellular antibodies, Tbet-PerCP-Cy5.5, Gata3-BV711, Rorγt-PE, Foxp3-APC, IFNγ-PE-Cy7, IL-4-BV421, IL-17A-APC-R700, and TGFβ-PE-CF594, IL-2- on a 4-laser BD LSRFortessa™. *See* Table 2 for suggested fluorochromes by instrument.

2.3 Enzyme-Linked Immunosorbent Assays (ELISA)/ Enzyme Immunoassay (EIA)

1. Capture antibody: Dilute to desired concentration in PBS-E (*see* **Note 4**). Store at 4 °C.
2. ELISA blocking buffer: 5% (w/v) BSA in PBS-E (*see* **Note 2**). Store at 4 °C.
3. Diluent solution: 1% (w/v) BSA in PBS-E (*see* **Note 2**). Store at 4 °C.
4. ELISA wash buffer: 0.05% (v/v) Tween-20 in PBS-E. Store at 4 °C.
5. Detection antibody: HRP-conjugated detection antibody (*see* **Note 4**). Dilute to desired concentration in Diluent solution. Do not include sodium azide in HRP-based detection antibody diluent as it inhibits HRP activity. Store at 4 °C.
6. ELISA substrate solution: 0.4 mg/mL o-phenylenediamine dihydrochloride (OPD), 0.4 mg/mL urea hydrogen peroxide, 0.05 M phosphate-citrate, and pH 5.0 (*see* **Note 5**). Determine the total volume of ELISA substrate solution that is required. Remove the number of required Sigma® Fast OPD (silver foil) and urea hydrogen peroxide (gold foil) tablets from the packet (stored at −20 °C) and allow to reach room temperature. In a bottle or centrifuge tube wrapped in aluminum foil, add one OPD and one urea hydrogen peroxide tablet to 20 mL of ultrapure water. Vortex to dissolve. Store at room temperature and use within 1 h of preparation.
7. ELISA stop solution: 100% (v/v) hydrochloric acid (*see* **Note 6**).

2.4 Multiplex Immunoassays

1. Multiplex immunoassay kit. For example, Bio-Plex PRO Human Chemokine Panel, 40-plex (Bio-Rad), or Human 42-Plex Human ProcartaPlex™ Panel 1 (Thermo Fisher Scientific). Prepare all reagents and samples as per the manufacturer's instructions.
2. Bio-Plex/Luminex system. Multiple instruments are on the market. Ensure the kit purchased is suitable for the instrument.
3. Handheld or automated magnetic separation wash station.
4. Bio-Plex System Validation Kit or Luminex Performance Verification Kit.
5. Bio-Plex Calibration Kit or Luminex Calibration Kit.
6. Microtiter plate shaker.

3 Methods

3.1 FACS

Perform all centrifugation steps at room temperature (unless indicated otherwise). To protect samples from light after fluorescent staining, wrap in aluminum foil.

3.1.1 Before Starting

1. Check the flow cytometer optical configuration—lasers and bandpass filter set up (Table 2). This will dictate the number and type of fluorochromes you can detect concurrently using your instrument. Multiple fluorochromes with the same spectra and detected by the same laser/filter cannot be co-labeled together in the same tube.
2. Have the brightest fluorochromes (e.g., PE, APC) for low-expression antigen and relatively weaker fluorochromes (e.g., PerCP, FITC) for highly expressed antigen (Table 2).

3.1.2 Preparation of Cells

1. Obtain desired cells or tissue, and prepare a single cell suspension in up to 15 mL PBS-E.
2. Centrifuge at 500 × *g* for 5 min to pellet cells, and discard supernatant.
3. Perform cell count using Trypan blue exclusion or Turk's white blood cell count (*see* Subheading 2.1).
4. Resuspend at 0.5–1 × 10^6 cells in 100 μL FACS Buffer per test (*see* **Notes 7** and **8**).
5. Optional: Block nonspecific binding to Fc receptors (*see* **Note 9**).

3.1.3 For Surface Antigen Staining

1. Add pre-titered amount of fluorochrome-conjugated antibody to each tube as appropriate (*see* **Note 10**). Unstained and control samples should be prepared to enable setup of flow cytometer (e.g., FSC vs SSC profile of fixed cell changes vs non-fixed; antibody specificity controls (*see* **Note 11**); and multi-fluorochrome compensation; **Note 12**). Pulse vortex and incubate for at least 30 min at 4 °C or on ice protected from light, with gentle agitation.
2. Wash cells by adding 500 μL FACS Buffer. Centrifuge at 500 × *g* for 5 min, and then discard supernatant.
3. Resuspend cells in 500 μL FACS fixation buffer. Pulse vortex and incubate for 30 min or overnight at 4 °C in the dark protected from light, with gentle agitation.
4. Wash cells by adding 500 μL FACS Buffer. Centrifuge at 500 × *g* for 5 min, and then discard supernatant (*see* **Note 13**).

3.1.4 For Intracellular Antigen Staining

1. Resuspend cell pellets in 300 μL FACS permeabilization buffer. Pulse vortex and incubate for 1 h at 4 °C or on ice protected from light, with gentle agitation.
2. Wash cells by adding 500 μL FACS permeabilization buffer. Centrifuge at 500 × *g* for 5 min, and then discard supernatant.
3. Resuspend cells in 100 μL FACS permeabilization buffer per tube. Add pre-titered amount of fluorochrome-conjugated antibody to each tube as appropriate for the detection of

intracellular antigen(s) (*see* **Note 10**). Pulse vortex and incubate for 45 min at 4 °C protected from light, with gentle agitation.

4. Add 500 μL FACS permeabilization buffer to each tube. Centrifuge at 500 × *g* for 5 min. Discard supernatant. If cells are likely to clump, load the sample onto the cell strainer cap of a 5 mL round-bottom polystyrene tube, test tube to ensure a single cell suspension.
5. Resuspend cells in 350 μL FACS buffer and acquire data on flow cytometer (*see* **Notes 14** and **15**).

3.2 Enzyme-Linked Immunosorbent Assays (ELISA)/ Enzyme Immunoassay (EIA)

1. Pipette 100 μL of a predetermined concentration of capture antibody into each required well of a 96-well polypropylene plate (*see* **Notes 16** and **17**). Incubate at room temperature for 3 h.
2. Wash wells with 300 μL of ELISA wash buffer, repeat five times (*see* **Notes 17** and **18**).
3. To prevent nonspecific binding, block wells with 200 μL of ELISA blocking buffer for 1 h at room temperature (*see* **Note 17**).
4. Wash wells as in **step 2**.
5. Load 50 μL of standards and neat or diluted samples. Incubate for 2 h at room temperature.
6. Wash wells as in **step 2**.
7. Add 50 μL of predetermined concentration of HRP-conjugated detection antibody (*see* **Notes 4** and **17**). Incubate for 2 h at room temperature.
8. Wash wells such as in **step 2**.
9. Add 100 μL of ELISA substrate solution to each well (*see* **Notes 5** and **17**). Incubate for 10–20 min at room temperature in the dark. Monitor to ensure the yellow-orange color does not overdevelop (*see* **Note 19**).
10. Read at 450 nm wavelength using spectrophotometer (*see* **Note 5**).
11. If required, add 25 μL of ELISA stop solution (*see* **Notes 6** and **19**), the solution will turn green. The acid will inactivate the enzyme stopping the reaction. Mix by gentle agitation or use a 5–10 s shake setting on the spectrophotometer to ensure even color development.
12. Read at 492 nm wavelength using spectrophotometer.

3.3 Multiplex Immunoassays

Unless otherwise specified, the buffers and diluted samples should be brought to room temperature before use. For agitation, seal the plate with fresh plastic film each time and wrap in aluminum foil to protect from light. All agitation is performed at 850 rpm (Bio-Plex) or 500 pm (Luminex) on a microtiter plate shaker at room temperature.

3.3.1 Before Starting

If using plasma, avoid using of heparin-based blood collection tubes as heparin-treated plasma may lyse red blood cells and absorb proteins in the assay. Avoid samples with lipemia or hemolyzed samples as they can interfere with the immunoassays by altering spectral readings and diluting, binding, or cross-reacting with the antigen of interest [46]. Such samples can be used if interference testing is performed.

Determine the total number of wells required for the experiment (including standards, blanks, controls, and samples) and calculate the volumes of coupled beads, detection antibody, and streptavidin-PE required. Seal non-required wells with plastic film for use at a later date.

3.3.2 General Protocol for Bio-Plex and Luminex Multiple Assays

1. Turn on the Bio-Plex or Luminex system and perform calibration (*see* **Note 20**). Warm-up of systems can take up to 30 min.
2. Prepare wash buffer.
3. Reconstitute and dilute the standards and controls (*see* **Notes 21** and **22**).
4. Dilute samples if required.
5. Vortex 1× antibody-coupled beads for 30 s (do not centrifuge) and load 50 μL into each required well of a 96-well polypropylene plate for standards, blanks, controls, and samples (*see* **Notes 17** and **23**).
6. Wash wells with 100 μL (Bio-Plex) or 150 μL (Luminex) of wash buffer, repeat two times.
7. Vortex standards, blanks (*see* **Note 24**), controls, and diluted samples for 5 s and load 50 μL (Bio-Plex) or 25 μL (Luminex) into appropriate wells changing the tip each time to prevent carryover. Seal the plate with film and wrap in foil. Incubate for 1–2 h with agitation.
8. Carefully remove foil and film, then wash wells with 100–150 μL of wash buffer, and repeat two times.
9. Vortex the 1× detection antibody for 5 s, and then add 25 μL of 1× detection antibody to required wells (*see* **Note 17**). Seal the plate with film and wrap in foil. Incubate for 30 min with agitation.
10. Wash wells as in **step 8**.
11. Vortex 1× streptavidin-PE, and then add 50 μL 1× streptavidin-PE to required wells (*see* **Note 17**). Seal with film and wrap in foil. Incubate for 10 min (Bio-Plex) or 30 min (Luminex) with agitation.

12. Wash wells such as in **step 8**.
13. Add 125 μL assay/reading buffer to required wells (*see* **Note 17**). Seal the plate with film and wrap in foil. Incubate for 30 s (Bio-Plex) or 5 min (Luminex) with agitation to resuspend the beads.
14. Carefully remove foil and film; ensure that all required wells contain buffer and acquire data on Bio-Plex or Luminex system. Consult the instrument and software manual for assay acquisition and analysis instructions.

4 Notes

1. The use of endotoxin-free glassware is highly recommended when acquiring data from (immune) cells. Endotoxins, also called lipopolysaccharides or LPS, are bacterial wall-derived components that cause nonspecific activation of immune cells, thereby confounding of experimental results. E-Toxa-Clean® concentrate is a strong alkali and can cause skin and eye irritation, wear appropriate PPE.
2. Optional: 0.05–0.1% (w/v) sodium azide may be added to FACS and ELISA buffers. Sodium azide is a preservative and acts to prevent bacterial growth within the laboratory and antibody solutions [47], as well to prevent loss of antigen signal through capping, shedding, or internalization of the antibody-antigen complex after binding. However, its use has been shown to activate cells and platelets [48] therefore should be tested by the end user to ensure it does not have a biological effect on the antigen of interest.
3. The FACS fixation and permeabilization buffers can be substituted for a commercially available fixation/permeabilization buffer kit. Use as per the manufacturer's instructions.
4. Serial dilution and titration of plasma/sera/supernatant samples and ELISA capture and detection antibodies should be performed to determine the optimal parameters for detection using the desired substrate.
5. Any of the substrates listed in Table 2 may be used for horseradish peroxidase. However, this will change the optical density wavelength. For example, replacing OPD (green after addition of acid stop solution) with TMB substrate requires the use of wavelength (blue) 370 nm before acid and (yellow) 652 nm after acid. Guides are available from most commercial company websites to aid in determining the most appropriate substrate.
6. Concentrated hydrochloric acid can be replaced by 2 N sulfuric acid or a commercially available ELISA Stop Solution. Volumes may differ due to differences in acid (H+) concentra-

tion and will need to be determined by the end user or as per manufacturer's instructions.

7. If using fewer than 500,000 cells, still use a minimum of 100 μL of FACS buffer. If using more than one million cells, scale up the FACS buffer and volume (i.e., maintain same concentration but in larger volume).
8. Steps for Subheadings 3.1.3 and 3.1.4 can be performed in conical (v-) bottom 96-well plates (NB: halve the listed reagent volumes), 1.7 mL microcentrifuge tubes, or 5 mL round-bottom polystyrene test tubes. If using a 96-well plate or microcentrifuge tubes, at Subheading 3.1.4, **step 5**, transfer the cells into 5 mL round polystyrene test tubes for data acquisition on the flow cytometer instrument.
9. Fc blocking controls are used to prevent false positives from occurring by eliminating nonspecific binding. To block nonspecific binding, preincubate cells for 20 min at 4 °C or on ice with an irrelevant Ig of the same clone and host species as the antibodies used for immunofluorescent staining. Alternatively, antibodies specific for the FcR I/II/III receptors or a commercially available blocking agent can be used. To avoid FcR receptor nonspecific binding, altogether purchase antibodies that are Fab or F(ab)2. These antibodies lack the constant (c) region of the antibody which is recognized by FcRs.
10. To maximize the FACS antigen-fluorochrome signal and minimize background noise (i.e., to optimize the signal-to-noise ratio), all antibodies in the single or multicolor panel should be titrated by the end user under the same conditions as required for the experimental samples. This will ensure optimal separation of positive and negative (background staining) populations while reducing antibody and therein cost. Starting with the company recommended concentration/test volume ("x") performs a twofold serial titration of 2×, 1×, 0.5×, 0.25×, 0.125×, and 0.0625× (six to eight dilutions are normally sufficient). Calculate the separation index and generate a scatterplot of signal index against the log antibody concentration. Signal index (SI) as defined by [49], where MFI is mean fluorescence intensity:

$$\mathrm{SI} = \frac{\left(\text{median MFI}_{\text{positive}} - \text{median MFI}_{\text{negative}}\right)}{\left[\left(\text{84th percentile median MFI}_{\text{negative}} - \text{median MFI}_{\text{negative}}\right)/\,0.995\right]}$$

The optimal concentration is therein the peak of the curve.

11. Antibody specificity controls: These controls are used to delineate the positive and negative cell populations. These are less important when the expression is bimodal (e.g., $CD3^{+}$ vs $CD3^{-}$), but where expression is on a spectrum (e.g., cytokines and

chemokines), antibody specific controls are required. Isotype controls are antibodies of the same isotype, fluorochrome conjugation, and fluorochrome-antibody ratio but lacking the antigen-binding site of the experimental antibody. Traditionally, they are used to determine the amount of signal that is attributable to nonspecific antibody binding (e.g., FcRs, **Note 8**). However, they have taken on less importance and have largely been replaced by the use of fluorochrome minus one (FMO) and biological controls (for detail, *see* ref. 50, 51). Our laboratory routinely uses the combination of isotype and biological controls and expresses the flow cytometric data as a fold change of stimulated/vehicle stimulated.

12. Compensation: Compensation is a process to remove confounding spectral overlap that leads to reduced sensitivity to delineate negative populations [52]. We recommend the use of compensation beads (e.g., BD™ CompBeads or Affymetrix eBioscience OneComp and UltraComp eBeads) that will bind your experimental antibodies, rather than fluorochrome-conjugated beads. These antibodies bind the κ light chain so will bind any antibody isotype of a particular host species (e.g., mouse, rat, rabbit). Compensation is typically required for the detection of FITC and PE if used on the same laser (Table 2; this can be avoided by using 561 nm laser for PE), or tandem dyes such as PE-Cy7, and to a lesser extent PE-Cy5, where emission is produced in two spectra.
13. Once fixed the cell pellet will be transparent. If at the end of your experiment you notice a marked loss of cells (total events) compared to your original cell numbers, increase the centrifugation of all postfixation wash steps to 10 min at 700 × *g* and/or reduce the deceleration (brake) speed to improve pelleting.
14. We routinely use a minimum of 10,000 events in our final gate to ensure our results are statistically meaningful. However, if detecting rare events, up to one to ten million events may need to be acquired.
15. Gating schemes and strategies should consider live gates (DRAQ7™, 7-AAD or PI negative, and Invitrogen Live/Dead™ fixable stain), doublet gates (FSC-a vs FSC-H), and fluorescence-detecting gates.
16. The surface of polystyrene 96-well plates will bind a range of proteins. However, to improve overall sensitivity of the ELSIA, use high binding plates as they bind four to five times more antibody than a low/medium binding plate (400–500 ng of IgG/cm^2 vs 100–200 ng of IgG/cm^2, respectively). The amount of antibody that binds to the polystyrene plate is proportional to the concentration and volume of the capture antibody applied so should be titrated by the end user to determine an optimal concentration for the desired ELISA conditions.

17. To reduce manual handling injury and improve assay reproducibility, use a reagent/pipetting reservoir and 8- or 12-well multichannel pipette. This will minimize time differences between the first and last loaded wells.
18. Manual plate washing: Gently load the wells with ELISA wash buffer to avoid dislodging the antibody or antigen-antibody complexes. Place a towel or paper towels on a bench top. Hold the plate with fingertips face up in the palm of the hand and in one fluid motion tip the contents onto the towel(s) and bang on towel(s) three times. Repeat for four times. Alternatively, hold the plate at a 20° angle and carefully decant the contents by pipette or replace manual wash steps with an automated plate washer using the same protocol.
19. The reaction should be read and/or stopped with acid before the optical density values exceed 2.0. If uncertain of the color development by the eye, before adding the acid stop solution, the absorbance can be read at multiple time points at 450 nm (or equivalent for other substrates). Once acid stop solution is added, the reactions cease, and no further color development will occur.
20. To standardize the fluorescent signal for reproducibility, calibration of the Bio-Plex or Luminex system should be performed daily or before use of the instrument. At a minimum calibration should be performed monthly even if the instrument is not in use.
21. The diluent used depends on the sample type used in the experiment. Refer to manufacturer's instructions.
22. Reconstitute the standards and controls at the same time to ensure that the incubation time is equal. This will improve assay reproducibility.
23. When pipetting coupled beads, only use a 200 μL pipette and tip and perform two transfers if required. The use of a 1000 μL pipette and tip will result in the loss of coupled beads in the dead volume of the tip which will not completely vacate during expulsion.
24. Blank wells should contain standard diluent.

Acknowledgments

Kelly J. McKelvey's work is supported by the National Health and Medical Research Council (NHMRC), Australia (CIA Jonathan M. Morris, grant number GNT1066606, 2014); Gaayathri Ariyakumar by Albert S. McKern Research Scholarship; and Sharon A. McCracken's by Ramsay Health Care, Australia.

References

1. Picot J et al (2012) Flow cytometry: retrospective, fundamentals and recent instrumentation. Cytotechnology 64(2):109–130
2. Hsu P, Nanan RK (2014) Innate and adaptive immune interactions at the fetal-maternal interface in healthy human pregnancy and preeclampsia. Front Immunol 5:125
3. Luppi P et al (2006) Preeclampsia activates circulating immune cells with engagement of the NF-kappaB pathway. Am J Reprod Immunol 56(2):135–144
4. Prins JR et al (2009) Preeclampsia is associated with lower percentages of regulatory T cells in maternal blood. Hypertens Pregnancy 28(3): 300–311
5. Wilczynski JR et al (2002) Cytokine secretion by decidual lymphocytes in transient hypertension of pregnancy and pre-eclampsia. Mediat Inflamm 11(2):105–111
6. Saito S et al (1999) Quantitative analysis of peripheral blood Th0, Th1, Th2 and the Th1:Th2 cell ratio during normal human pregnancy and preeclampsia. Clin Exp Immunol 117(3):550–555
7. Sasaki Y et al (2007) Proportion of peripheral blood and decidual CD4(+) CD25(bright) regulatory T cells in pre-eclampsia. Clin Exp Immunol 149(1):139–145
8. Sacks GP et al (1998) Normal pregnancy and preeclampsia both produce inflammatory changes in peripheral blood leukocytes akin to those of sepsis. Am J Obstet Gynecol 179(1): 80–86
9. Rieger L et al (2009) Specific subsets of immune cells in human decidua differ between normal pregnancy and preeclampsia-a prospective observational study. Reprod Biol Endocrinol 7:132
10. Stallmach T et al (1999) Aberrant positioning of trophoblast and lymphocytes in the feto-maternal interface with pre-eclampsia. Virchows Arch 434(3):207–211
11. de Groot CJ et al (2010) Preeclampsia is associated with increased cytotoxic T-cell capacity to paternal antigens. Am J Obstet Gynecol 203(5):496.e1–496.e6
12. Huang SJ et al (2008) Pre-eclampsia is associated with dendritic cell recruitment into the uterine decidua. J Pathol 214(3):328–336
13. Darmochwal-Kolarz D et al (2003) Myeloid and lymphoid dendritic cells in normal pregnancy and pre-eclampsia. Clin Exp Immunol 132(2):339–344
14. Estensen ME et al (2015) Elevated inflammatory markers in preeclamptic pregnancies, but no relation to systemic arterial stiffness. Pregnancy Hypertens 5(4):325–329
15. Austgulen R et al (1997) Increased maternal plasma levels of soluble adhesion molecules (ICAM-1, VCAM-1, E-selectin) in preeclampsia. Eur J Obstet Gynecol Reprod Biol 71(1): 53–58
16. Kim S-Y et al (2004) Maternal serum levels of VCAM-1, ICAM-1 and E-selectin in preeclampsia. J Korean Med Sci 19(5):688–692
17. Saito S et al (1999) Increased T-helper-1-type immunity and decreased T-helper-2-type immunity in patients with preeclampsia. Am J Reprod Immunol 41(5):297–306
18. Darmochwal-Kolarz D et al (1999) T helper 1- and T helper 2-type cytokine imbalance in pregnant women with pre-eclampsia. Eur J Obstet Gynecol Reprod Biol 86(2):165–170
19. Kocyigit Y et al (2004) Changes in serum levels of leptin, cytokines and lipoprotein in pre-eclamptic and normotensive pregnant women. Gynecol Endocrinol 19(5):267–273
20. Luppi P, Deloia JA (2006) Monocytes of preeclamptic women spontaneously synthesize pro-inflammatory cytokines. Clin Immunol 118(2–3):268–275
21. Sunder-Plassmann G et al (1989) Increased serum activity of interleukin-2 in patients with pre-eclampsia. J Autoimmun 2(2):203–205
22. Jonsson Y et al (2006) Cytokine mapping of sera from women with preeclampsia and normal pregnancies. J Reprod Immunol 70(1–2):83–91
23. Vince GS et al (1995) Interleukin-6, tumour necrosis factor and soluble tumour necrosis factor receptors in women with pre-eclampsia. Br J Obstet Gynaecol 102(1):20–25
24. Conrad KP, Miles TM, Benyo DF (1998) Circulating levels of immunoreactive cytokines in women with preeclampsia. Am J Reprod Immunol 40(2):102–111
25. Madazli R et al (2003) Maternal plasma levels of cytokines in normal and preeclamptic pregnancies and their relationship with diastolic blood pressure and fibronectin levels. Acta Obstet Gynecol Scand 82(9):797–802
26. Velzing-Aarts FV et al (2002) High serum interleukin-8 levels in afro-caribbean women with pre-eclampsia. Relations with tumor necrosis factor-alpha, duffy negative phenotype and von Willebrand factor. Am J Reprod Immunol 48(5):319–322
27. Kupferminc MJ et al (1994) Tumor necrosis factor-α is elevated in plasma and amniotic fluid of patients with severe preeclampsia. Am J Obstet Gynecol 170(5):1752–1759

28. Heyl W et al (2005) Increased soluble VCAM-1 serum levels in preeclampsia are not correlated to urinary excretion or circadian blood pressure rhythm. J Perinat Med 33(2): 144–148
29. Budak E et al (1998) Vascular cell adhesion molecule-1 (VCAM-1) and leukocyte activation in pre-eclampsia and eclampsia. Int J Gynaecol Obstet 63(2):115–121
30. Daniel Y et al (1999) A selective increase in plasma soluble vascular cell adhesion molecule-1 levels in preeclampsia. Am J Reprod Immunol 41(6):407–412
31. Siddiqui AH et al (2010) Angiotensin receptor agonistic autoantibody is highly prevalent in preeclampsia. Hypertension 55(2):386
32. Hubel CA et al (2007) Agonistic angiotensin II type 1 receptor autoantibodies in postpartum women with a history of preeclampsia. Hypertension 49(3):612
33. LaMarca B et al (2008) Autoantibodies to the angiotensin type I receptor in response to placental ischemia and tumor necrosis factor α in pregnant rats. Hypertension 52(6): 1168–1172
34. LaMarca B et al (2009) Hypertension in response to autoantibodies to the angiotensin II type I receptor (AT1-AA) in pregnant rats. Hypertension 54(4):905
35. Branch DW et al (1994) Pre-eclampsia and serum antibodies to oxidised low-density lipoprotein. Lancet 343(8898):645–646
36. Kestlerová A et al (2012) Immunological and biochemical markers in preeclampsia. J Reprod Immunol 96(1–2):90–94
37. do Prado AD et al (2010) Association of anticardiolipin antibodies with preeclampsia: a systematic review and meta-analysis. Obstet Gynecol 116(6):1433–1443
38. Yamamoto T et al (1996) Anti-phospholipid antibodies in preeclampsia and their binding ability for placental villous lipid fractions. J Obstet Gynaecol Res 22(3):275–283
39. Saghafi N et al (2014) Evaluation of selected thrombotic factors among pregnant women with preeclampsia and normal pregnant women. Iran J Reprod Med 12(12):793–798
40. Crowther JR, Angarita L, Anderson J (1990) Evaluation of the use of chromogenic and fluorogenic substrates in solid-phase enzyme linked immunosorbent assays (ELISA). Biologicals 18(4):331–336
41. Blais BW et al (2004) Comparison of fluorogenic and chromogenic assay systems in the detection of Escherichia coli O157 by a novel polymyxin-based ELISA. Lett Appl Microbiol 39(6):516–522
42. duPont NC et al (2005) Validation and comparison of luminex multiplex cytokine analysis kits with ELISA: determinations of a panel of nine cytokines in clinical sample culture supernatants. J Reprod Immunol 66(2):175–191
43. Leng SX et al (2008) ELISA and multiplex technologies for cytokine measurement in inflammation and aging research. J Gerontol A Biol Sci Med Sci 63(8):879–884
44. Salem M et al (2015) Flow cytometric assessment of endothelial and platelet microparticles in preeclampsia and their relation to disease severity and Doppler parameters. Hematology 20(3):154–159
45. Martinez-Fierro ML et al (2015) Plasma cancer biomarker multiplex screening and the risk of subsequent preeclampsia. Int J Cardiol 179:58–60
46. Dimeski G (2008) Interference testing. Clin Biochem Rev 29(Suppl 1):S43–S48
47. Chang S, Lamm SH (2003) Human health effects of sodium azide exposure: a literature review and analysis. Int J Toxicol 22(3):175–186
48. Russo I et al (2008) Sodium azide, a bacteriostatic preservative contained in commercially available laboratory reagents, influences the responses of human platelets via the cGMP/PKG/VASP pathway. Clin Biochem 41(4–5): 343–349
49. Telford WG et al (2009) Green fiber lasers: an alternative to traditional DPSS green lasers for flow cytometry. Cytometry A 75A(12): 1031–1039
50. Maecker HT, Trotter J (2006) Flow cytometry controls, instrument setup, and the determination of positivity. Cytometry A 69A(9):1037–1042
51. Hulspas R et al (2009) Considerations for the control of background fluorescence in clinical flow cytometry. Cytometry B Clin Cytom 76B(6):355–364
52. Roederer M (2001) Spectral compensation for flow cytometry: visualization artifacts, limitations, and caveats. Cytometry 45(3):194–205

Chapter 8

Methods to Enrich Exosomes from Conditioned Media and Biological Fluids

Shayna Sharma, Katherin Scholz-Romero, Gregory E. Rice, and Carlos Salomon

Abstract

Exosomes are nano-vesicles which can transport a range of molecules including but not limited to proteins and miRNA. This ability of exosomes renders them useful in cellular communication often resulting in biological changes. They have several functions in facilitating normal biological processes such as immune responses and an involvement in pregnancy. However, they have also been linked to pathological conditions including cancer and pregnancy complications such as preeclampsia. An understanding for the role of exosomes in preeclampsia is based on the ability to purify and characterize exosomes. There have been several techniques proposed for the enrichment of exosomes such as ultracentrifugation, density gradient separation, and ultrafiltration although there is no widely accepted optimized technique. Here we describe a workflow for isolating exosomes from cell-conditioned media and biological fluids using a combination of centrifugation, buoyant density, and ultrafiltration approaches.

Key words Extracellular vesicles, Exosomes, Isolation, Characterization, Density gradient separation, Ultracentrifugation, Ultrafiltration

1 Introduction

Pregnancy is often associated with several complications that result in both maternal and placental inflammation such as gestational diabetes mellitus (GDM) and preeclampsia [1]. Preeclampsia is characterized as a new diagnosis of hypertension during pregnancy in addition to proteinuria—abnormal amounts of protein present in the urine of patients [2]. Approximately 7% of pregnant women worldwide have pregnancies complicated with preeclampsia [3]. However, the causes underlying preeclampsia remain unclear although several risk factors have been postulated. These include obesity, chronic hypertension, and genetic factors. The lack of understanding surrounding preeclampsia results in increased maternal-fetal morbidity and mortality [1]. Therefore, it is essential that

Padma Murthi and Cathy Vaillancourt (eds.), *Preeclampsia: Methods and Protocols*, Methods in Molecular Biology, vol. 1710,
https://doi.org/10.1007/978-1-4939-7498-6_8, © Springer Science+Business Media LLC 2018

novel techniques which are informative and minimally invasive be examined to better understand the disease.

This demand for novel diagnostic techniques has brought extracellular vesicles (EVs), specifically exosomes to the forefront. Exosomes are small membranous vesicles of an endocytic origin. They are approximately 100 nm in diameter with a density between 1.13 and 1.19 g/mL in a sucrose gradient [4, 5]. Exosome biogenesis begins with an inward budding of the plasma membrane leading to the formation of early endosome [6]. The early endosome then matures to a late endosomal stage which is characterized by a change in structure toward a more spherical morphology. The late endosome then becomes a multivesicular body (MVB) which can be distinguished by the presence of intraluminal vesicles (ILVs) [7]. These ILVs are formed by the inward budding of the MVB membrane. The MVB can then fuse with the plasma membrane leading to the release of these ILVs which are now termed exosomes. Due to the endocytic origin, exosomes provide a capture of the environment within the cell and are therefore highly informative.

However, one of the major challenges remains the standardization of an isolation technique for exosomes [4]. Exosomes can be isolated from a variety of samples such as cell-conditioned media, plasma, serum, and other bodily fluids using a range of different methods such as sequential ultracentrifugation, density gradient separation, ultrafiltration, and commercial kits [8, 9].

Differential and sequential ultracentrifugation is often used to discard dead cells, cellular debris, and large vesicles. The gravitation force or speed at which the sample is centrifuged and the amount of time required often depends on the starting sample as different samples have varying levels of contamination. The centrifugation often begins at a low speed of approximately $10{,}000 \times g$ which is gradually increased to reach an ultracentrifugation speed of approximately $100{,}000 \times g$ [10]. However, the $100{,}000 \times g$ pellet is often contaminated with vesicles of varying sizes, and thus to enrich the pellet with vesicles of interest, i.e., exosomes, further processing is required.

2 Materials

Prepare and store all reagents at room temperature unless indicated otherwise. Adjustment of the volume of solutions may be required depending on the number of samples to be processed (*see* **Note 1**).

2.1 Materials and Reagents

1. Starting sample (cell-conditioned media (CCM)/biological fluid) (*see* **Note 2**).
2. Centrifuge tubes (*see* **Note 3**).

3. Glass Pasteur pipettes.
4. 0.2 μm syringe filter.
5. 10 mL syringe.
6. Needle (18G × 1.5″).
7. 15 mL 100 kDa ultrafiltration tubes.
8. Refrigerated centrifuge (*see* **Note 4**).
9. 10 mL glass ultracentrifugation tubes.
10. 14 × 80 mm polypropylene ultracentrifugation tubes.
11. Ultracentrifuge.
12. 70iti fixed angle ultracentrifuge rotor (*see* **Note 5**).
13. High-speed centrifuge.
14. R15A Fixed Angle Rotor.
15. SW41Ti swinging ultracentrifuge rotor (*see* **Note 6**).
16. Phosphate-buffered saline (PBS).

2.2 Solutions

1. 0.25 M sucrose/10 M Tris (pH 7.5) stock solution: To prepare 200 mL, combine 17.115 g of UltraPure Sucrose (molecular weight, 342.30) with 0.24 g of Trizma base (molecular weight, 121.14) in a sterile bottle. Add 170 mL of ultrapure water into the bottle. Stir the solution for a few minutes and check the pH of the solution. If the pH is higher than 7.5, add a few drops of hydrochloric acid (HCl) to reach the desired pH of 7.5. Finally, add enough ultrapure water to the solution to reach a total volume of 200 mL.
2. 40%/20%/10%/5% w/v sucrose solutions: Take four 50 mL centrifugation tubes and label them, 40%, 20%, 10%, and 5%, respectively. Use the 0.25 M sucrose/10 M Tris stock solution in conjunction with the OptiPrep™ density gradient medium (60% w/v) according to Table 1 to prepare the w/v solutions.

3 Methods

Before beginning, refer to **Notes 7–11**.

3.1 Isolation of Exosomes from Biological Fluids (Fig. 1)

3.1.1 Ultracentrifugation

1. Dilute 1 mL of the biological fluid (e.g., plasma) with 1 mL of PBS to get a total of 2 mL in a microcentrifuge tube (*see* **Note 12**).
2. Centrifuge the diluted sample at 2000 × *g* for 30 min (4 °C) (*see* **Notes 13** and **14**).
3. Carefully (avoiding the pellet) transfer the supernatant to a new microcentrifuge tube.

Table 1
w/v solution preparation for OptiPrep™ density gradient separation

w/v solutions	OptiPrep™ density gradient medium (mL)	0.25 M sucrose/10 nM Tris
40%	26.67	13.33
20%	13.33	26.67
10%	6.67	33.33
5%	3.33	36.67

4. Resuspend the pellet (large extracellular vesicles and proteins) in 500 μL of PBS and store at −80 °C (*see* **Note 15**).
5. Centrifuge the supernatant at 12,000 × *g* for 45 min (4 °C).
6. Carefully (avoiding the pellet) transfer the supernatant to the glass ultracentrifugation tubes.
7. Resuspend the pellet (large vesicles and other contaminants) in 500 μL of PBS and save at −80 °C.
8. Top up the supernatant in the glass ultracentrifugation tubes with PBS to get a total of 10 mL (*see* **Notes 16** and **17**).
9. Place the glass ultracentrifugation tubes into the 70iti fixed angle ultracentrifuge rotor (*see* Table 2).
10. Place the rotor into the ultracentrifuge and centrifuge at 100,000 × *g* for 2 h (4 °C) (*see* **Note 18**).
11. Carefully remove the glass centrifuge tubes from the rotor (*see* **Note 19**).
12. Discard the supernatant from the glass ultracentrifuge tubes and save the visible pellet resuspended in 500 μL of PBS in a microcentrifuge tube.
13. Store the pellet at −80 °C until further processing (*see* **Note 20**).

3.1.2 OptiPrep™ Density Gradient Separation (Fig. 2)

1. Prepare the discontinuous gradient by firstly placing 3 mL of the 40% w/v sucrose solution into the polypropylene ultracentrifugation tube (*see* **Notes 21** and **22**).
2. On top of the 40% w/v solution, carefully, drop by drop, layer 3 mL of the 20% w/v sucrose solution (*see* **Notes 23** and **24**).
3. Add carefully, drop by drop, 3 mL of the 10% w/v sucrose solution.
4. Add carefully, drop by drop, 2.5 mL of the 5% w/v sucrose solution.

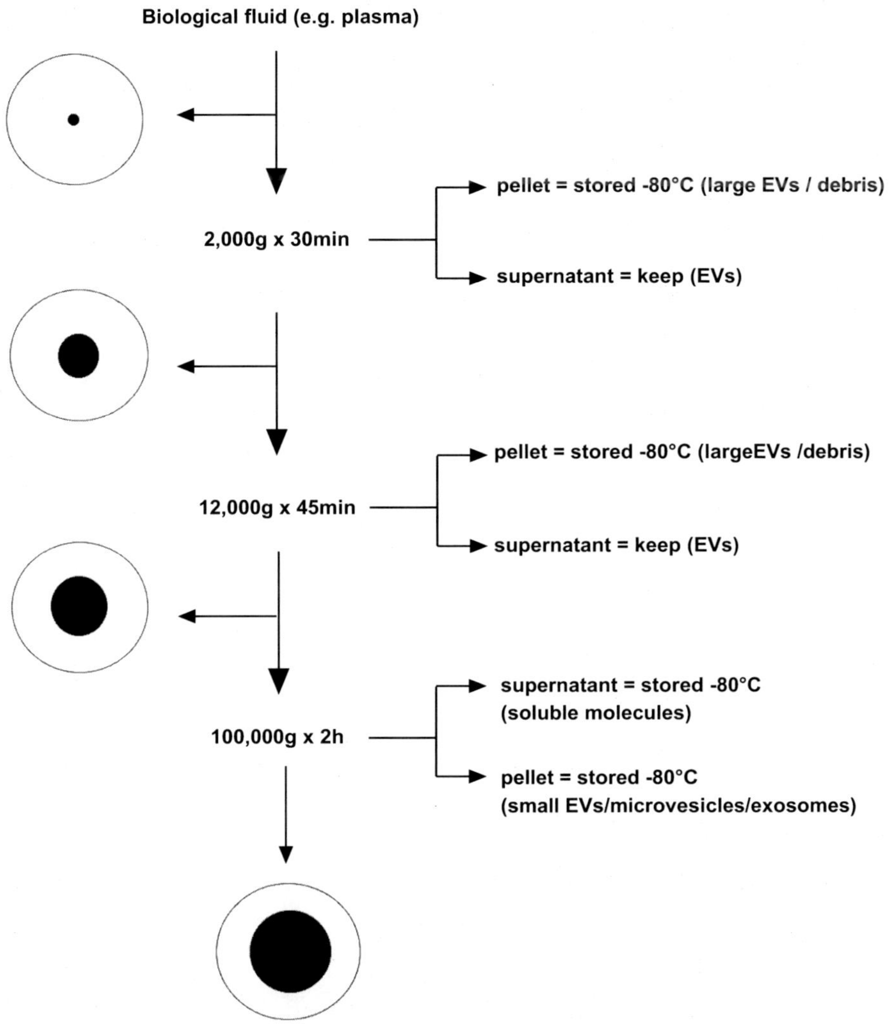

Fig. 1 Enrichment of small vesicles. A flowchart of the ultracentrifugation process leading to the 100,000 g pellet. Circles represent the ratio exosomes (*black*)/non-exosomes vesicles (*white*). *EVs* extracellular vesicles

Table 2
Rotor details

Rotor	Fixed angle (FA)/ swinging bucket (SW)	RCF (g)	Time (minutes)
R15A Hitachi	Fixed angle	12,000	10
70iti rotor	Fixed angle	100,000	120
SW41Ti rotor	Swinging bucket	100,000	1200

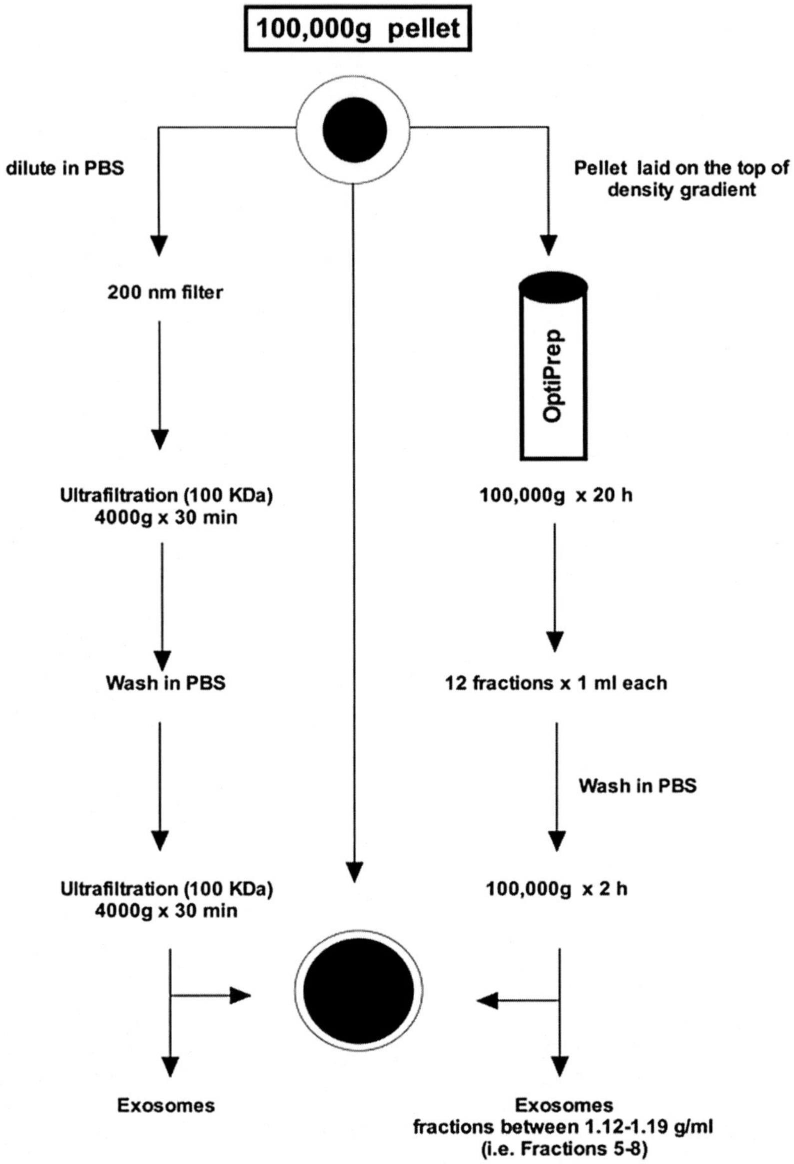

Fig. 2 Enrichment of exosomes vesicles. A flowchart of the OptiPrep™ density gradient and ultrafiltration separation methods used to further purify the 100,000 × *g* pellet. Circles represent the ratio exosomes (*black*)/non-exosomes vesicles (*white*)

5. Layer 500 μL of the 100,000 × *g* pellet obtained from ultracentrifugation on to the discontinuous sucrose gradient.
6. Carefully, place the polypropylene ultracentrifugation tubes into the SW41Ti swinging ultracentrifuge rotor.
7. Place the rotor into the ultracentrifuge and centrifuge at 100,000 × *g* for 20 h (4 °C).

8. Carefully remove the polypropylene tubes from the rotor.
9. Starting at the top of the tube, collect 1 mL of the solution and place into a glass ultracentrifugation tube (*see* **Notes 25** and **26**).
10. Collect another 1 mL of the solution and place into a new glass ultracentrifugation tube.
11. Repeat the above step for a total of 12 times to obtain 12 fractions (12 glass ultracentrifugation tubes).
12. Top up all the glass ultracentrifugation tubes with PBS to get a total of 10 mL per tube.
13. Place the glass ultracentrifugation tubes into the 70iti fixed angle ultracentrifuge rotor and place the rotor into the ultracentrifuge.
14. Centrifuge at 100,000 × *g* for 2 h (4 °C).
15. Discard the supernatant from each glass centrifuge tube and save each pellet in separate microcentrifuge tubes by resuspending in 500 μL of PBS at −80 °C (*see* **Note 27**).

3.1.3 Ultrafiltration

1. Resuspend the 500 μL of the 100,000 g pellet in 9.5 mL of PBS to get a total of 10 mL.
2. Remove the lid of the 100 kDa ultrafiltration tube and place the 0.2 μm syringe filter on top of the tube (*see* **Notes 28** and **29**).
3. Collect the 10 mL of the resuspended pellet using the drawing syringe and needle.
4. Pass the resuspended pellet through the 0.2 μm syringe filter into the ultrafiltration tube.
5. Add 5 mL of PBS to the ultrafiltration tube to get a total of 15 mL.
6. Centrifuge the ultrafiltration tube at 4000 × *g* for 30 min using the refrigerated centrifuge with a fixed angle rotor.
7. Collect the liquid from the interphase using the glass Pasteur pipettes (retentate—liquid that has not passed through the filters).
8. Save the retentate at −80 °C (Fig. 3).

3.2 Isolation of Exosomes from Conditioned Media

3.2.1 Ultracentrifugation (Cell-Conditioned Media)

1. Transfer the cell-conditioned media to a centrifuge tube (e.g., 50 mL) (*see* **Note 2**).
2. Centrifuge the cell-conditioned media at 800 × *g* for 10 min (4 °C) using the refrigerated centrifuge with a fixed angle rotor to discard dead cells and cell debris.
3. Collect the supernatant and discard the cell pellet.
4. Centrifuge the supernatant at 2000 × *g* for 10 min (4 °C) using the refrigerated centrifuge with a fixed angle rotor.

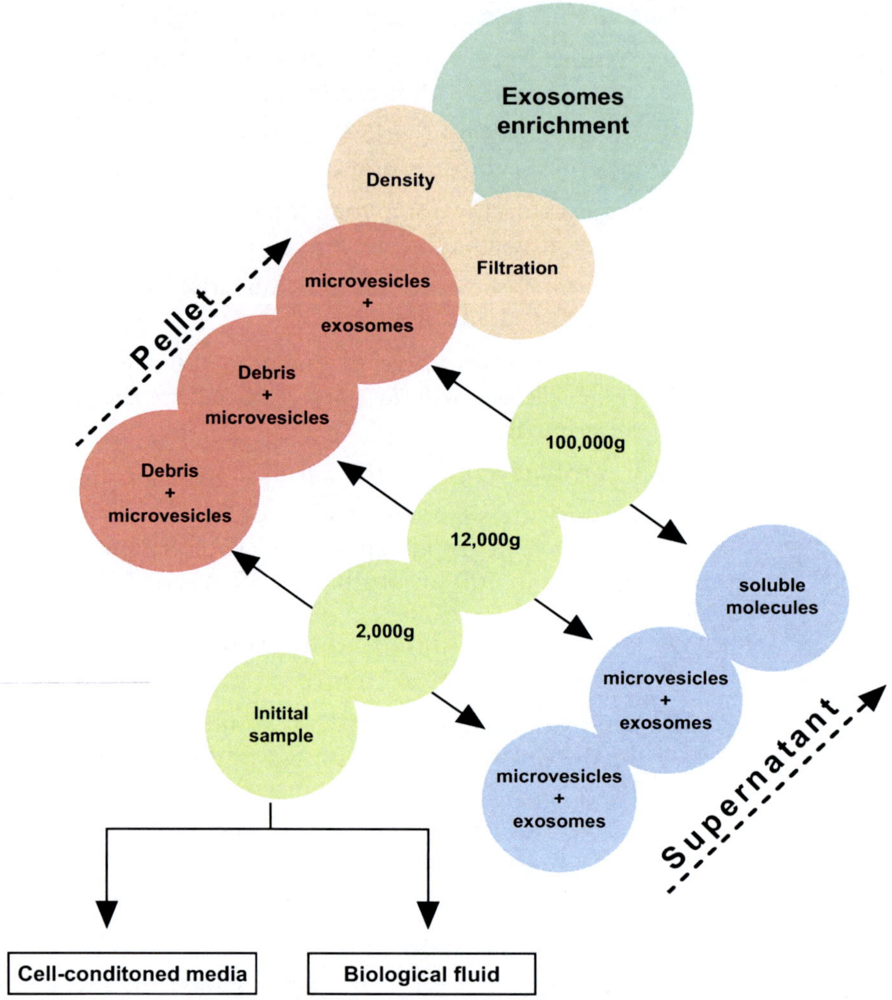

Fig. 3 A comparison of the pellets and supernatant obtained after each sequential centrifugation step. The process of obtaining enriched exosomes from the starting sample is shown along with the stages at which contaminants are removed through sequential centrifugation. The figure shows the presence of several types of vesicles in the pellets obtained after centrifugation and that these vesicles are different to the vesicles present in the supernatant obtained after centrifugation. Furthermore, it is shown that two processes can be used to acquire enriched exosomes from the 100,000 × *g* pellet

5. Carefully (avoiding the pellet) transfer the supernatant to a new centrifuge tube.
6. Resuspend the pellet (large extracellular vesicles and proteins) in 500 μL of PBS and store at −80 °C.
7. Centrifuge the supernatant at 12,000 × *g* for 10 min (4 °C) using the R15A Fixed Angle Rotor and the high-speed centrifuge.

8. Carefully (avoiding the pellet) transfer the supernatant to the glass ultracentrifugation tubes.
9. Repeat **steps 7–13** from Subheading 3.1.1.

3.2.2 OptiPrep™ Density Gradient Separation (Cell-Conditioned Media)

Repeat **steps 1–15** from Subheading 3.1.2.

3.2.3 Ultrafiltration (Cell-Conditioned Media)

1. Resuspend the 500 μL of the 100,000 × *g* pellet in 9.5 mL of PBS to get a total of 10 mL.
2. Remove the lid of the 100 kDa ultrafiltration tube and place the 0.2 μm syringe filter on top of the tube (*see* **Note 29**).
3. Collect the 10 mL of the resuspended pellet using the drawing syringe and needle.
4. Pass the resuspended pellet through the 0.2 μm syringe filter into the ultrafiltration tube.
5. Add 5 mL of PBS to the ultrafiltration tube to get a total of 15 mL.
6. Centrifuge the ultrafiltration tube at 4000 × *g* for 30 min using the refrigerated centrifuge with a fixed angle rotor.
7. After the centrifugation, collect the liquid from the interphase using the glass Pasteur pipettes (retentate—liquid that has not passed through the filters).
8. Save the retentate at −80 °C.

4 Notes

1. Different sample types require different sample preparation. Often biological fluids such as plasma, serum, saliva, cyst fluid, and ascites have a high yield of exosomes from a low volume of starting sample, e.g., 1 mL [9]. However, cell-conditioned media requires a large volume (e.g., 150 mL) of starting sample to obtain a high yield of exosomes.
2. To obtain cell-specific exosomes from cell-conditioned media, cells must be incubated with serum-free media for approximately 48 h. However, if the origin of the exosomes is not important, cells can be incubated with media containing serum. Briefly, cells can be cultured to approximately 90% confluence and then washed and incubated for 48 h with serum-free media. After 48 h, the cell-conditioned media can be isolated and processed.
3. Samples with larger volumes will require large volume (e.g., 50 mL) centrifuge tubes for the centrifugation steps.

4. When using large volumes of samples in centrifuge tubes, a refrigerated centrifuge for large volumes can be used to perform the initial centrifugation steps.
5. Exosome isolation is highly dependent on the centrifugation speed and time as well as the type of rotor used for isolation. Two commonly used rotors include the swinging bucket rotors and the fixed angle rotors. The fixed angle rotor maintains a secure position for the samples, while the swinging bucket rotor allows for samples to be horizontal to the rotational axis during centrifugation [11]. Table 2 shows details for the rotors used in the protocols in this chapter.
6. The swinging bucket rotor has a longer sedimentation path length which results in decreased pelleting ability compared to the fixed angle rotor [11, 12]. The sedimentation path length is the longest distance that a particle has to travel with particles originally at the meniscus of the tube in a swinging rotor, and for a fixed angle rotor, it is the tube wall closest to the rotation axis [12].
7. Perform all steps at room temperature and all centrifugation steps at 4 °C. When working with biological fluids, ensure that all samples are kept on ice to prevent degradation and, in the case of plasma, coagulation of blood.
8. Although the workflow uses plasma and cell-conditioned media as the starting material, it is applicable to a wide range of starting samples (including serum, urine, milk, and other biological fluids). However, when using different fluids such as cell-conditioned media, the protocol varies and this is visible when the two workflows are compared. When using sample such as cell-conditioned media, a preliminary centrifugation step at 800 × *g* for 10 min must be performed to discard dead cells and cell debris.
9. A paper by Witwer et al. compares different starting samples and the preparation methods for these starting samples [13]. It has been shown that different groups work with a range of different starting volumes [14].
10. In addition to density gradient separation and ultrafiltration, other techniques such as size-exclusion chromatography (SEC), magnetic bead separation, affinity separation, flow fractionation, fluorescence-activated cell sorting (FACS), precipitation techniques, and high-throughput/high-pressure liquid chromatography have also been reported in literature [14].
11. Biological fluid samples should be diluted in PBS to increase sample volume and decrease the amount of starting material required to obtain a high yield of vesicles.

12. Extracellular vesicles (EVs) are a broad term which encompass vesicles of approximate diameter between 30 and 5000 nm [11]. Vesicles within this size range can be found in most of the starting samples, and therefore it is essential that vesicles that are not of interest (non-exosomal vesicles) be discarded using sequential centrifugation steps.
13. Gravitational force (g) or relative centrifugation force (RCF) is the speed at which a sample is centrifuged, expressed in terms of gravitational force.
14. Low-speed centrifugations up to 2000 × *g* allow for the pelleting of apoptotic bodies which usually have a size range between 80 and 5000 nm and are released by dying cells [11, 12].
15. Centrifugation speeds between 10,000 and 20,000 × *g* pellet microvesicles (100–1000 nm) which bud off the plasma membrane of functional cells [11].
16. Ensure that all glass centrifugation tubes have similar weight to allow the rotor to be balanced.
17. Put a mark on the glass ultracentrifugation tube, and place that mark facing outward from the rotor to identify the location of the pellet after centrifugation.
18. A speed of approximately 100,000 × *g* is required to pellet exosomes; however, increasing the speed greatly can result in other aggregated proteins being isolated, thus resulting in a contaminated pellet. The pellet obtained through density gradient separation contains less proteins per particle compared to ultracentrifugation indicating that density gradient separation results in a purer pellet with less protein contamination [15]. Therefore, the protocol outlined in this chapter uses an ultracentrifugation speed of 100,000 × *g*.
19. If the pellet is not visible, approximately 500 μL of liquid should be left at the bottom of the ultracentrifugation tube.
20. The yield of exosomes obtained after isolation does not change significantly regardless of whether fresh or frozen plasma is used as the starting material [16]. Furthermore, there are no morphological differences in the obtained vesicles as determined using electron microscopy. It has also been noted that exosomal miRNA remains stable over long periods of time and yield is similar when compared to miRNA extracted from exosomal samples. Ge et al. (2014) showed that exosomal miRNA remained stable for up to 5 years when stored at different temperatures (4 °C, −20 °C, and −80 °C). Comparatively, circulating RNA in plasma was significantly degraded when stored at 4 °C, and long-term storage also led to degradation [17].
21. Either a continuous or discontinuous gradient can be used for density gradient separation although discontinuous gradients

are commonly used due to ease of preparation. A continuous gradient can be obtained by layering a low percentage sucrose or iodixanol solution (e.g., 5%) on top of a high percentage solution (e.g., 30%) and using a magnetic platform to create the continuous gradient (refer to Chen et al. (2013) for detailed methodology) [8]. The protocol outlined here uses a discontinuous gradient.

22. Particles with lower density than the sample medium travel opposite the centrifugal force toward the top, whereas particles with higher density travel parallel to the centrifugal force toward the bottom. However, particles that are larger in size travel at a greater speed.
23. Ensure that the different w/v sucrose solutions are added slowly and drop by drop so that a difference in density is visible through the separation of the solutions in the same polypropylene tube.
24. Avoid shaking the polypropylene tubes to prevent the gradients from mixing.
25. Keep the pipette tip close to the top of the fraction to prevent collecting two separate fractions.
26. Change pipette tips when collecting a new fraction.
27. The fractions which are believed to contain the exosomes depending on density can be combined.
28. The filters in the ultrafiltration tube should be cleaned and rehydrated as per manufacturer's instructions before use.
29. The ultrafiltration device used here had a nominal molecular weight limit of 100 kDa indicating that it would exclude proteins of molecular weight 100,000 Da. However, depending on interest, ultrafiltration devices with different cut-offs can also be used.

Acknowledgment

CS was in receipt of a Lions Medical Research Foundation Fellowship. This study was supported by the Lions Medical Research Foundation, UQ ECR Award, Royal Brisbane and Women's Foundation, Diabetes Australia, and UQ-Ochsner Seed Grant. The ISO17025 accredited research facility was supported by grants from Therapeutics Innovation Australia and the National Collaborative Research Infrastructure Strategy.

This review is supported partly by funding from the Lions Medical Research Foundation (LMRF), The University of Queensland, and Fondo Nacional de Desarrollo Científico y Tecnológico (FONDECYT 1170809), Chile.

References

1. Paredes V, Espinoza-Caicedo JA, Salazar-Pousada D, Escobar GS, Pérez-López FR, Chedraui P (2016) Lower placental growth factor and higher free β-hCG and PAPP-A levels in the fetal circulation of near-term pregnancies complicated with severe preeclampsia. Gynecol Endocrinol 33:79–81. https://doi.org/10.1080/09513590.2016.1241228
2. Powe CE, Levine RJ, Karumanchi SA (2011) Preeclampsia, a disease of the maternal endothelium: the role of antiangiogenic factors and implications for later cardiovascular disease. Circulation 123(24):2856–2869. https://doi.org/10.1161/circulationaha.109.853127
3. Ramesh K, Gandhi S, Rao V (2014) Socio-demographic and other risk factors of pre eclampsia at a tertiary care hospital, Karnataka: case control study. J Clin Diagn Res 8(9):JC01–JC04. https://doi.org/10.7860/JCDR/2014/10255.4802
4. Raposo G, Stoorvogel W (2013) Extracellular vesicles: exosomes, microvesicles, and friends. J Cell Biol 200(4):373–383. https://doi.org/10.1083/jcb.201211138
5. Colombo M, Raposo G, Thery C (2014) Biogenesis, secretion, and intercellular interactions of exosomes and other extracellular vesicles. Annu Rev Cell Dev Biol 30:255–289. https://doi.org/10.1146/annurev-cellbio-101512-122326
6. Beach A, Zhang H-G, Ratajczak MZ, Kakar SS (2014) Exosomes: an overview of biogenesis, composition and role in ovarian cancer. J Ovarian Res 7:14. https://doi.org/10.1186/1757-2215-7-14
7. Kowal J, Tkach M, Théry C (2014) Biogenesis and secretion of exosomes. Current Opin Cell Biol 29:116–125. https://doi.org/10.1016/j.ceb.2014.05.004
8. Chen CY, Hogan MC, Ward CJ (2013) Purification of exosome-like vesicles from urine. Methods Enzymol 524:225–241. https://doi.org/10.1016/b978-0-12-397945-2.00013-5
9. Lobb RJ, Becker M, Wen Wen S, Wong CSF, Wiegmans AP, Leimgruber A, Möller A (2015) Optimized exosome isolation protocol for cell culture supernatant and human plasma 4:27031
10. Hata T, Murakami K, Nakatani H, Yamamoto Y, Matsuda T, Aoki N (2010) Isolation of bovine milk-derived microvesicles carrying mRNAs and microRNAs. Biochem Biophys Res Commun 396(2):528–533. https://doi.org/10.1016/j.bbrc.2010.04.135
11. Cvjetkovic A, Lotvall J, Lasser C (2014) The influence of rotor type and centrifugation time on the yield and purity of extracellular vesicles. J Extracell Vesicles 3. https://doi.org/10.3402/jev.v3.23111
12. Livshits MA, Khomyakova E, Evtushenko EG, Lazarev VN, Kulemin NA, Semina SE, Generozov EV, Govorun VM (2015) Isolation of exosomes by differential centrifugation: theoretical analysis of a commonly used protocol. Sci Rep 5:17319. https://doi.org/10.1038/srep17319. http://www.nature.com/articles/srep17319#supplementary-information
13. Witwer KW, Buzás EI, Bemis LT, Bora A, Lässer C, Lötvall J, Nolte-'t Hoen EN, Piper MG, Sivaraman S, Skog J, Théry C, Wauben MH, Hochberg F (2013) Standardization of sample collection, isolation and analysis methods in extracellular vesicle research. J Extracell Vesicles 2:2013
14. Gardiner C, Di Vizio D, Sahoo S, Théry C, Witwer KW, Wauben M, Hill AF (2016) Techniques used for the isolation and characterization of extracellular vesicles: results of a worldwide survey. J Extracell Vesicles 5:32945
15. Van Deun J, Mestdagh P, Sormunen R, Cocquyt V, Vermaelen K, Vandesompele J, Bracke M, De Wever O, Hendrix A (2014) The impact of disparate isolation methods for extracellular vesicles on downstream RNA profiling. J Extracell Vesicles 3. https://doi.org/10.3402/jev.v3.24858
16. Sarker S, Scholz-Romero K, Perez A, Illanes SE, Mitchell MD, Rice GE, Salomon C (2014) Placenta-derived exosomes continuously increase in maternal circulation over the first trimester of pregnancy. J Transl Med 12:204. https://doi.org/10.1186/1479-5876-12-204
17. Ge Q, Zhou Y, Lu J, Bai Y, Xie X, Lu Z (2014) miRNA in plasma exosome is stable under different storage conditions. Molecules 19(2):1568–1575. https://doi.org/10.3390/molecules19021568

Chapter 9

Isolation and Characterization of Extracellular Vesicles from Ex Vivo Cultured Human Placental Explants

Mancy Tong and Lawrence W. Chamley

Abstract

Ex vivo culture of human placental explants has long allowed placentologists to study the milieu of soluble factors secreted by the human placenta throughout gestation while retaining the correct three-dimensional structure of the placental villi. Here, we detail the placental explant culture method employed in our laboratory to collect extracellular vesicles which are known to be released by the human placenta throughout pregnancy from 6 weeks of gestation. Using this method, at least three different populations of placental extracellular vesicles can be simultaneously collected from each placental sample, allowing for comparative analysis of the cargos and downstream effects of the different types of extracellular vesicles produced by the human placenta.

Key words Vesicle, Trophoblastic debris, Microparticle, Explant culture, Placenta

1 Introduction

In addition to the secretion of hormones and other soluble factors, the production of extracellular vesicles by the human placenta has recently been recognized as a novel mode of feto-maternal communication that is important for both physiological adaptations during normal human pregnancy [1–4] and the pathophysiology of obstetric diseases such as preeclampsia [5–8]. The effects of placental extracellular vesicles on recipient cells are likely to be mediated by their protein, lipid, and nucleic acid cargos [9].

As the outermost surface of the human placenta is covered by the multinucleated syncytiotrophoblast, a large range of extracellular vesicles can be produced by the human placenta, ranging in size from macro-vesicles (20–150 μm), to microvesicles (100–1000 nm), to exosomes and other nano-vesicles (20–100 nm) [10, 11]. While placental extracellular vesicles have been detected in the blood of pregnant women from as early as 6 weeks of gestation, their levels in the circulation are much lower than that of maternal platelet-derived and endothelial cell-derived extracellular vesicles [12].

Padma Murthi and Cathy Vaillancourt (eds.), *Preeclampsia: Methods and Protocols*, Methods in Molecular Biology, vol. 1710, https://doi.org/10.1007/978-1-4939-7498-6_9,

Therefore, it has been challenging to isolate circulating placental extracellular vesicles for downstream analysis. This is compounded by a lack of robust placenta-specific markers that can be used for the purification of placenta-derived extracellular vesicles from the blood [13, 14]. Therefore, in order to characterize placental extracellular vesicles to better understand their potential functions and to identify novel markers for these extracellular vesicles, most current studies have isolated extracellular vesicles from human placentae ex vivo.

In the literature, placental macro- and nano-vesicles have predominately been collected by culturing villous placental explants in a static and minimally disruptive system for 24–96 h and isolating the extracellular vesicles by differential centrifugation [9]. In contrast, three methods have been commonly reported for the collection of placental microvesicles: (1) mechanical dissection/disruption, (2) placental explant culture, and (3) placental perfusion. Depending on the method used to collect placental microvesicles, their cargo and downstream effects can be drastically different [15–17], and it is now established that mechanical disruption of placental villi is a poor method for collecting physiologically relevant microvesicles [17].

For the collection of extracellular vesicles from intact term placentae, both placental explant culture and placental perfusion methods can be used, while only the placental explant culture method can be used to isolate extracellular vesicles from first trimester placentae as these placentae are often damaged and lack the depth of villous tissue required to perform perfusion. Chapter 14 has detailed the principles and methods of placental perfusion; thus, this chapter will describe the placental explant culture method in detail and how this can be employed to isolate different size fractions of extracellular vesicles simultaneously from the same placental sample by sequential centrifugation. Finally, the characterization of the total protein content as well as the shape and size of extracellular vesicles by electron microscopy and nanoparticle tracking analysis, respectively, will be described.

2 Materials

Prepare all solutions using ultrapure water and analytical grade reagents.

2.1 Placental Explant Culture

1. Phosphate-buffered saline (PBS): 120 mM NaCl, 2.7 mM KCl, 1.5 mM Na_2HPO_4, and 8 mM KH_2PO_4 (pH 7.4). Dissolve 8.09 g NaCl, 0.2 g KCl, 0.2 g KH_2PO_4, and 1.14 g Na_2HPO_4 in 900 mL of ultrapure water and adjust pH to 7.4 using HCl. Make up the total volume to 1 L and sterilize by autoclaving. Store at room temperature.

2. Sterile petri dishes (10 cm diameter).
3. Sterile forceps and scalpels.
4. Advanced DMEM/F12 medium: Supplement sterile medium with 2% fetal bovine serum (*see* **Note 1**) and 1% penicillin/streptomycin in a laminar flow hood (v/v). Store this placental culture medium at 4 °C.
5. Plastic inserts with a 400 μm mesh: Sterilize between use by leaving in 1% bleach for 1 h, leaving in disinfectant (*see* **Note 2**) for 72 h, and storing in 70% ethanol at room temperature until required. 1 h before use, the required number of inserts should be air-dried in a sterile tissue culture hood.
6. 12-well sterile culture plates.
7. Micropore tape.
8. Tissue culture incubator set at 37 °C and 5% CO_2.
9. 10× PBS: Dissolve 8.09 g NaCl, 0.2 g KCl, 0.2 g KH_2PO_4, and 1.14 g Na_2HPO_4 in 100 mL ultrapure water and sterilize by autoclaving. Store at room temperature.
10. Antihuman CD45 Dynabeads (*see* **Note 3**) and suitable magnet.
11. Blood tube rotator.

2.2 Sequential Centrifugation

1. 0.2 μm filtered sterile PBS.
2. Digital balance that is accurate to 0.001 g.
3. Polycarbonate tubes suitable for ultracentrifugation up to 100,000 × *g*.
4. Ultracentrifuge with a fixed-angle rotor that can reach over 100,000 × *g*.

2.3 Electron Microscopy

1. Uranyl acetate: 2% (w/v) in ultrapure water and filtered. Store at room temperature in the dark.
2. Formvar-coated copper mesh grids.
3. Parafilm.
4. Hardened ashless filter paper.
5. Lamp.
6. Transmission electron microscope.

2.4 Nanoparticle Tracking Analysis

1. 0.2 μm filtered sterile PBS.
2. 1 mL syringes.
3. Ethanol: 10% (v/v) in ultrapure water.
4. NanoSight nanoparticle tracking analysis system (*see* **Note 4**).

2.5 Extraction of Total Protein

Prepare radioimmunoprecipitation (RIPA) buffer: 50 mM Tris (pH 7.4), 150 mM NaCl, 1% sodium deoxycholate (w/v), 0.1% SDS (w/v), 1% Nonidet P40 substitute (w/v), and 1 mM PMSF with protease inhibitor (*see* **Note 5**).

3 Methods

After the collection of placentae from the clinic, minimize contamination by carrying out all procedures in a laminar flow hood, and sterilize all reagents and equipment used for tissue culture by autoclaving, 70% ethanol, or filtration through a 0.2 μm filter. Carry out all procedures at room temperature unless otherwise specified.

3.1 Placental Explant Culture

1. 1 h before the collection of placentae, start to dry plastic inserts in a laminar flow hood that you will subsequently use to process the placenta.
2. For first trimester placentae, wash placentae in sterile PBS to remove as much of the contaminating maternal blood as possible, and dissect away blood clots and placental membranes. For mid−/late-gestation placentae, dissect and discard the top 2 mm of the maternal aspect of the placenta, which contains maternal decidual tissue, and dissect out approximately 2cm^3 of the underlying villous placental tissue. To increase the representativeness of sampling, usually at least three areas of the mid−/late-gestation placenta are sampled ranging from the center of the placenta to the periphery, resulting in at least 6cm^3 of placental villous tissue. Rinse thoroughly in sterile PBS (*see* **Note 6**).
3. After sufficient washing, further dissect the villous placental tissue into explants of approximately 400 mg (*see* **Note 7**). Four placental explants usually generate sufficient extracellular vesicles for physical characterization and protein collection.
4. By this time, the inserts should have dried and can be placed in a 12-well culture plate, creating two compartments (Fig. 1). Place placental explants in the inserts in the upper compartment, and add 3 mL of supplemented advanced DMEM/F12 medium into each well. This should be sufficient to cover the placental explant (Fig. 1).
5. If you are investigating the effects of various reagents (e.g., preeclamptic serum) on the composition, size, or number of extracellular vesicles extruded, these reagents should be added at this stage, with the appropriate controls. When adding such reagents, take care to avoid overly diluting the base medium, and if using human serum, as a general rule, this should make

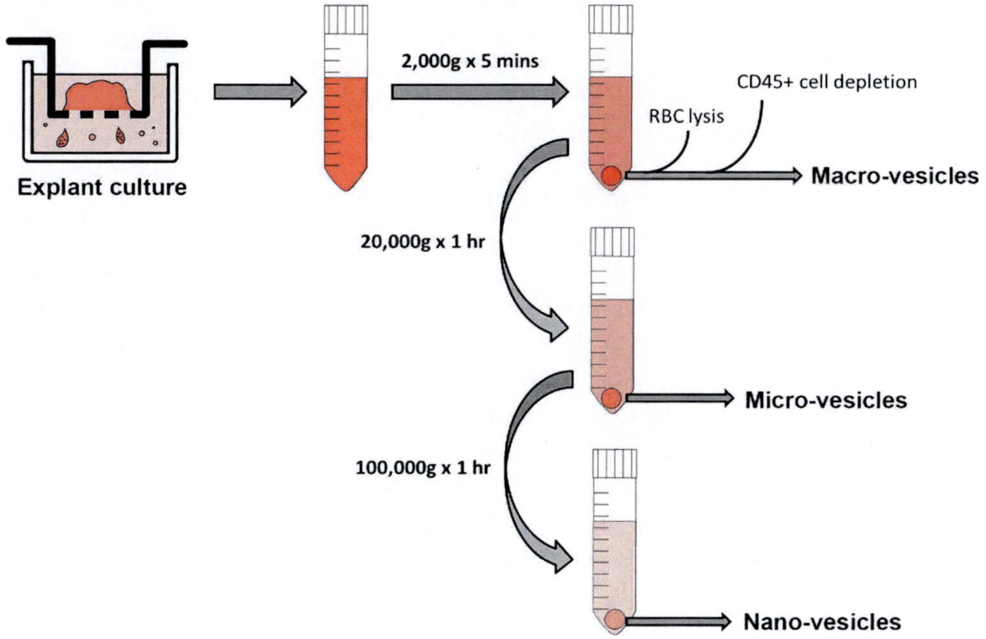

Fig. 1 Schematic representation of the workflow for preparing macro-, micro-, and nano-vesicles from placental explants

up less than 20% of the total volume of the culture medium to avoid toxicity. We also always include a set of untreated explants as an additional control.

6. Seal culture plates with micropore tape (*see* **Note 8**).
7. Culture placental explants in an incubator set at 37 °C and 5% CO_2. In our work, we have frequently cultured placental explants at ambient oxygen levels for 16 h, but culture conditions can be easily manipulated in this system (*see* **Note 9**). We have also previously reported that culture oxygen conditions (2, 8 and 20%) did not significantly affect the number and size of micro- and nano-vesicles extruded from first trimester human placentae [11].

3.2 Sequential Centrifugation

1. After 16 h of culture, lift the inserts, each containing a placental explant, out from the wells of the 12-well plate, taking care to decant as much of the culture medium from around the placental explant as possible back into the well.
2. Mix the culture medium in each well by pipetting, and collect the culture medium from all placental explants (in the four culture wells) into one sterile tube.

3. Centrifuge at 2000 × *g* for 5 min at 4 °C to sediment the placental macro-vesicles and other contaminating cells (red and white blood cells) from the culture medium (Fig. 1). Carefully decant the supernatant resulting from this centrifugation step into a sterile polycarbonate ultracentrifugation tube (*see* **Note 10**), and store at 4 °C for up to 48 h prior to ultracentrifugation to isolate the micro- and nano-vesicles.
4. After decanting, resuspend the pellet, containing placental macro-vesicles and contaminating red and white blood cells, in the remaining ~200 μL of supernatant by gently tapping the base of the tube.
5. Remove contaminating red blood cells by adding in 9 mL sterile water and inverting to create a hypotonic environment. After 10 s, restore isotonic conditions by adding 1 mL sterile 10× PBS and inverting to mix (*see* **Note 11**).
6. Centrifuge the tube again at 2000 × *g* for 5 min at 4 °C. This time, the pellet should look white as most red blood cells should be lysed (*see* **Note 12**).
7. Discard the supernatant and the pellet is again resuspended by gentle tapping in the residual PBS.
8. Contaminating white blood cells can be removed by the addition of antihuman CD45 Dynabeads. To do this, add 800 μL sterile PBS into the tube (making the total volume approximately 1 mL) and add 10 μL of Dynabeads into the tube (*see* **Note 13**).
9. Incubate the tubes for 1 h at 4 °C on a blood tube rotator.
10. Insert the tube into a suitable magnet, which traps the Dynabeads against the wall of the tube, and after 10 s, transfer the supernatant containing placental macro-vesicles into a sterile 1.5 mL tube.
11. Centrifuge tubes at 8000 × *g* for 5 min at 4 °C, and after removal of the supernatant by pipetting, the pellet contains the placental macro-vesicle fraction which should be resuspended in the relevant buffer or media.
12. While the placental macro-vesicle fraction is being purified, placental microvesicles can also be simultaneously isolated from the supernatant collected in **Step 3**. To isolate placental microvesicles, the supernatant collected in **Step 3** is centrifuged at 20,000 × *g* for 1 h at 4 °C (Fig. 1; *see* **Note 14**).
13. The resulting pellet containing the placental microvesicle fraction should be kept in the fridge, while placental nano-vesicles are isolated from the supernatant. The supernatant from the 20,000 × *g* centrifugation step (**Step 12**) should be decanted into a new sterile polycarbonate tube that is rated for ultracentrifugation at 100,000 × *g* and centrifuged at 100,000 × *g* for

1 h at 4 °C to collect the placental nano-vesicle fraction (Fig. 1).

14. For all vesicle pellets, supernatant that was not completely decanted is removed using a pipette after resting the tubes upright for 5 min at room temperature.
15. Depending on the downstream assay, different solutions can be used to resuspend the vesicle pellets.

3.3 Electron Microscopy

1. Resuspend pellets of extracellular vesicles in ultrapure water by repeat pipetting with a 1 mL and 200 μL micropipette at least 20 times each (*see* **Notes 15–17**).
2. Mix thoroughly and pipette 20 μL of sample onto parafilm.
3. Gently overlay a formvar-coated copper mesh grid onto this droplet to coat the surface for 2 min at room temperature.
4. Carefully wick off excess solution with hardened ashless filter paper, and transfer the copper grid onto a droplet of 2% uranyl acetate for 2 min at room temperature.
5. Carefully wick off excess solution with hardened ashless filter paper, and transfer the copper grid onto a droplet of ultrapure water for 2 min.
6. Repeat **Step 5** to remove excess stain, and after wicking off excess solution with hardened ashless filter paper, allow grids to dry at room temperature under a lamp.
7. Sample-coated copper grids are stored sample side up at room temperature and viewed by transmission electron microscopy within 2 h.

3.4 Nanoparticle Tracking Analysis

1. Resuspend pellets of extracellular vesicles in 1 mL of 0.2 μm filtered PBS using a 1 mL pipette.
2. Turn on the NanoSight system and flush 10 mL of ultrapure water through the tubing and gasket.
3. Then flush 5 mL of filtered PBS through the system and dry the system by suction.
4. Mix vesicles well and dilute in filtered PBS (*see* **Note 18**). The system requires 1 mL of sample for analysis.
5. Mix the sample well before loading it all into a 1 mL syringe, without bubbles.
6. Connect the syringe to the NanoSight system inlet, and rapidly load 500 μL of the sample into the NanoSight system (*see* **Note 19**).
7. Vesicles should now be apparent on the NanoSight computer, and the focus can be adjusted on the NanoSight machine such that the majority of vesicles have sharp boundaries and perhaps

one halo around them. This is the plane that will be recorded and analyzed by the NanoSight software.

8. The sample is now ready to be analyzed and the temperature of the stage should be set, usually at 25 °C. In our work, we have typically taken three 30 s recordings of each sample volume, and this is automatically controlled by running a script (Table 1). The NanoSight system that we use (NanoSight NS300) can also be set up with a syringe pump system which allows samples to be constantly flowing during the recording (*see* **Note 20**). An example of a script that can be used for analyzing flowing vesicles is provided in Table 1.
9. After the first set of recordings and analysis, advance the sample by 100 μL in the syringe and do another set of recordings. To obtain representative counts, at the end of this recording, we advanced the sample and counted it three more times, resulting in a total of five sets of readings (15 recordings of 30 s in total).
10. The average vesicle concentration, mean, and modal size of each set of readings were recorded, and from this, the final average concentration, mean, and modal size of all five sets of readings can be calculated (*see* **Note 21**).
11. Taking into account the dilutions performed, the total number of extracellular vesicles in the samples can be calculated, and we typically normalize this value to the weight of the original placental explants or the protein content of the placental explants (*see* **Note 22**).

3.5 Extraction of Total Protein

1. Make fresh RIPA buffer (Table 2) and store on ice.
2. Resuspend pellets of extracellular vesicles in 100 μL of RIPA buffer by vigorous pipetting (*see* **Note 23**).

Table 1
Examples of scripts that can be used on the NanoSight system

Static system	Flow system
SETTEMP 25 REPEATSTART CAPTURE 30 DELAY 10 REPEAT 2 PROCESSSINGLESETTING EXPORTRESULTS	SETTEMP 25 REPEATSTART LOAD 20 DELAY 30 CAPTURE 30 DELAY 10 REPEAT 2 PROCESSSINGLESETTING EXPORTRESULTS

Table 2
Composition of stock solutions to make radioimmunoprecipitation assay (RIPA) buffer

RIPA stock	Composition/recipe	Volume to add to make 2 mL RIPA
Tris/NaCl (pH 7.4)	1.21 g Tris and 1.753 g NaCl in 100 mL H_2O	1 mL
NP-40	1 mL NP-40 in 9 mL H_2O	200 μL
Sodium deoxycholate	1 g in 9 mL H_2O	200 μL
SDS	0.5 g in 50 mL H_2O	200 μL
Protease inhibitor	1 tablet in 10 mL H_2O	390 μL
PMSF	0.348 g in 10 mL isopropanol	10 μL

NaCl, sodium chloride; NP-40, nonidet P-40; SDS, sodium dodecyl sulfate; PMSF, phenylmethylsulfonyl fluoride

3. Transfer extracellular vesicles into a cold 1.5 mL tube and incubate on ice for 10 min with intermittent pipetting.
4. Directly store protein lysates of extracellular vesicles at −80 °C.

4 Notes

1. In some studies, fetal bovine serum is first diluted 1:1 in fresh media and ultracentrifuged up to 120,000 × g for 18 h to remove endogenous extracellular vesicles before being used to supplement culture media [18, 19]. However, recent studies have shown that culture with media supplemented with extracellular vesicle-depleted fetal bovine serum reduced cell proliferation compared to culture with traditional media [20, 21].
2. 5% TriGene™ can be used as a disinfectant to sterilize plastic inserts for reuse.
3. We only have experience using human anti-CD45 Dynabeads to remove white blood cells, but other magnetic beads may also be used, with the concentration adjusted as recommended by the manufacturer.
4. A NanoSight NS300 system equipped with a 405 nm laser and an sCMOS camera was used. This system is required for the detection of smaller extracellular vesicles.
5. In order to quickly make fresh RIPA buffer each time, stock solutions can be prepared (Table 2). All stock solutions are

stored at room temperature except for the protease inhibitor, which is stored at 4 °C for up to a month, and PMSF, which is stored at −20 °C for up to 3 months. Sodium deoxycholate should be stored at room temperature in the dark.

6. For first trimester placentae, usually 3–5 PBS washes are sufficient, but for later gestation placentae, 10–20 washes may be required depending on the volume used. Rinse tissue until the effluent isn't red anymore.
7. Explants from later gestation placentae can be cut into four smaller pieces to further open up the structure to allow the release of extruded extracellular vesicles into the culture medium.
8. Micropore tape is used to seal the system so that the plate and inserts stay together, but oxygen can still freely flow through into the culture system.
9. In the current literature, the concentration of oxygen used for placental explant culture varies from 2 to 20% oxygen. In general, lower oxygen concentrations are used for first trimester placentae. The length of time for placental explant culture also varies between 24 and 96 h in different studies.
10. Ultracentrifuge tubes can be sterilized and reused by making sure the pellet has been removed, thoroughly washing the tubes with water, and spraying with 70% ethanol. Tubes should be dried in a laminar flow hood. Before UV exposure, take care to read the specifications of the tubes to determine whether this would weaken the tube strength. We do not expose our tubes to UV rays.
11. In our experience, removal of red blood cells by water lysis does not damage placental macro-vesicles.
12. The red blood cell lysis step may need to be repeated up to three times to remove red blood cells from macro-vesicle preparations from mid−/late-gestation placentae.
13. Invert and ensure the stock Dynabeads solution is well mixed before use.
14. It is important to balance the tubes for centrifugation to within 0.01 × g using 0.2 μm filtered sterile PBS to prevent potential damage to the ultracentrifuge and rotor.
15. For electron microscopy, samples must be resuspended in salt-free solutions to prevent crystals from forming when the copper mesh grid dries.
16. Whether resuspending vesicles in water for electron microscopy has any effect on vesicle morphology is unclear but within

3 h, micro- and nano-vesicles can still be observed under electron microscopy suggesting that these vesicles are resistant to hypotonic lysis.

17. For the visualization of vesicles by electron microscopy, less is more as excess loading onto the copper mesh grids will break the coating present. In our experience, extracellular vesicles from 4 first trimester placental explants need to be resuspended in at least 2 mL of ultrapure water to be dilute enough for visualization.
18. From four placental explants, carefully do a 1:1000 dilution of the 1 mL of collected extracellular vesicles as a starting dilution for analysis on the NanoSight system. Check the dynamic range of the NanoSight system used to adjust sample dilution as required.
19. Rapidly infusing the sample into the NanoSight system will trigger and turn on the laser and camera for detection.
20. Analysis of extracellular vesicles under flow conditions technically increases the volume measured and therefore should be more representative and accurate. However, in our previous work, we have found that the current NanoSight 3.0 software insufficiently adjusts for flow rate, causing inaccurate measurements [22].
21. The measured concentration tends to reduce during the later analyses from any sample, potentially due to settling of the vesicles. Therefore, always try to complete recordings for each vesicle sample as quickly as possible, and if required, outliers can be removed before calculating the final averages.
22. Protein content of the placental explants can be obtained by homogenizing the placental explant in 1 mL of fresh RIPA buffer and performing a BCA assay following the manufacturer's instructions.
23. Placental nano-vesicles are particularly hard to resuspend in small volumes of RIPA buffer, so sometimes it is easier to partially scrap off the pellet using the pipette tip before pipetting vigorously to break apart the pellet and to mix.

Acknowledgments

Mancy Tong is a recipient of the University of Auckland Health Research Doctoral Scholarship and the Freemasons Postgraduate Scholarship.

References

1. Abrahams VM, Straszewski-Chavez SL, Guller S, Mor G (2004) First trimester trophoblast cells secrete Fas ligand which induces immune cell apoptosis. Mol Hum Reprod 10(1):55–63
2. Frangsmyr L, Baranov V, Nagaeva O, Stendahl U, Kjellberg L, Mincheva-Nilsson L (2005) Cytoplasmic microvesicular form of Fas ligand in human early placenta: switching the tissue immune privilege hypothesis from cellular to vesicular level. Mol Hum Reprod 11(1):35–41. https://doi.org/10.1093/molehr/gah129
3. Stenqvist AC, Nagaeva O, Baranov V, Mincheva-Nilsson L (2013) Exosomes secreted by human placenta carry functional Fas ligand and TRAIL molecules and convey apoptosis in activated immune cells, suggesting exosome-mediated immune privilege of the fetus. J Immunol 191(11):5515–5523. https://doi.org/10.4049/jimmunol.1301885
4. Taylor D, Akyol S, Gercel-Taylor C (2006) Pregnancy-associated exosomes and their modulation of T cell signaling. J Immunol 176(3):1534–1542
5. Baig S, Kothandaraman N, Manikandan J, Rong L, Ee KH, Hill J, Lai CW, Tan WY, Yeoh F, Kale A, LL S, Biswas A, Vasoo S, Choolani M (2014) Proteomic analysis of human placental syncytiotrophoblast microvesicles in preeclampsia. Clin Proteomics 11(1):40. https://doi.org/10.1186/1559-0275-11-40
6. Shomer E, Katzenell S, Zipori Y, Sammour RN, Isermann B, Brenner B, Aharon A (2013) Microvesicles of women with gestational hypertension and preeclampsia affect human trophoblast fate and endothelial function. Hypertension 62(5):893–898. https://doi.org/10.1161/HYPERTENSIONAHA.113.01494
7. Chen Y, Huang Y, Jiang R, Teng Y (2012) Syncytiotrophoblast-derived microparticle shedding in early-onset and late-onset severe pre-eclampsia. Int J Gynaecol Obstet 119(3):234–238. https://doi.org/10.1016/j.ijgo.2012.07.010
8. Shen F, Wei J, Snowise S, DeSousa J, Stone P, Viall C, Chen Q, Chamley L (2014) Trophoblast debris extruded from preeclamptic placentae activates endothelial cells: a mechanism by which the placenta communicates with the maternal endothelium. Placenta 35(10):839–847. https://doi.org/10.1016/j.placenta.2014.07.009
9. Tong M, Chamley LW (2015) Placental extracellular vesicles and feto-maternal communication. Cold Spring Harb Perspect Med 5(3):a023028. https://doi.org/10.1101/cshperspect.a023028
10. Chamley LW, Holland OJ, Chen Q, Viall CA, Stone PR, Abumaree M (2014) Review: where is the maternofetal interface? Placenta 35(Suppl):S74–S80. https://doi.org/10.1016/j.placenta.2013.10.014
11. Tong M, Kleffmann T, Pradhan S, Johansson CL, DeSousa J, Stone PR, James JL, Chen Q, Chamley LW (2016) Proteomic characterization of macro-, micro- and nano-extracellular vesicles derived from the same first trimester placenta: relevance for feto-maternal communication. Hum Reprod 31(4):687–699. https://doi.org/10.1093/humrep/dew004
12. Lok CA, Van Der Post JA, Sargent IL, Hau CM, Sturk A, Boer K, Nieuwland R (2008) Changes in microparticle numbers and cellular origin during pregnancy and preeclampsia. Hypertens Pregnancy 27(4):344–360. https://doi.org/10.1080/10641950801955733
13. VanWijk MJ, Nieuwland R, Boer K, van der Post JA, VanBavel E, Sturk A (2002) Microparticle subpopulations are increased in preeclampsia: possible involvement in vascular dysfunction? Am J Obstet Gynecol 187(2):450–456
14. Tannetta DS, Dragovic RA, Gardiner C, Redman CW, Sargent IL (2013) Characterisation of syncytiotrophoblast vesicles in normal pregnancy and pre-eclampsia: expression of Flt-1 and endoglin. PLoS One 8(2):e56754. https://doi.org/10.1371/journal.pone.0056754
15. Gupta AK, Holzgreve W, Hahn S (2008) Decrease in lipid levels of syncytiotrophoblast micro-particles reduced their potential to inhibit endothelial cell proliferation. Arch Gynecol Obstet 277(2):115–119. https://doi.org/10.1007/s00404-007-0425-2
16. Gupta AK, Holzgreve W, Huppertz B, Malek A, Schneider H, Hahn S (2004) Detection of fetal DNA and RNA in placenta-derived syncytiotrophoblast microparticles generated in vitro. Clin Chem 50(11):2187–2190. https://doi.org/10.1373/clinchem.2004.040196
17. Gupta AK, Rusterholz C, Huppertz B, Malek A, Schneider H, Holzgreve W, Hahn S (2005) A comparative study of the effect of three different syncytiotrophoblast micro-particles preparations on endothelial cells. Placenta 26(1):59–66. https://doi.org/10.1016/j.placenta.2004.04.004

18. Shelke GV, Lasser C, Gho YS, Lotvall J (2014) Importance of exosome depletion protocols to eliminate functional and RNA-containing extracellular vesicles from fetal bovine serum. J Extracell Vesicles 3. https://doi.org/10.3402/jev.v3.24783
19. Thery C, Amigorena S, Raposo G, Clayton A (2006) Isolation and characterization of exosomes from cell culture supernatants and biological fluids. Curr Protoc Cell Biol Chapter 3:Unit 3 22. https://doi.org/10.1002/0471143030.cb0322s30
20. Aswad H, Jalabert A, Rome S (2016) Depleting extracellular vesicles from fetal bovine serum alters proliferation and differentiation of skeletal muscle cells in vitro. BMC Biotechnol 16:32. https://doi.org/10.1186/s12896-016-0262-0
21. Eitan E, Zhang S, Witwer KW, Mattson MP (2015) Extracellular vesicle-depleted fetal bovine and human sera have reduced capacity to support cell growth. J Extracell Vesicles 4:26373. https://doi.org/10.3402/jev.v4.26373
22. Tong M, Brown OS, Stone PR, Cree LM, Chamley LW (2016) Flow speed alters the apparent size and concentration of particles measured using NanoSight nanoparticle tracking analysis. Placenta 38:29–32. https://doi.org/10.1016/j.placenta.2015.12.004

Chapter 10

Optimized Specific Isolation of Placenta-Derived Exosomes from Maternal Circulation

Andrew Lai, Omar Elfeky, Gregory E. Rice, and Carlos Salomon

Abstract

Exosomes are small (~100 nm) vesicles that carry a wide range of molecules including proteins, RNAs, and DNA. Exosomes are secreted from a wide range of cells including placental cells. Interestingly, exosomes secreted from placental cells have been identified in maternal circulation as early as in 6 weeks of gestation, and their concentration increases with the gestational age. While there is growing interest in elucidating the role of exosomes during normal and complicated pregnancies (such as preeclampsia), progress in the field has been delayed because of the inability to isolate placental exosomes from maternal circulation. Therefore, here we describe a workflow to isolate placental exosomes from maternal circulation.

Key words Exosomes, Preeclampsia, Immunoaffinity isolation, Placenta

1 Introduction

Preeclampsia (PE), along with its consequential diseases, is one of the most significant complications of pregnancy, as it is responsible for almost 40% of premature births and occurs in 3–5% of pregnancies [1]. PE is diagnosed after the twentieth week of gestation, and complications of the condition include placental abruption, coagulopathy, renal failure, uteroplacental insufficiency, and eclampsia [2]. Currently, there is no effective antenatal treatment of PE; the only definitive treatment is delivery of the fetus. Therefore, establishing and developing methods to predict the development of PE earlier in the pregnancy can help provide better care for the mother and fetus as well as possibly lead to a reduced prevalence of the disease.

Recently, tissue-specific extracellular vesicles (EVs) have been studied as diagnostic tools of PE [3–5]. EVs are subcategorized into subgroups by factors such as origin and size. Exosomes are a specific type of EVs that are categorized by their size and endosomal origin and have been found to incorporate specific molecules in response to the microenvironment milieu [6]. Exosomes measure between 40 and 100 nm and have a very stable lipid bilayer, which is the result

Padma Murthi and Cathy Vaillancourt (eds.), *Preeclampsia: Methods and Protocols*, Methods in Molecular Biology, vol. 1710, https://doi.org/10.1007/978-1-4939-7498-6_10, © Springer Science+Business Media LLC 2018

of the inward budding of multivesicular bodies [7]. Exosomes have been found to contain a diverse array of signaling molecules, however little is known about the mechanism by which they are packaged. These signaling molecules are thought to be released from the parent cell into the exosome following the exocytotic fusion of the multivesicular bodies with the cell membrane. Once the exosome is released into the extracellular space, some exosomes have the capability to travel along the systemic circulation to interact with distant tissues in the body as a form of non-hormonal signaling or communication. Since the exosomes are in the systemic circulation, they present an opportunity for the development of a noninvasive biopsy of the tissue of origin, which presents a new approach to the development of screening and diagnostic tests [6].

Recently, we have been able to obtain an enriched exosome fraction with minimal contribution from other EVs using the well-established and validated method of buoyant density centrifugation and used that to establish that placental derived exosomes are present in the maternal circulation and that their concentration increases as the pregnancy progresses [8–10]. There are no studies, however, that have isolated specific placental exosomes from maternal circulation.

Invading human leukocyte antigen-G+ (HLA-G+) extravillous trophoblasts (EVT) are key players in the anchoring of the placenta, the opening of the uterine spiral arteries, and the prevention of maternal immune attacks on foreign fetal and placental tissues [11, 12]. They are found at the tips of anchoring villi (columnar EVT) from which they detach and subsequently adhere to proteins in the extracellular matrix and travel through decidual tissue (interstitial EVT) to invade the uterine spiral arteries and lead to endothelial dysfunction by replacing the endothelial cell layer (endovascular EVT). At early gestation, EVT plug is in direct contact with the maternal circulation; therefore, EVT-derived exosomes may be present in maternal circulation. Placental-derived exosomes have been found to have syncytiotrophoblast-specific proteins, placental alkaline phosphatase, PLAP. Furthermore, studies have identified the presence of PLAP+ exosomes only in the circulation of pregnant women [9, 13]. Here we described a method to isolate placental exosomes from maternal circulation by immunoaffinity capture using anti-HLA-G and anti-PLAP-coated beads to isolate exosomes secreted from extravillous trophoblast cells (HLA-G+) and syncytiotrophoblast (PLAP+), respectively.

2 Materials

1. Phosphate buffered saline (PBS).
2. Rabbit anti-HLA-G antibody.
3. Rabbit anti-placental alkaline phosphatase (PLAP) antibody.

4. Protein A agarose beads.
5. Dimethylformamide (DMF).
6. Disuccinimidyl suberate (DSS).
7. Elution buffer: 0.1 M glycine-HCl pH 2.8.
8. Neutralization buffer: 1 M Tris pH 8.0.
9. Radioimmunoprecipitation assay buffer (RIPA buffer).
10. Bolt™ SDS-PAGE system: Bolt™ 4–12% Bis-Tris Plus gels, 10 wells; 10× Bolt® Sample Reducing Agent; 4× Bolt® LDS Sample Buffer; 20× Bolt® MOPS SDS Running Buffer.
11. Pierce™ Silver Stain Kit.
12. Trans-Blot® Turbo™ Transfer System.
13. Tris-buffered saline with 0.1% v/v Tween 20 (TBST): 50 mM Tris–Cl, pH 7.5, 150 mM NaCl.
14. Odyssey blocking buffer in Tris-buffered saline.
15. Anti-rabbit IgG (H + L) (DyLight™ 800 4× PEG Conjugate).

3 Methods

3.1 Binding of Antibody to Protein A Agarose Beads

1. For each reaction, transfer 20 μL of protein A-coated bead slurry into a 0.2 mL centrifuge tube (*see* **Note 1**).
2. Briefly centrifuge (~2690 × *g*), carefully remove supernatant, and wash with 1× PBS. Repeat this washing process once. Aspirate the final PBS wash (*see* **Note 2**).
3. Dilute 10 μg of anti-HLA-G or 10 μg of anti-PLAP antibody to a final volume of 100 μL using the 20× PBS and water. Reserve 5 μL as the input antibody for post-binding analysis on an SDS-PAGE.
4. Transfer diluted antibody solution to the beads and incubate the antibody solution with beads at room temperature for 60 min with rotation.
5. Briefly centrifuge (~2690 × *g*) and aspirate antibody solution from beads and reserve 5 μL for analysis.
6. Wash beads with 100 μL of 1× PBS, centrifuge, and remove supernatant for analysis.

3.2 Cross-Linking the Bound Antibodies to Protein A Agarose Beads

1. Weigh out 2 mg of DSS (*see* **Note 3**) in a 0.5 mL centrifuge tube, and add 217 μL of dried DMF (*see* **Note 4**). Briefly vortex.
2. Dilute stock DSS solution ten times with DMF (2.5 mM).
3. Add 2.5 μL of 20× PBS, 9 μL of 2.5 mM DSS, and 38.5 μL of H_2O to the beads.

4. Incubate with rotation at room temperature for 1 h.
5. Wash twice with 100 μL elution buffer. After each wash, a sample was retained. This is to confirm the success of the cross-linking reaction.
6. Verify samples from **step 3** in Subheading 3.1 (input), **step 5** in Subheading 3.1 (unbound), **step 6** in Subheading 3.1 (wash), and **step 5** in Subheading 3.2 (elution 1, elution 2) for the presence/absence of the anti-HLA-G or anti-PLAP antibody by separation using the Bolt™ SDS-PAGE system and subsequent silver staining of the resulting gel. If the reaction was successful, the antibody should only be detected in the input sample. Expected results are shown in Fig. 1.
7. Optional: Perform titration experiments on the antibody-conjugated beads by serial dilution using agarose beads (*see* **Note 5**).

3.3 Incubation of Exosome with Antibody-Conjugated Agarose Beads

1. Exosomes were previously isolated from 500 μL plasma using a combination of differential ultracentrifugation followed by ultrafiltration (*see* **Note 6**).
2. Dilute 5 μL of exosomes to a final volume of 100 μL with PBS. Make an additional replicate sample as the starting exosome (sample input in Fig. 1).
3. Add diluted exosome to the antibody-conjugated beads and incubate overnight at 4 °C with rotation.
4. After incubation, reserve the supernatant from each tube (unbound exosomes) for analysis with NTA and Western blot (sample unbound in Fig. 1).
5. Wash with 100 μL of PBS and reserve (sample wash in Fig. 1).
6. To elute bound exosomes, add 90 μL of 0.1 M glycine-HCl pH 2.8 to the beads. Centrifuge and transfer the supernatant to tubes containing 10 μL of 1 M Tris pH 8.0 to neutralize the pH (sample elution 1 in Fig. 1).
7. Repeat the elution process once (sample elution 2 in Fig. 1).

3.4 Quantitative Western Blotting Using the Odyssey System

1. To assess whether the enrichment of HLA-G- or PLAP-positive exosomes were successful, samples will need to be interrogated for the presence/absence of HLA-G or PLAP using Western blotting.
2. Mix 11.25 μL of each sample from Subheading 3.3 (load, unbound, wash, elution 1 and 2) with 5 μL of RIPA buffer, 2.5 μL of Sample Reducing Agent, and 6.25 μL of LDS Sample Buffer (*see* **Note 7**).
3. Heat each sample at 70 °C for 10 min and resolve on a 4–12% Bis-Tris Plus SDS-PAGE gel using MOPS SDS running buffer at 200 V.

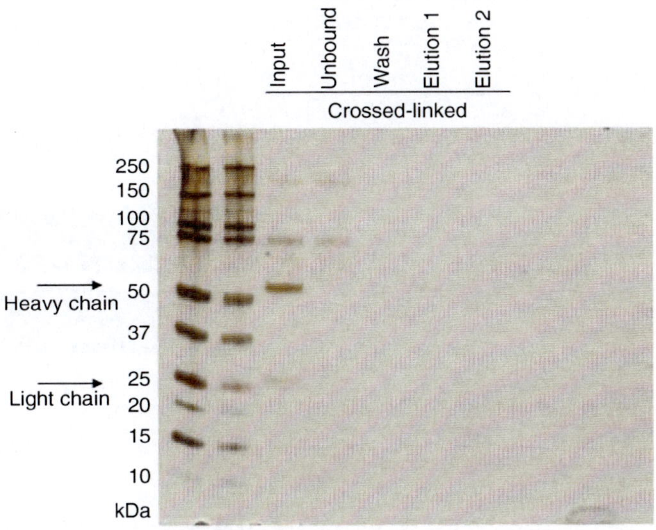

Fig. 1 Verification of cross-linking of the anti-HLA-G or PLAP antibody to protein A agarose beads. Anti-HLA-G antibody samples obtained from preincubation (input) and postincubation with protein A agarose beads (unbound). The beads were washed once with PBS (wash) and twice with a low pH buffer (elution 1 and 2). All samples were separated based on molecular weight using SDS-PAGE, and the resulting gel was stained with silver

4. Transfer the resolved proteins onto an activated polyvinylidene difluoride (PVDF) membrane using the turbo-mixed molecular weight setting on the Trans-Blot® Turbo™ Transfer System (*see* **Note 8**).
5. Block membrane with 5 mL of Odyssey blocking buffer (OBB) for 1 h at room temperature with shaking.
6. Dilute 5 μL of anti-HLA-G or anti-PLAP antibody in 5 mL of OBB, and incubate blot overnight at 4 °C with shaking.
7. Remove primary antibody and wash blot three times with Tris-buffered saline with 0.1% v/v Tween 20 (TBST) for 5 min each.
8. Dilute 0.66 μL of anti-rabbit secondary conjugated with Dylight® 800 in 10 mL of OBB.
9. Incubate blot with diluted antibody for 1 h in room temperature with shaking.
10. Remove secondary antibody, and wash blot six times with Tris-buffered saline with 0.1% v/v Tween 20 (TBST) for 5 min each (*see* **Note 9**).
11. Scan blot with the Li-cor Odyssey system.
12. Quantify the bands corresponding to the HLA-G or PLAP using the Image Studio™ software. Expected results are shown in Fig. 2.

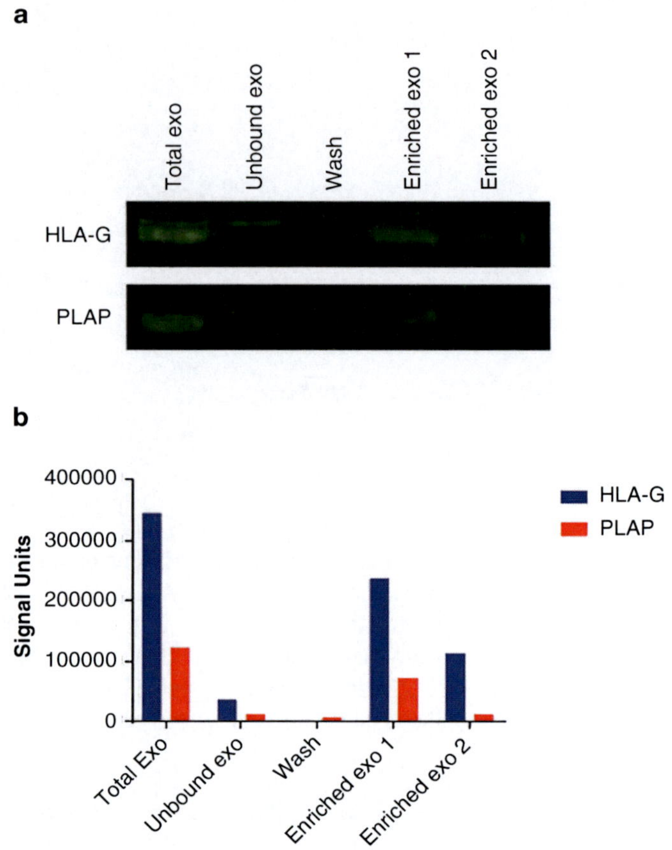

Fig. 2 Confirmation of the isolation of HLA-G positive or PLAP exosome from maternal circulation using Western blotting. A mixed population of exosomes (total exosomes) was incubated with anti-HLA-G (**a**) or anti-PLAP (**b**) conjugated beads. A sample was taken postincubation (unbound exosomes) and the beads washed once with PBS (wash). Bound exosomes to the beads were eluted by low pH (enriched exosomes 1 and 2). *Upper level*: the resulting blot was interrogated with an anti-HLA-G or anti-PLAP antibody. *Lower level*: each band was quantified using Image Studio™ software

4 Notes

1. For antibodies raised in mouse, protein G agarose should be used. This is due to protein G having a higher affinity for mouse antibodies compared to protein A. In addition, non-purified sources of antibodies can also be used, such as from ascites fluid or conditioned medium. However, due to difficulties in quantifying the amount of antibody, a purification step should ideally be performed initially using protein A or G agarose.
2. A simple method to completely remove the supernatant without disturbing the beads pellet is by the use of a rolled up wipers.

3. Alternative cross-linking reagents such as the water-soluble bis(sulfosuccinimidyl)suberate (BS3) can also be used.
4. Use fresh DMF or alternatively, store DMF with molecular sieves to remove any water present.
5. Titration experiments should be performed due to the large excess of antibodies conjugated to a small volume of beads. The beads can be diluted with protein A agarose, or as a cheaper alternative, sepharose beads.
6. Exosomes can be isolated using several methods [14–20]. This protocol has been designed to enrich placental exosomes from a total exosomes population. Therefore, this workflow can be used to enrich placental exosomes after exosomes isolation from maternal plasma.
7. The inclusion of the RIPA buffer in the sample mix is to ensure the complete disruption of the exosomes.
8. Trans-Blot® Turbo™ Transfer System is based on the transfer of proteins using semidry chemistries. Using the turbo setting, a complete transfer can be conducted in 7 min. Alternative wet-based transfer methods can also be used.
9. For a cleaner Western blot with a lower background, a final wash with TBS for 5 min can also be performed. This will remove any residual Tween which can increase background signals.

Acknowledgment

CS was in receipt of a Lions Medical Research Foundation Fellowship. This study was supported by The Lions Medical Research Foundation, UQ ECR award, Royal Brisbane and Women's Foundation, Diabetes Australia, and UQ-Ochsner Seed Grant. The ISO17025 accredited research facility was supported by grants from Therapeutics Innovation Australia and the National Collaborative Research Infrastructure Strategy.

This review is supported partly by funding from the Lions Medical Research Foundation (LMRF), The University of Queensland, and Fondo Nacional de Desarrollo Científico y Tecnológico (FONDECYT 1170809), Chile.

References

1. Kuklina EV, Ayala C, Callaghan WM (2009) Hypertensive disorders and severe obstetric morbidity in the United States. Obstet Gynecol 113(6):1299–1306
2. Ananth CV, Keyes KM, Wapner RJ (2013) Pre-eclampsia rates in the United States, 1980-2010: age-period-cohort analysis. Brit Med J 347:f6564
3. Xiao DY, Ohlendorf J, Chen YL, Taylor DD, Rai SN, Waigel S et al (2012) Identifying mRNA, MicroRNA and protein profiles of melanoma exosomes. PLoS One 7(10):e46874

4. Rabinowits G, Gercel-Taylor C, Day JM, Taylor DD, Kloecker GH (2009) Exosomal MicroRNA: a diagnostic marker for lung cancer. Clin Lung Cancer 10(1):42–46
5. Tannetta DS, Dragovic RA, Gardiner C, Redman CW, Sargent IL (2013) Characterisation of syncytiotrophoblast vesicles in normal pregnancy and pre-eclampsia: expression of Flt-1 and endoglin. PLoS One 8(2):e56754
6. Mitchell MD, Peiris HN, Kobayashi M, Koh YQ, Duncombe G, Illanes SE et al (2015) Placental exosomes in normal and complicated pregnancy. Am J Obstet Gynecol 213(4):S173–S181
7. Colombo M, Raposo G, Thery C (2014) Biogenesis, secretion, and intercellular interactions of exosomes and other extracellular vesicles. Annu Rev Cell Dev Biol 30:255–289
8. Salomon C, Scholz-Romero K, Sarker S, Sweeney E, Kobayashi M, Correa P et al (2015) Gestational diabetes mellitus is associated with changes in the concentration and bioactivity of placenta-derived exosomes in maternal circulation across gestation. Diabetes 65:598
9. Sarker S, Scholz-Romero K, Perez A, Illanes SE, Mitchell MD, Rice GE et al (2014) Placenta-derived exosomes continuously increase in maternal circulation over the first trimester of pregnancy. J Transl Med 12:204
10. Salomon C, Torres MJ, Kobayashi M, Scholz-Romero K, Sobrevia L, Dobierzewska A et al (2014) A gestational profile of placental exosomes in maternal plasma and their effects on endothelial cell migration. PLoS One 9(6):e98667
11. Goldman-Wohl DS, Ariel I, Greenfield C, Hanoch J, Yagel S (2000) HLA-G expression in extravillous trophoblasts is an intrinsic property of cell differentiation: a lesson learned from ectopic pregnancies. Mol Hum Reprod 6(6):535–540
12. Hara N, Fujii T, Yamashita T, Kozuma S, Okai T, Taketani Y (1996) Altered expression of human leukocyte antigen G (HLA-G) on extravillous trophoblasts in preeclampsia: immunohistological demonstration with anti-HLA-G specific antibody "87G" and anti-cytokeratin antibody "CAM5.2". Am J Reprod Immunol 36(6):349–358
13. Salomon C, Torres MJ, Kobayashi M, Scholz-Romero K, Sobrevia L, Dobierzewska A et al (2014) A gestational profile of placental exosomes in maternal plasma and their effects on endothelial cell migration. PLoS One 9(6):e98667
14. Taylor DD, Zacharias W, Gercel-Taylor C (2011) Exosome isolation for proteomic analyses and RNA profiling. Methods Mol Biol 728:235–246
15. Kalra H, Adda CG, Liem M, Ang CS, Mechler A, Simpson RJ et al (2013) Comparative proteomics evaluation of plasma exosome isolation techniques and assessment of the stability of exosomes in normal human blood plasma. Proteomics 13(22):3354–3364
16. Schageman J, Zeringer E, Li M, Barta T, Lea K, Gu J et al (2013) The complete exosome workflow solution: from isolation to characterization of RNA cargo. Biomed Res Int 2013:253957
17. Ban JJ, Lee M, Im W, Kim M (2015) Low pH increases the yield of exosome isolation. Biochem Biophys Res Commun 461(1):76–79
18. Li M, Rai AJ, DeCastro GJ, Zeringer E, Barta T, Magdaleno S et al (2015) An optimized procedure for exosome isolation and analysis using serum samples: application to cancer biomarker discovery. Methods 87:26–30
19. Lobb RJ, Becker M, Wen SW, Wong CS, Wiegmans AP, Leimgruber A et al (2015) Optimized exosome isolation protocol for cell culture supernatant and human plasma. J Extracell Vesicles 4:27031
20. Thery C, Amigorena S, Raposo G, Clayton A (2006) Isolation and characterization of exosomes from cell culture supernatants and biological fluids. Curr Protoc Cell Biol Chapter 3:Unit 3.22

Chapter 11

Proteomics Method to Identification of Protein Profiles in Exosomes

Andrew Lai, Vyjayanthi Kinhal, Zarin Nuzhat, Ramkumar Menon, Gregory E. Rice, and Carlos Salomon

Abstract

Exosomes are membrane-bound nanovesicles that transport molecular signals (e.g., proteins) between cells and are released from a wide range of cells, including the human placenta. Interestingly, the levels of exosomes present in maternal circulation are higher in preeclamptic pregnancies and their protein content profile change in response to the microenvironment milieu. Through the discovery of candidate biomarkers, mass spectrometry (MS)-based proteomics may provide a better understanding of the pathophysiology underlying pregnancy-associated disorders. With advances in sample preparation techniques, computational methodologies, and bioinformatics, MS-based proteomics have addressed the challenge of identifying and quantifying thousands of proteins and peptides from a variety of complex biological samples. Despite increasing interest in biomarker diagnostics, the complex nature of biological matrices (e.g., plasma) poses a challenge for candidate biomarker discovery. Here we describe a workflow to prepare exosomes for proteomic analysis.

Key words Proteomics, Mass spectrometry, Extracellular vesicles, Exosomes, Biological markers

1 Introduction

Preeclampsia (PE) is a common disorder characterized by the onset of hypertension and proteinuria at or after approximately 20 weeks of gestation in a normally non-hypertensive woman [1]. Preeclampsia is also associated with impaired placentation, resulting in poor extravillous trophoblast (EVT) invasion and impaired remodeling of the spiral arteries [2–4], resulting in fetal malnutrition [3]. Additionally, this elevates the risk of perinatal morbidity and mortality. Early detection of the disease is necessary for monitoring its progression and improving patient outcomes. Thus, there is a compelling need for innovative and minimally invasive tests for predicting disease risk and early disease detection. As such

Andrew Lai and Vyjayanthi Kinhal contributed equally to this work.

Padma Murthi and Cathy Vaillancourt (eds.), *Preeclampsia: Methods and Protocols*, Methods in Molecular Biology, vol. 1710, https://doi.org/10.1007/978-1-4939-7498-6_11, © Springer Science+Business Media LLC 2018

there have been increasing efforts to identify early biomarkers of preeclampsia, as well as other disorders of pregnancy.

The secretome is comprised of proteins secreted by a cell, tissue, or organism [5]. Secretomes are present in a wide variety of biological fluids and cell-culture-conditioned media (CCM). They exist as either soluble proteins arising from classical secretory pathways, transmembrane proteins from proteolytic shedding of ectodomains, or membrane-bound extracellular vesicles (EVs). Notably, EVs represent a putative source of biomarkers [6].

Secreted from cells under physiological and pathological conditions, EVs have been isolated from a diverse range of biological fluids, including blood plasma and serum, breast milk, urine, and cerebrospinal fluid [7, 8]. The increasing interest in EV structure and function stems from their high abundance in physiological fluids and their ubiquitous secretion from multiple cell types. Additionally, the proteomes of EVs may be specific to their cell of origin, as they retain unique markers of their origin (i.e., specific membrane proteins). Proteomic profiling of EVs enriched with disease-associated proteins may enable the utilization of EVs as diagnostic markers of disease. Furthermore, proteomic profiling may elucidate the role of the EV proteome in pathogenesis. Thus, the EV proteome holds great promise for diagnostic, prognostic, and therapeutic purposes).

Despite these advantages, it is well established that some cell types are dominant sources of EVs [9], and the concentration of these EVs and associated proteins can vary by several orders of magnitude [5, 7, 10]. This can reduce the detection of rare EV subpopulations and related proteins from less abundant cell types. Additionally, the isolation of membrane-bound proteins in the "bottom-up" fashion, which involves the analysis of enzymatically digested proteomes, is extremely difficult [5]. Thus, focusing on a specific subpopulation of EVs (e.g., exosomes) may be more useful for biomarker discovery.

"EV" is an umbrella term that encompasses several types of vesicles including exosomes, microvesicles, and apoptotic vesicles [8]. Variation in EV isolation methods across the research community often results in the extraction of multiple types of EVs with overlapping physical features (e.g., vesicle diameter and membrane markers). This makes it difficult to isolate and proteomically profile homogeneous EV subpopulations. Although we are specifically interested in exosomes, the workflow detailed in this chapter can be applied to a variety of vesicular structures. Therefore, we will be using the term "EV" to refer to all vesicles of interest isolated from a variety of biological matrices.

The sensitivity and overall quality of mass spectrometric analysis of proteolytically derived peptides is highly dependent on optimal sample preparation [11–13] (*see* **Note 1**). Proteomic analysis of EVs presents several sample-specific challenges. The presence of various types of EVs and high-abundance proteins in the source media (e.g., plasma vs. CCM) can contaminate the EV isolate [14].

Furthermore, the multistep nature of EV isolation (e.g., repeated ultracentrifugation steps) can result in reduced EV recovery and, consequently, a low protein yield [7, 14, 15].

Proteomic analysis of complex) secretomes can be further improved by fractionation at the peptide or protein level, which "simplifies" complex peptide mixtures and enables the identification and quantitation of more, often rare, peptides [16–18]. Fractionation may also provide addition information, such as molecular weight and isoelectric point. When combined with MS data, this information can be used to confirm peptide-spectrum matches and improve peptide identification [19]. There are numerous methods of peptide fractionation, including strong cation exchange (SCX) chromatography [20, 21], SDS-PAGE [19, 22], and peptide isoelectric focusing [23–25]. This chapter will focus on OFFGEL isoelectric focusing, where peptides are fractionated according to their isoelectric point along an immobilized pH gradient strip [26]. The resulting fractions are in the liquid phase, making collection simpler than with traditional gels (e.g., gel electrophoresis) [27]. This liquid-phase recovery of peptide fractions makes OFFGEL fractionation directly compatible with liquid-phase workflows such as liquid chromatography-tandem mass spectrometry (LC-MS/MS) [22].

Thus, the primary aim of this chapter is to establish a robust EV preparation protocol for proteomic profiling within the context of a bottom-up proteomics workflow (*see* **Note 2**).

2 Materials

2.1 Reagents

1. Trifluoretic acid (TFA).
2. Acetonitrile (ACN) (LC grade).
3. Formic acid.
4. Acetic acid (glacial; $C_2H_4O_2$).
5. Dithiothreitol (DTT) (AR grade).
6. Iodoacetic acid (IAA) (AR grade).
7. Ammonium bicarbonate (anhydrous; NH_4HCO_3).
8. Trypsin (MS grade).
9. RIPA lysis buffer.
10. Empore octadecyl C18 47 mm solid-phase extraction disks.
11. Poros R3.
12. Ultrapure water (DNase and RNase free).
13. GELoader tips.
14. 200 μL tips (with 2–3 mm removed).
15. Combitip (1.25 mL).

16. LoBind protein tubes (1.5 mL).
17. Parafilm M sealing) foil.
18. Vacuum centrifuge.
19. 9 mm clear glass screw thread vials.
20. Incubator (37 °C and 60 °C).
21. Mineral oil (cover fluid).
22. 100% isopropanol.
23. 100% methanol.
24. 100% formic acid.
25. OFFGEL buffer (GE Healthcare, pH 3–10 NL).
26. Agilent 3100 OFFGEL fractionator machine.
27. OFFGEL electrode pads.
28. Agilent OFFGEL starter kit (white tray, electrodes, 24 translucent well frame, cover seal).
29. OFFGEL dry strip pH 3–10 NL 24 cm (GE Healthcare, Immobiline Dry Strip).
30. Tweezers.

2.2 Solutions

Prepare and store all reagents at room temperature (unless indicated otherwise). Prepare all solutions using analytical grade reagents and high-performance liquid chromatography (HPLC) grade water. Adjustment of the volume of the solutions listed below may be required) according to the number of samples.

2.2.1 Reduction

1. 1 M NH_4HCO_3 solution (Solution 1): Add 100 mL of water to a sterile glass beaker or graduated cylinder. Weigh 79 g NH_4HCO_3 and transfer to the cylinder. Add 900 mL of water to make up to 1 L. Shelf life: store the solution at 4 °C for up to 1 month.
2. 50 mM NH_4HCO_3, pH 8 (Solution 2): Add 9.5 mL of water to a 10 mL tube. Add 0.5 mL of 1 M NH_4HCO_3 solution (Solution 1). Vortex to mix and store at room temperature. Shelf life: solution must be prepared daily.
3. 1 M DTT solution (Solution 3): Add 100 μL of water to a sterile LoBind tube. Weigh 15 mg of DTT and transfer to the tube. Vortex to dissolve and store at room temperature. Shelf life: solution must be prepared daily.
4. 20 mM DTT in 100 mM NH_4HCO_3 solution (Solution 4): Add 880 μL water to a LoBind tube. Add 100 μL of 1 M NH_4HCO_3 solution (Solution 1). Add 20 μL of 1 M DTT solution (Solution 3). Vortex to mix and store at room temperature. Shelf life: solution must be prepared daily.

2.2.2 Alkylation

100 mM IAA in 100 mM NH_4HCO_3 solution (Solution 5): Add 900 μL water to a LoBind tube. Weigh 18.5 mg IAA and transfer to the tube. Vortex to dissolve. Add 100 μL 1 M NH_4HCO_3 (Solution 1). Vortex to mix and store in the dark until ready to use. Shelf life: solution must be prepared immediately before use (*see* **Note 3**).

2.2.3 Tryptic Digestion

1. 50 mM $C_2H_4O_2$ solution (Solution 6): Measure 3.0025 g of $C_2H_4O_2$ and add to 1 L of water (adjust volumes depending on number of samples). Mix well and store at 4 °C. Shelf life: indefinite.
2. Trypsin stock solution (1 μg/μL; Solution 7): Reconstitute 100 μg of trypsin as per the manufacturer's method to a final concentration of 1 μg/μL (i.e., 100 μg trypsin +100 μL 50 mM $C_2H_4O_2$). Aliquot into 5 and 10 μL volumes and store at −20 °C (for up to 1 month) or −70 °C (long term).
3. 1:1 NH_4HCO_3 + ACN solution) (Solution 8): Combine 50 μL of 1 M NH_4HCO_3 (Solution 1) and 50 μL of 100% ACN in a LoBind tube. Vortex to mix. Shelf life: solution must be prepared daily.
4. Trypsin working solution (0.5 μg/μL; Solution 9): Combine equal volumes of trypsin stock solution (Solution 7) and 1:1 NH_4HCO_3 + ACN solution (Solution 8) to give a working solution of trypsin with a final concentration of 0.5 μg/μL (*see* **Note 4**).

2.2.4 Desalting

1. Poros R3 slurry: Add 1 mL of methanol to a LoBind tube. Weigh 50 mg of Poros R3 beads and transfer to the tube. Vortex to mix well.
2. 0.1% (v/v) TFA in H_2O: Combine 100 mL of water and 100 μL TFA in a sterile bottle. Shake to mix well. Shelf life: store at room temperature for up to 1 month.
3. 0.1% (v/v) formic acid in ACN: Combine 100 mL of ACN and 100 μL formic acid in a sterile bottle. Shake to mix well. Shelf life: store at room temperature for up to 1 month.
4. 0.1% (v/v) formic acid in H_2O: Combine 100 mL of water and 100 μL formic acid in a sterile bottle. Shake to mix well. Shelf life: store at room temperature for up to 1 month.

2.2.5 OFFGEL

1. OFFGEL stock solution (1.25×): In a clean 10 mL tube, combine 5 mL of MilliQ water and 60 μL of OFFGEL buffer. Vortex to mix and store on ice during use. Shelf life: excess solution can be stored at −20 °C for later use (up to 1 month).
2. OFFGEL strip rehydration buffer: In a clean LoBind tube, mix 480 μL of the OFFGEL stock solution (1.25×) and 720 μL

MilliQ water. Vortex to mix and store on ice during use. Shelf life: solution must be prepared daily (*see* **Note 5**).

3. OFFGEL peptide recovery) solution: In a clean 10 mL tube, combine 5 mL methanol, 4.9 mL MilliQ water and 100 μL of formic acid. Vortex to mix and store on ice during use. Shelf life: solution must be prepared daily (*see* **Note 6**).

3 Methods

Perform all procedures at room temperature unless otherwise indicated. The following workflow is applicable to a wide range of protein-containing matrices (including pregnancy-associated biological fluids and tissues).

3.1 Reduction

1. Add an equal volume of RIPA buffer to the EV sample and sonicate for 30 min at 30 °C. Final sample + RIPA volume should be approximately 100 μL (*see* **Notes 2** and 7).
2. Combine 100 μL of sample with 100 μL of 50 mM NH_4HCO_3 (Solution 2).
3. Add 10 μL of solution 4 (20 mM DTT in 100 mM NH_4HCO_3) to the sample (*see* **Note 8**).
4. Pipette up and down to mix well.
5. Incubate at 60 °C for 1 h.

3.2 Alkylation

1. Add 10 μL of solution 5 (100 mM IAA in 100 mM NH_4HCO_3) to each sample (*see* **Note 9**).
2. Incubate in the dark at 37 °C for 1 h.

3.3 Tryptic Digestion

1. Add 2 μL of solution) 9 (trypsin 0.5 μg/μL) to each sample. Vortex briefly to mix.
2. Cover samples with Parafilm to prevent evaporation and incubate at 37 °C overnight (*see* **Note 10**).

3.4 Desalting of Protein Digestates

1. Following incubation, add 100 μL 0.1% (v/v) formic acid in H_2O to each sample in preparation for LC-MS/MS.
2. Punch out 1–2 pieces of Empore C18 membrane using a cut down 200 μL pipette tip (*see* **Note 11**; Fig. 1).
3. Transfer the membrane to a GELoader tip using a needle or another GELoader tip. Ensure the membrane is compressed down with no spaces (Fig. 2).
4. Vortex the Poros R3 slurry to resuspend the particles. Pipette 5 μL of the slurry on top of the membrane piece (*see* **Note 12**).

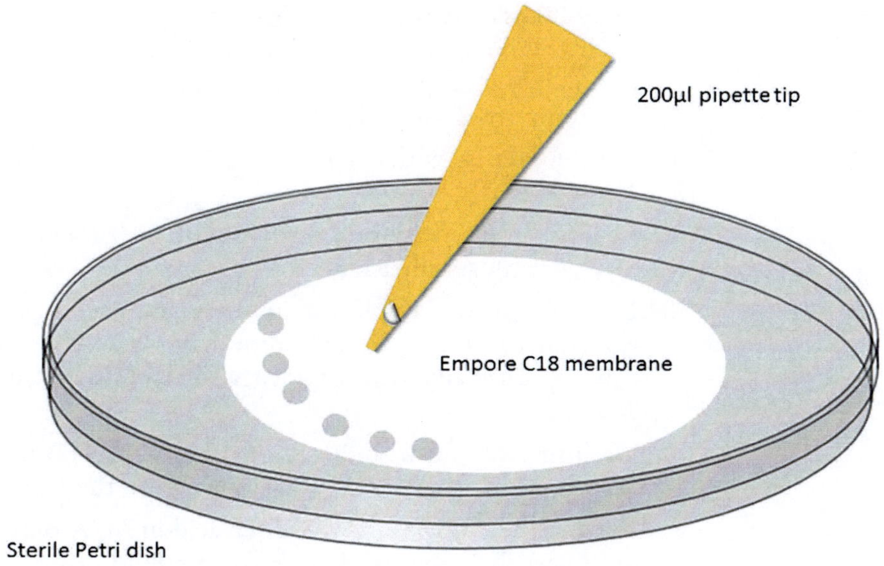

Fig. 1 Punch out the Empore) C18 membrane using a cut down 200 μL pipette tip in a sterile Petri dish or surface

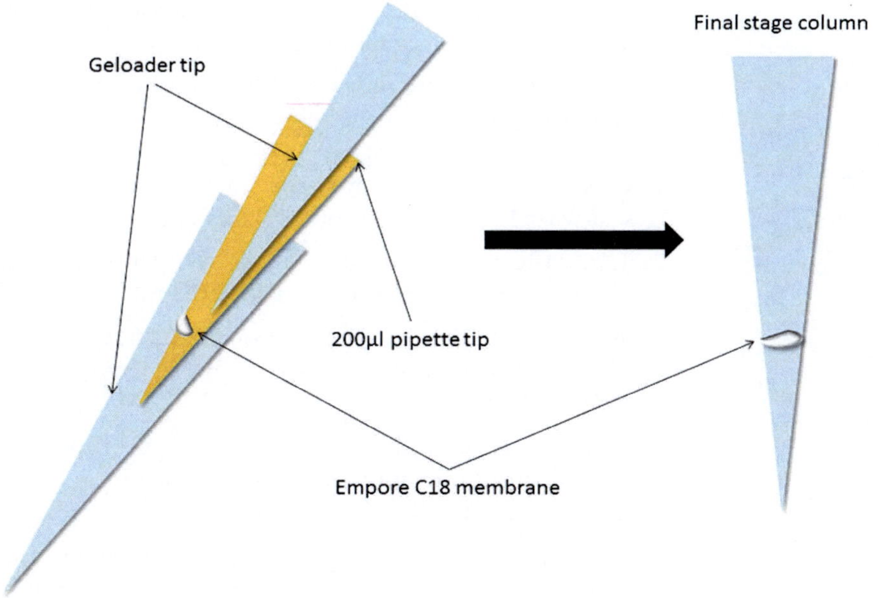

Fig. 2 Transfer the membrane to a GELoader tip using a needle or another GELoader tip. Ensure the membrane is compressed down into the final stage column with no spaces

5. Load 20 μL of 0.1% (v/v) formic acid in ACN on top of the microcolumn and shake by hand to move the fluid down on to the membrane. Press the fluid through the column with the Combitip (*see* **Note 13**).
6. Repeat **Step 4** with 20 μL of 0.1% (v/v) TFA in H_2O (*see* **Note 14**).
7. Acidify samples with an equal volume of 0.1% (v/v) TFA in H_2O. Vortex briefly to mix.
8. Load 40 μL of sample on to the column and press slowly through the Empore membrane using a Combitip. Repeat this step until all of the samples has been pushed through (*see* **Note 15**).
9. Wash the column with 20 μL of 0.1% (v/v) TFA in H_2O and leave approximately 1 μL of the solvent on the membrane.
10. Load 15 μL of 0.1% (v/v) formic acid in ACN on to the column and shake by hand to move the fluid down. Using the Combitip, elute the peptides slowly into a LoBind) tube.
11. Repeat **Step 9** with an additional 15 μL of 0.1% (v/v) formic acid in ACN. Final volume of purified peptides should be approximately 30 μL.
12. Dry the samples in a vacuum centrifuge at 45 °C for 1–2 h (or until all fluid has evaporated).
13. Store the dried peptides at −20 °C until ready for OFFGEL fractionation.

3.5 OFFGEL Fractionation

3.5.1 Day 1

1. Clean the OFFGEL tray, translucent well frames, and cover seal with 100% isopropanol, 70% ethanol, and MilliQ water.
2. Clean the electrodes with 100% isopropanol and MilliQ water. Do not clean the electrodes with ethanol.
3. Reconstitute the dried peptides with 1.16 mL of MilliQ water. Vortex thoroughly and pulse spin at maximum speed for 1 min. Transfer the contents to a clean 10 mL tube.
4. Add 1 mL of MilliQ water to the same tube. Vortex thoroughly and pulse spin at maximum speed for 1 min. Transfer the contents to the 10 mL tube.
5. Add 1.44 mL of the OFFGEL stock solution 1.25× to the same tube. Vortex well and pulse spin at maximum speed for 1 min. Transfer the contents to the clean 10 mL tube. The final volume should be approximately 3.6 mL. Store the peptide solution on ice.
6. Store the OFFGEL) apparatus as per the manufacturer's instructions.
7. Remove the plastic backing from a new OFFGEL dry strip and place in a lane on the tray. Ensure that the "+" sign is

positioned to the left of the tray, and the serial number is upside down and unreadable (*see* **Note 16**).

8. Place the translucent well frame on top of the gel strip and clip down tightly.
9. Add 40 μL of the rehydration buffer to each of the 24 wells from alternating ends of the lane (*see* **Note 17**).
10. Using sterile tweezers, dip four electrode pads into the strip rehydration buffer and place on top of the exposed gel strip ends. Ensure there are two pads stacked on top of each other at each end of the gel strip.
11. Place a cover seal over the well frame and allow 15 min for the gel to swell.
12. Add 150 μL of the reconstituted peptide solution to each well from alternating ends of the well. If there is an insufficient volume of peptide solution to fill all the wells, redistribute the solution from neighboring wells and finish to 150 μL with the rehydration buffer.
13. Place the cover seal over the well frame to prevent contamination.
14. Rehydrate the electrode pads with 10 μL of the rehydration buffer.
15. Place the white tray on to the OFFGEL fractionation machine and pipette 200 μL mineral oil on to the left side and 400 μL on the right side. Ensure oil is pipetted directly onto the electrode pads. Wait 3 min before adding 200 μL mineral to each side. Wait 3 min and add 200 μL to the left hand side. Thus, each end of the lane (containing the electrode pads) should have 600 μL of mineral oil (*see* **Note 18**).
16. Fix the left electrode by placing the two hooks on the white tray and swing down to clip) the electrode into place. Ensure the electrodes are in contact with the electrode pad.
17. Fix the right electrode to the white tray. Ensure this electrode is in direct contact with the OFFGEL apparatus (touching the gray metal plate) before clipping into place.
18. Switch the machine on and close the OFFGEL lid.
19. Select the appropriate focusing method. For 24-well peptide fractionations, we use the OG24PE01 focusing method.
20. Ensure the following starting values are set on the machine: Method: OG24PE01; Volt Hour [kVh]: 50kVh; Voltage [V]: 4500 V; Current [μA]: 50 μA; Power [mW]: 200 mW; Time [h:min]: 100:00.
21. Start the fractionation and allow machine to run for 50kVh (approximately 20–24 h). (*see* **Note 19**; Fig. 3).

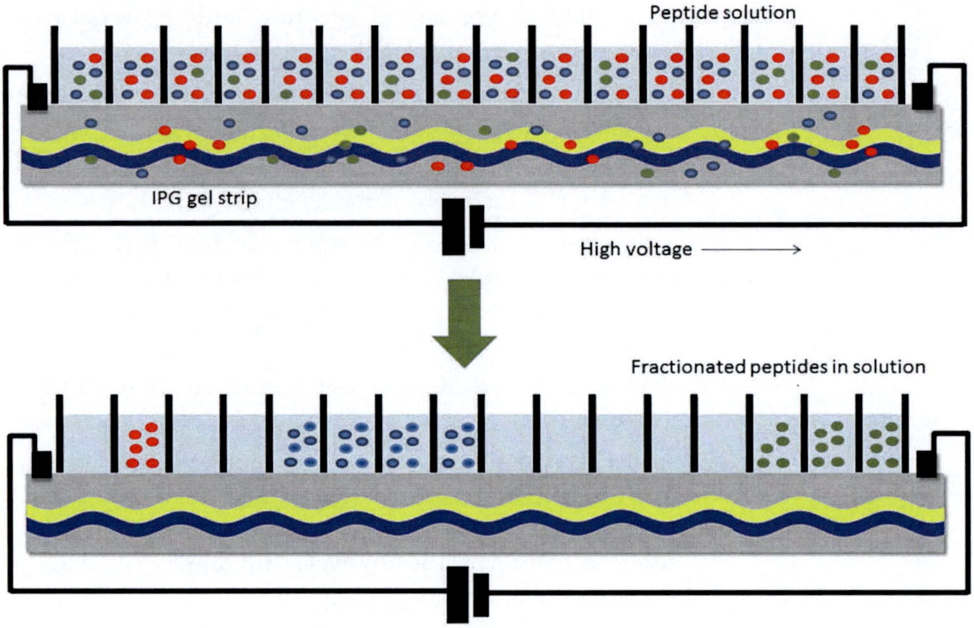

Fig. 3 Following the addition) of equal volumes of the peptide sample into all wells in the frame, a high voltage is applied to the ends of the gel strip. This causes the peptide molecules to migrate through the gel strip until they are positioned where the pH equals the isoelectric point (pI) of the molecule. The electric field also extends into the liquid phase, where the peptides are suspended. This ensures the molecules remain suspended in solution at their respective pI even after the fractionation run is complete. Do not turn off the fractionator until you are ready to collect the peptide fractions

3.5.2 Day 2

1. The run is finished when the electrodes are flashing. Do not turn off the machine until you are ready to collect the peptide fractions (*see* **Note 20**).
2. Prepare 24 sterile LoBind tubes and label 1–24. Keep the lids closed to minimize the risk of contamination by other proteins (*see* **Note 21**).
3. Turn the machine off, open the lid, and remove the white tray.
4. Carefully remove the cover seal from the 24-well translucent frame (*see* **Note 22**).
5. Using a new pipette) tip each time, collect the peptide fraction from each well and transfer to the appropriately labeled LoBind tube (*see* **Notes 23** and **24**).
6. Using a new pipette tip every 6–8 wells, transfer 150 μL of the OFFGEL peptide recovery solution into each well and let sit for 15 min. Using a new pipette tip each time, collect the recovery solution from each well and transfer to the respective LoBind tube.
7. Repeat the previous step twice. Finally, the peptides should be resuspended in ~450 μL of the peptide recovery solution.

8. Using a vacuum centrifuge, dry the samples down at 45 for approximately 4–5 h or until all liquid has evaporated from the tubes.
9. Store dried peptides at −20 °C until further processing (*see* **Note 25**).

3.5.3 Preparing Peptides for LC-MS/MS Analysis

1. To prepare samples for spectral acquisition, reconstitute the dried peptides in 40 μL of 0.1% (v/v) formic acid in H_2O.
2. Vortex samples for 1 min each to mix thoroughly.
3. Pulse spin at maximum speed for 1–3 min at 4 °C.
4. Transfer the reconstituted peptides to glass vials and store at 4 °C for analysis.

4 Notes

1. Careful sample handling, at both the protein and peptide level, is essential for successful MS analysis. Wear gloves at all times to ensure samples are not contaminated by other proteins (e.g., keratins).
2. When working with EVs, ensure samples have been treated with RIPA buffer to lyse all vesicles. Lysis of EVs ensures that a greater number of peptides are extracted and identified.
3. Iodoacetic acid (IAA) is light sensitive and unstable. To preserve its activity, solutions containing IAA must be prepared immediately before use. Ideally, the alkylation step should be performed in a low-light or dark environment.
4. Excess trypsin working solution can be frozen (in 20 μL aliquots) for later use. Thawed portions (i.e., after one freeze-thaw cycle) should be discarded after use).
5. Depending on how many samples are being fractionated, volumes may have to be doubled.
6. The OFFGEL peptide recovery solution is required on Day 2 of the procedure. Ensure the solution is made before use, ideally under a safety cabinet or fume hood. Wear gloves at all times to prevent contamination by other proteins (e.g., keratins).
7. Lysis of nanovesicles ensures that a greater number of peptides are extracted and identified.
8. Dithiothreitol (DTT) is a reducing agent, which reduces the disulfide bonds of proteins and prevents the formation of new disulfide bonds between cysteine residues of proteins. DTT does this by converting the disulfide bonds into free sulfhydryl groups [28].

9. Iodoacetamide (IAA) is an alkylating agent. IAA reacts with the free sulfhydryl groups of cysteine residues to form S-carboxyamidomethyl-cysteine, which cannot be oxidized again to form disulfide bonds. Thus, IAA prevents protein refolding after DTT treatment and maximizes trypsin's access to cleavage sites within the protein.

10. Following incubation with trypsin, if samples are not undergoing the desalting process immediately, use a vacuum centrifuge to dry samples completely and store at −20 °C until further processing. Once desalting has begun, it cannot be paused until the sample has been completely processed and dried down for OFFGEL fractionation. Desalting can be a lengthy process (particularly when working with a large number of samples), so it is best to dry samples after tryptic digestion and resume desalting samples in batches at your convenience.

11. It is best to punch out the Empore membrane on a sterile surface, in order to prevent contamination with other proteins or detergents. A sterile Petri dish (cleaned with acetonitrile and MilliQ water) can be used to prepare and store the membrane. It is also best to avoid sharing the membrane (and all other LC-MS/MS reagents) with multiple users to avoid contamination.

12. The slurry will not always settle on top of the membrane and may settle on the sides of the GELoader tip. This is not a problem as it will be washed down) on to the membrane when other reagents are added in the following steps.

13. Ensure 1–2 μL of solvent remains above the Empore membrane. Do not allow the column to run dry.

14. This step ensures the removal of ACN traces and equilibrates the Empore membrane. Ensure that 1–2 μL of solvent remains in the column so that the membrane is well conditioned and does not run dry.

15. Adjust the volume of sample added according to the size of the Combitip and GELoader tips used. Ensure that the Combitip is not touching the sample. Press the Combitip with gentle and steady pressure to ensure unidirectional flow of the sample. In this step, peptides will bind to the Poros R3 and the C18 material embedded in the Empore membrane. The flow through can be discarded.

16. If you are not using all lanes, start with loading samples from the middle lanes of the tray outward.

17. Ensure the pipette tip does not touch the gel strip and avoid bubble formation. To minimize the risk of contamination, change pipette tips every 6–8 wells.

18. Ensure that the waiting times are strictly observed. Premature addition of mineral oil can result in the end wells overflowing. This could cause oil leakage contamination of peptide samples.
19. If the run time is greater than 24 h, ensure the electrode pads are replaced every 24 h. Remove the old pads. Dip the new pads in rehydration buffer or deionized water before placing them in the tray grooves. If run stops, replace the electrode pads and replenish the mineral oil (cover fluid) to a level no higher than ½ to ¾ height of the tray groove. Run the samples again for 18–20 h.
20. Do not turn the machine off until you are ready to collect the peptide fractions as this will cause peptides to migrate back to their starting positions. This is because the electric field running through the gel also extends into the liquid phase, where the peptides are suspended, thereby ensuring the peptide molecules remain suspended in solution at their respective pI even after the fractionation run is complete.
21. Wear gloves at all times.
22. Take care when removing the cover seal. Do not lift the well frames and avoid contaminating the fractions with mineral oil.
23. Avoid aspirating the gel when collecting fractions. When collecting fractions, we have) found that leaning the pipette tip against the well frame prevents gel aspiration. Additionally, do not lean over the peptide fraction – sit at a reasonable distance away from the apparatus in order to prevent contamination by other proteins (i.e., keratins).
24. During peptide fractionation, it is normal for some wells to have reduced liquid levels or no liquid in them at all. If there is no liquid visible in a well, simply move on to the peptide recovery step (**Step 5** of Subheading 3.5.2).
25. If possible, try to minimize the storage period for dried peptides.

Acknowledgments

CS was in receipt of a Lions Medical Research Foundation Fellowship. This study was supported by The Lions Medical Research Foundation, UQ ECR award, Royal Brisbane and Women's Foundation, Diabetes Australia, and UQ-Ochsner Seed Grant. The ISO17025 accredited research facility was supported by grants from Therapeutics Innovation Australia and the National Collaborative Research Infrastructure Strategy.

This review is supported partly by funding from the Lions Medical Research Foundation (LMRF), The University) of Queensland and Fondo Nacional de Desarrollo Científico y Tecnológico (FONDECYT 1170809), Chile.

References

1. Shu C, Liu Z, Cui L, Wei C, Wang S, Tang JJ, Cui M, Lian G, Li W, Liu X, Xu H, Jiang J, Lee P, Zhang DY, He J, Ye F (2014) Protein profiling of preeclampsia placental tissues. PLoS One 9(11):e112890. https://doi.org/10.1371/journal.pone.0112890
2. Ghulmiyyah L, Sibai B (2012) Maternal mortality from preeclampsia/eclampsia. Semin Perinatol 36(1):56–59. https://doi.org/10.1053/j.semperi.2011.09.011
3. Mikat B, Gellhaus A, Wagner N, Birdir C, Kimmig R, Koninger A (2012) Early detection of maternal risk for preeclampsia. ISRN Obstet Gynecol 2012:172808. https://doi.org/10.5402/2012/172808
4. Tranquilli AL, Dekker G, Magee L, Roberts J, Sibai BM, Steyn W, Zeeman GG, Brown MA (2014) The classification, diagnosis and management of the hypertensive disorders of pregnancy: a revised statement from the ISSHP. Pregnancy Hypertens 4(2):97–104. https://doi.org/10.1016/j.preghy.2014.02.001
5. Raimondo F, Morosi L, Chinello C, Magni F, Pitto M (2011) Advances in membranous vesicle and exosome proteomics improving biological understanding and biomarker discovery. Proteomics 11(4):709–720. https://doi.org/10.1002/pmic.201000422
6. Diehl HC, Stuhler K, Klein-Scory S, Volmer MW, Schoneck A, Bieling C, Schmiegel W, Meyer HE, Schwarte-Waldhoff I (2007) A catalogue of proteins released by colorectal cancer cells in vitro as an alternative source for biomarker discovery. Proteomics Clin Appl 1(1):47–61. https://doi.org/10.1002/prca.200600491
7. Kreimer S, Belov AM, Ghiran I, Murthy SK, Frank DA, Ivanov AR (2015) Mass-spectrometry-based molecular characterization of extracellular vesicles: lipidomics and proteomics. J Proteome Res 14(6):2367–2384. https://doi.org/10.1021/pr501279t
8. Tannetta D, Dragovic R, Alyahyaei Z, Southcombe J (2014) Extracellular vesicles and reproduction-promotion of successful pregnancy. Cell Mol Immunol 11(6):548–563. https://doi.org/10.1038/cmi.2014.42
9. Gyorgy B, Szabo TG, Pasztoi M, Pal Z, Misjak P, Aradi B, Laszlo V, Pallinger E, Pap E, Kittel A, Nagy G, Falus A, Buzas EI (2011) Membrane vesicles, current state-of-the-art: emerging role of extracellular vesicles. Cell Mol Life Sci 68(16):2667–2688. https://doi.org/10.1007/s00018-011-0689-3
10. Law KP, Han TL, Tong C, Baker PN (2015) Mass spectrometry-based proteomics for preeclampsia and preterm birth. Int J Mol Sci 16(5):10952–10985. https://doi.org/10.3390/ijms160510952
11. Anagnostopoulos AK, Tsangaris GT (2013) Proteomics advancements in fetomaternal medicine. Clin Biochem 46(6):487–496. https://doi.org/10.1016/j.clinbiochem.2012.10.011
12. Rappsilber J, Ishihama Y, Mann M (2003) Stop and go extraction tips for matrix-assisted laser desorption/ionization, nanoelectrospray, and LC/MS sample pretreatment in proteomics. Anal Chem 75((3)):663
13. Kussmann M, Nordhoff E, Rahbek-nielsen H, Haebel S, Rossel-larsen M, Jakobsen L, Gobom J, Mirgorodskaya E, Kroll-kristensen A, Palm|| L, Roepstorff P (1997) Matrix-assisted laser desorption/ionization mass spectrometry sample preparation techniques designed for various peptide and protein analytes. J Mass Spectrom 32(6):593–601. https://doi.org/10.1002/(SICI)1096-9888(199706)32:6<593::AID-JMS511>3.0.CO2-D
14. Lobb RJ, Becker M, Wen SW, Wong CS, Wiegmans AP, Leimgruber A, Moller A (2015) Optimized exosome isolation protocol for cell culture supernatant and human plasma. J Extracell Vesicles 4:27031. https://doi.org/10.3402/jev.v4.27031
15. Schageman J, Zeringer E, Li M, Barta T, Lea K, Gu J, Magdaleno S, Setterquist R, Vlassov AV (2013) The complete exosome workflow solution: from isolation to characterization of RNA cargo. Biomed Res Int 2013:253957. https://doi.org/10.1155/2013/253957
16. Rideau A, Besson D, Boissard A, Coqueret O, Guette C (2013) Two-step OFFGEL approach for effective peptide separation compatible with iTRAQ labeling. Proteomics

13(22):3261–3266. https://doi.org/10.1002/pmic.201300161

17. Lam HT, Josserand J, Lion N, Girault HH (2007) Modeling the isoelectric focusing of peptides in an OFFGEL multicompartment cell. J Proteome Res 6(5):1666–1676. https://doi.org/10.1021/pr0606023
18. Hubner NC, Ren S, Mann M (2008) Peptide separation with immobilized pI strips is an attractive alternative to in-gel protein digestion for proteome analysis. Proteomics 8(23-24):4862–4872. https://doi.org/10.1002/pmic.200800351
19. Shapiro AL, Vinuela E, Maizel JV Jr (1967) Molecular weight estimation of polypeptide chains by electrophoresis in SDS-polyacrylamide gels. Biochem Biophys Res Commun 28(5):815–820
20. Choudhary G, Horvath C (1996) Ion-exchange chromatography. Methods Enzymol 270:47–82
21. Peng J, Elias JE, Thoreen CC, Licklider LJ, Gygi SP (2003) Evaluation of multidimensional chromatography coupled with tandem mass spectrometry (LC/LC-MS/MS) for large-scale protein analysis: the yeast proteome. J Proteome Res 2(1):43–50
22. Jafari M, Primo V, Smejkal GB, Moskovets EV, Kuo WP, Ivanov AR (2012) Comparison of in-gel protein separation techniques commonly used for fractionation in mass spectrometry-based proteomic profiling. Electrophoresis 33(16):2516–2526. https://doi.org/10.1002/elps.201200031
23. Chen J, Lee CS, Shen Y, Smith RD, Baehrecke EH (2002) Integration of capillary isoelectric focusing with capillary reversed-phase liquid chromatography for two-dimensional proteomics separation. Electrophoresis 23(18):3143–3148. https://doi.org/10.1002/1522-2683(200209)23:18<3143::aid-elps3143>3.0.co;2-7
24. Michel PE, Reymond F, Arnaud IL, Josserand J, Girault HH, Rossier JS (2003) Protein fractionation in a multicompartment device using off-gel isoelectric focusing. Electrophoresis 24(12):3–11. https://doi.org/10.1002/elps.200390030
25. Chenau J, Michelland S, Sidibe J, Seve M (2008) Peptides OFFGEL electrophoresis: a suitable pre-analytical step for complex eukaryotic samples fractionation compatible with quantitative iTRAQ labeling. Proteome Sci 6:9. https://doi.org/10.1186/1477-5956-6-9
26. Mostovenko E, Hassan C, Rattke J, Deelder AM, van Veelen PA, Palmblad M (2013) Comparison of peptide and protein fractionation methods in proteomics. EuPA Open. Proteomics 1:30–37. http://dx.doi.org/10.1016/j.euprot.2013.09.001
27. Horth P, Miller CA, Preckel T, Wenz C (2006) Efficient fractionation and improved protein identification by peptide OFFGEL electrophoresis. Mol Cell Proteomics 5(10):1968–1974. https://doi.org/10.1074/mcp.T600037-MCP200
28. Gundry RL, White MY, Murray CI, Kane LA, Fu Q, Stanley BA, Van Eyk JE (2009) Preparation of proteins and peptides for mass spectrometry analysis in a bottom-up proteomics workflow. Curr Protoc Mol Biol Chapter 10:Unit10.25. https://doi.org/10.1002/0471142727.mb1025s88

Chapter 12

Harvesting and Characterization of Syncytial Nuclear Aggregates Following Culture of First Trimester Human Placental Explants

Priyadarshini Pantham and Lawrence W. Chamley

Abstract

There is currently no effective method to study multinucleated trophoblast debris extruded from the syncytiotrophoblast into the maternal circulation. In Chapter 9, an in vitro placental explant culture model to generate trophoblast debris was described. Here, we detail the method utilized to isolate individual large multinucleated syncytial nuclear aggregates (SNAs) that are extruded from the syncytiotrophoblast following the culture of first trimester human placental explants. Syncytial nuclear aggregates have been observed in the peripheral maternal circulation as early as 6 weeks' gestation and may play a role in tolerating the maternal immune system during pregnancy. Conversely, aberrant cell death processes in the syncytiotrophoblast due to various maternal factors leading to the extrusion of SNAs that are altered in nature have been implicated in the development of preeclampsia. The methods described herein allow for the isolation and harvest of SNAs without other types of extruded trophoblast debris and can be used to investigate the effect of various maternal factors on the nature of SNAs extruded from the placenta in vitro.

Key words Syncytial nuclear aggregates, Trophoblastic debris, Explant culture, Placenta

1 Introduction

Transport of the trophoblast debris from the placenta is known as "trophoblast deportation." This phenomenon was first described and associated with preeclamptic pregnancies nearly 120 years ago by the German pathologist Georg Schmorl. He observed large multinucleated trophoblastic fragments trapped in the pulmonary vessels of 14 out of 17 women who had died of eclampsia. These fragments were not observed in the pulmonary circulation of normal pregnant women that had died of other causes, leading Schmorl to propose that this finding was related to the development of preeclampsia [1]. It is now accepted that the phenomenon of extrusion of trophoblast debris is a feature of normal pregnancies and that the amount of debris is increased in preeclampsia [2–4].

Padma Murthi and Cathy Vaillancourt (eds.), *Preeclampsia: Methods and Protocols*, Methods in Molecular Biology, vol. 1710,
https://doi.org/10.1007/978-1-4939-7498-6_12, © Springer Science+Business Media LLC 2018

Throughout pregnancy, a variety of trophoblast debris, ranging in size from nanometers to tens of micrometers, and encompassing, in order of increasing size, syncytiotrophoblast microvillous membrane microparticles (STBMs, >100 nm), mononuclear cytotrophoblasts (25 μm), and multinucleated syncytial nuclear aggregates (SNAs) (25–200 μm) are continuously extruded from the placental syncytiotrophoblast into the maternal blood [1, 5, 6]. There are differences in the literature in the nomenclature of the structures referred to here as "syncytial nuclear aggregates." These structures are variously termed syncytial knots and syncytial sprouts, among other names [7, 8]. This confusion may arise from the methods of study employed by different researchers [9]. Syncytial knots and syncytial sprouts may represent different populations of multinucleated structures with different functionalities that bud off from the syncytiotrophoblast; however both these structures are defined as histological features of placentae, and the phrases do not refer to the structures that have been extruded from the placenta [7]. For the sake of simplicity, multinucleated syncytial aggregates that have been extruded from the placenta will be referred to as "syncytial nuclear aggregates" (SNAs) herein.

Trophoblast deportation is a difficult phenomenon to study, since thus far there is no effective method to harvest trophoblast debris from the maternal blood in substantial numbers [3]. An in vitro model of trophoblast death and extrusion of trophoblast debris has been established to study the nature of extruded mononuclear and multinucleated trophoblast debris and the mechanisms of their clearance in normal and pathological conditions [10]. Placental explants are cultured in Netwell® inserts with 400 μm mesh bottoms, which allows trophoblast debris of a range of sizes to pass into the bottom of the culture well. This method allows for the examination of placental explants, SNAs and other trophoblast debris extruded from the placenta, as well as placental culture media under different culture conditions [10]. This model has been utilized to investigate the effect of various factors implicated in the development of preeclampsia on the extrusion of trophoblast debris from the syncytiotrophoblast [11–14].

2 Materials

All solutions must be prepared using ultrapure water and analytical grade reagents.

2.1 Harvesting of Syncytial Nuclear Aggregates Following Culture of Human Placental Explants

1. Phosphate-buffered saline (PBS): 120 mM NaCl, 2.7 mM KCl, 1.5 mM Na_2HPO_4, and 8 mM KH_2PO_4 (pH 7.4). Dissolve 8.09 g NaCl, 0.2 g KCl, 0.2 g KH_2PO_4, and 1.14 g Na_2HPO_4 in 900 mL of ultrapure water and adjust pH to 7.4 using HCl. Make up the total volume to 1 L and sterilize by autoclaving. Add 1 tablet of complete EDTA-free protease

inhibitor cocktail (Sigma-Aldrich, catalog no: 11873580001) per 50 mL of PBS for use to harvest and store SNAs. Store at room temperature.

2. Sterile culture dishes (60 and 35 mm).
3. Sterile forceps.
4. Dual-stage glass micropipette puller.
5. Glass capillaries (1 mm outer diameter × 0.58 mm inner diameter) pulled to a fine point using a glass puller and sterilized by autoclaving.
6. Micromanipulator system with pneumatic injector and injection holder.
7. Inverted microscope with movable stage that can accommodate 60 and 35 mm diameter culture plates.
8. Manual cell counter.

2.2 Extraction of Proteins and Bicinchoninic Assay to Quantify Protein Yield from Syncytial Nuclear Aggregates Using RIPA Buffer

1. Radioimmunoprecipitation (RIPA) assay buffer: 50 mM Tris, pH 4, 150 nM NaCl, 1% Nonidet P40, 1% sodium deoxycholate, 0.1% sodium dodecyl sulfate (SDS), 5× cOmplete EDTA-free protease inhibitor cocktail, and 1 mM phenylmethanesulfonylfluoride.
2. Ultrasonic bath.
3. BCA protein assay kit.
4. Incubator set at 37 °C.
5. Microplate spectrophotometer.

2.3 Immunostaining of Syncytial Nuclear Aggregates

1. Pre-cleaned microscope slides.
2. Poly-L-lysine.
3. Dako pen.
4. Microscope coverslips.
5. Aquatex.
6. Normal goat serum.
7. Lithium carbonate (store at room temperature).
8. 3-Amino-9-ethylcarbazole (AEC+) substrate-chromogen (store at 4 °C).
9. Hematoxylin (Gills No. 2) (store at room temperature).
10. Phosphate-buffered saline (PBS).
11. Humidity chamber.
12. Primary antibody.
13. Biotin-conjugated secondary antibody.
14. Streptavidin-conjugated horseradish peroxidase.
15. Microscope.

3 Methods

3.1 Harvesting of Syncytial Nuclear Aggregates Following Culture of Human Placental Explants

1. Culture placental explants dissected from first trimester human placenta in 6-well plates following the protocol described in Chapter 9.
2. If the effects of various reagents on SNAs are being investigated (e.g., immune factors such as antibodies or interleukins), they should be added along with appropriate controls and untreated controls at the time point of interest.
3. Culture of one untreated placental explant of approximately 400 mg and 2 cm^3 generates an average of ~20 SNAs.
4. Following culture in the appropriate conditions described in the Chapter 9, remove each Netwell® insert containing a placental explant using forceps, taking care to decant as much of the culture medium from around the placental explant as possible back into the well.
5. Pipette to mix the culture medium in each well in order to agitate the trophoblast debris that may have settled at the bottom of the culture well.
6. Aspirate the culture medium containing trophoblast debris from two culture wells at a time (3 mL from each well), giving a total volume of 6 mL into a sterile culture dish (dish 1, 60 mm).
7. Turn on the microscope and the micromanipulator system connected to the pneumatic injector system (*see* **Notes 1–3**).
8. Attach a glass capillary that has been pulled to create a pointed end to the injection holder (*see* **Note 4**).
9. Flush the glass capillary with up to 50 μL of sterile PBS at least five times each by aspirating and ejecting the PBS (*see* **Note 5**).
10. Affix the culture dish (dish 1) containing the cell culture medium with the trophoblast debris securely to the moveable stage of the inverted microscope.
11. Adjust the focus of the inverted microscope so that the large trophoblast debris settled at the bottom of the culture dish is clearly visible.
12. Using the rotating adjustable clamp attached to the injection holder, lower the pointed end of the glass capillary into the center of the culture dish.
13. Aspirate SNAs up to the inner third of the glass capillary.
14. Eject SNAs into a separate sterile culture dish (dish 2, 35 mm) containing 1 mL of sterile PBS with complete EDTA-free protease inhibitor cocktail stored on ice.
15. Collect SNAs starting from the center of the culture dish moving outward until the whole area of the culture dish is covered.

16. Once SNAs are transferred from the culture dish containing culture medium (dish 1) to a separate sterile culture dish containing sterile PBS with complete EDTA-free protease inhibitor cocktail (dish 2) stored on ice, collect the SNAs once again following **steps 11–15** into a new sterile culture dish (dish 3, 35 mm) containing 1 mL of sterile PBS with complete EDTA-free protease inhibitor cocktail.
17. Count the SNAs in culture dish 3 manually using a cell counter.
18. Transfer the SNAs in 1 mL of sterile PBS with complete EDTA-free protease inhibitor cocktail tablets into a microcentrifuge tube (*see* **Note 6**).

3.2 Extraction of Proteins and Bicinchoninic Assay to Quantify Protein Yield from Syncytial Nuclear Aggregates Using RIPA Buffer

1. Centrifuge microcentrifuge tubes containing a minimum of ~100 SNAs in a minicentrifuge at 17,000 × *g* for 15 min at 4 °C, and discard supernatant (*see* **Note 7**).
2. Add 100 μL of RIPA buffer to the microcentrifuge tubes containing SNAs, and pipette vigorously on ice for 5 min.
3. Sonicate samples using an ultrasonic bath for 1 min at 250 V, 50 Hz.
4. Centrifuge samples at 17,000 × *g* at 4 °C for 10 min, remove lysate, and store at −80 °C.
5. Use the bichinchoninic assay (BCA) to estimate the protein quantity of pooled, lysed SNAs, using the BCA protein assay kit (*see* **Note 8**). The basis of this assay is that BCA forms a purple complex with cuprous ions in an alkaline medium, known as the biuret reaction [15]. This complex is stable and exhibits a strong absorbance at 562 nm, and the color increases in a linear manner with increasing protein concentrations.
6. Prepare the bovine serum albumin standards from 2 mg/mL stock by diluting the standard provided in the kit in a fivefold dilution series of 25–2000 μg/mL using the diluent RIPA buffer.
7. Dilute the lysate from SNAs 2.5-fold to provide an end volume of 50 μL. Add 25 μL of samples and standards to a 96-well plate. Add 2% w/v cupric acid solution to BCA solution in a 1:50 ratio, and add 25 μL of this mixture to each well.
8. Incubate the well in the dark at 37 °C for 30 min, and read the absorbance at 562 nm using a spectrophotometer.
9. Construct a standard curve and calculate the protein concentration of the lysate from SNAs.

3.3 Immunostaining of Syncytial Nuclear Aggregates

1. Collect SNAs using the micromanipulator connected to the inverted microscope system as described in Subheading 3.1.
2. Immediately after collection, using a pipette tip, smear 100 μL of PBS containing SNAs onto poly-L-lysine-coated slides.

3. Allow slides to air-dry overnight (*see* **Note 9**).
4. Using a Dako pen, draw a ring around the cell smear (*see* **Note 10**).
5. Wash slides with distilled water once, once Dako ring is dry.
6. Block slides using 10% normal goat serum in PBS and incubate for 1 h at room temperature in a humidity chamber.
7. Tip off block solution, and add 100 μL of primary antibody or irrelevant control antibody to each slide and incubate for 1 h at room temperature.
8. Wash slides three times using PBS.
9. Incubate smears with 100 μL of biotin-conjugated secondary antibody for 1 h at room temperature.
10. Wash slides three times using PBS.
11. Incubate smears with 100 μL of streptavidin-conjugated horseradish peroxidase for 1 h at room temperature.
12. Wash slides three times using PBS.
13. Add 100 μL of the substrate AEC (3-amino-9-ethylcarbazole) to smears and incubate for 3–20 min depending upon the color development.
14. Counterstain slides using Gills II hematoxylin for 30–60 s and dip in a 1% lithium carbonate solution.
15. Wash slides with distilled water and mount coverslips using Aquatex.
16. Allow slides to dry overnight. SNAs can be visualized using a microscope at magnifications of 10× and 20× (Fig. 1, *see* **Note 11**).

4 Notes

1. A Nikon/Narishige NT V-88-V3 Micromanipulator system connected to a Nikon Eclipse Ti inverted microscope was utilized to isolate individual SNAs that were extruded from placental explants and had passed through the mesh of the Netwell® into the lower chamber of the culture wells following culture.
2. The micromanipulator system consisted of a pneumatic microinjector (IM-9C), which utilizes air pressure to aspirate and eject liquid, connected to an injection holder with a rotating adjustable clamp allowing for range of motion.
3. The IM-9C pneumatic injector consists of a plunger with a depth of 53 mm and allows for full rotation of approximately 6 mm.

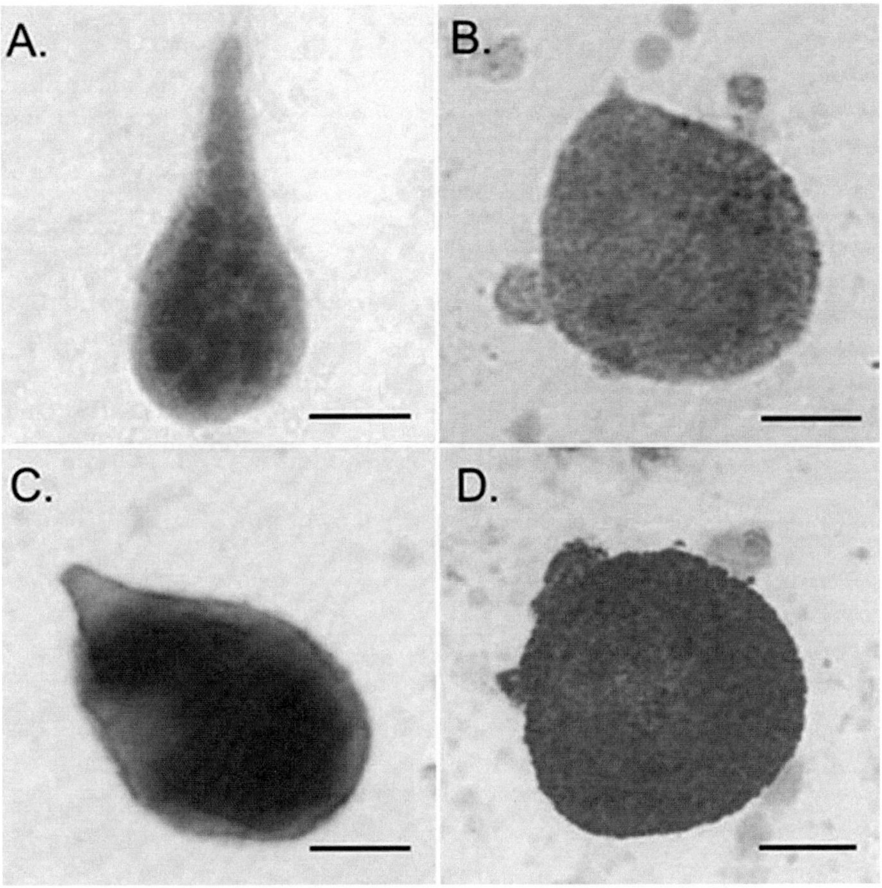

Fig. 1 (**a**) Syncytial nuclear aggregates (SNAs) stained with an irrelevant control rabbit IgG (grade score of 0) and (**b–d**) SNAs stained with calreticulin at different levels—grade score of 1 (**b**), grade score of 2 (**c**), and grade score of 3 (**d**). Scale bars represent 20 μm

4. Glass capillaries were pulled using the single pull setting in order to create a capillary with a fine point that was large enough to allow SNAs to pass through it. If the tip of the capillary is too long, it can be broken off gently prior to autoclaving and sterilization.
5. Care must be taken not to aspirate liquid through the capillary into the injection holder and the tubing, which connects the injection holder to the multi-use valve of the pneumatic injector. If this occurs, flush with 70% ethanol and allow to dry overnight before use again.
6. Syncytial nuclear aggregates collected for proteolysis can be stored at −80 °C until proteolysis, thawed on ice, and pooled prior to proteolysis.

7. After centrifugation of the SNAs prior to proteolysis with RIPA buffer, the pellet in the microcentrifuge tube should be visible under a microscope at 20× magnification in order to have a measureable amount of protein using the lysis method described in this chapter.
8. To minimize the amount of lysate from SNAs used to measure protein concentration, the Micro BCA protein assay kit may be used.
9. Syncytial nuclear aggregates collected for immunostaining must be processed and smeared on slides immediately without freezing.
10. Begin the immunohistochemistry protocol immediately the next day after the SNAs are smeared on the slides and allowed to air-dry overnight.
11. SNAs were visualized using a Nikon E400 microscope at magnifications of 10× and 20×.

Acknowledgment

This study was funded by the Marsden Fund of the Royal Society of New Zealand. P.P. is a recipient of The University of Auckland Health Research Doctoral Scholarship.

References

1. Schmorl G (1893) Pathologisch-anatomische Untersuchungen über Puerperal-Eklampsie. Vogel, Würzburg
2. Chua S, Wilkins T, Sargent I, Redman C (1991) Trophoblast deportation in pre-eclamptic pregnancy. Br J Obstet Gynaecol 98(10):973–979
3. Johansen M, Knight M, Maher EJ, Smith K, Sargent IL (1995) An investigation of methods for enriching trophoblast from maternal blood. Prenat Diagn 15(10):921
4. Attwood HD, Park WW (1961) Embolism to the lungs by trophoblast. J Obstet Gynecol 68:611–617
5. Johansen M, Redman CW, Wilkins T, Sargent IL (1999) Trophoblast deportation in human pregnancy—its relevance for pre-eclampsia. Placenta 20(7):531–539
6. Mincheva-Nilsson L, Nagaeva O, Chen T, Stendahl U, Antsiferova J, Mogren I, Hernestal J, Baranov V (2006) Placenta-derived soluble MHC class I chain-related molecules down-regulate NKG2D receptor on peripheral blood mononuclear cells during human pregnancy: a possible novel immune escape mechanism for fetal survival. J Immunol 176(6):3585–3592
7. Burton G, Jones C (2009) Syncytial knots, sprouts, apoptosis, and trophoblast deportation from the human placenta. Taiwan J Obstet Gynecol 48(1):28
8. Cantle SJ, Kaufmann P, Luckhardt M, Schweikhart G (1987) Interpretation of syncytial sprouts and bridges in the human placenta. Placenta 8(3):221
9. Askelund K, Chamley L (2011) Trophoblast deportation part I: review of the evidence demonstrating trophoblast shedding and deportation during human pregnancy. Placenta 32(10):716–723
10. Abumaree MH, Stone PR, Chamley LW (2006) An in vitro model of human placental trophoblast deportation/shedding. Mol Hum Reprod 12(11):687
11. Chen L, Liu B, Zhao H, Stone P, Chen Q, Chamley L (2010) IL-6, TNFalpha and TGFbeta promote nonapoptotic trophoblast deportation and subsequently causes endothelial cell activation. Placenta 31(1):75

12. Chen Q, Guo F, Jin HY, Lau S, Stone P, Chamley L (2012) Phagocytosis of apoptotic trophoblastic debris protects endothelial cells against activation. Placenta 33(7):548–553. https://doi.org/10.1016/j.placenta.2012.03.007
13. Chen Q, Stone PR, McCowan LM, Chamley LW (2006) Phagocytosis of necrotic but not apoptotic trophoblasts induces endothelial cell activation. Hypertension 47(1):116
14. Chen Q, Viall C, Kang Y, Liu B, Stone P, Chamley L (2009) Anti-phospholipid antibodies increase non-apoptotic trophoblast shedding: a contribution to the pathogenesis of pre-eclampsia in affected women? Placenta 30(9):767–773
15. Smith P, Krohn R, Hermanson G, Mallia A, Gartner F, Provenzano M, Fujimoto E, Goeke N, Olson B, Klenk D (1985) Measurement of protein using bicinchoninic acid. Anal Biochem 150(1):76

Chapter 13

Use of GATA3 and TWIST1 Immunofluorescence Staining to Assess In Vitro Syncytial Fusion Index

Severine A. Degrelle and Thierry Fournier

Abstract

In human placenta, the multinucleated syncytiotrophoblast (ST) allows all the exchanges between the maternal and fetal circulation and is also the site of placental hormonal functions. Absence or disturbances of ST formation are associated with a defect or pathologies of pregnancy such as preeclampsia (PE) and intrauterine growth retardation (IUGR). All along pregnancy, the ST is regenerated by fusion of underlying mononucleated villous cytotrophoblasts (VCT). The protocol described here provides details on how GATA3 or TWIST1 immunostaining and analysis can be used to easily assess the in vitro differentiation of human placental cytotrophoblast.

Key words Immunofluorescence, GATA3, TWIST1, Fusion index, Trophoblast, Syncytiotrophoblast, Human placenta

1 Introduction

The maintenance of healthy fetal development is highly dependent on proper placental growth throughout pregnancy. During the process of placenta formation, mononucleated villous cytotrophoblasts (VCT) either (1) proliferate and differentiate into highly invasive extravillous cytotrophoblasts (EVCT), which can invade the maternal endometrium and remodel the spinal arteries, or (2) fuse and form the continuous, multinucleated syncytiotrophoblast (ST). The ST, which forms the outermost surface of the placenta chorionic villi, is located at the interface between maternal and fetal circulation. This multinucleated layer regulates gas and nutrient exchanges, possesses intensive endocrine functions, and provides immunological support to the fetus. A better understanding of the process of differentiation and fusion of VCT to form the ST is essential because disturbance of this regulation is thought to be associated with pregnancy disorders such as preeclampsia (PE) and intrauterine growth retardation (IUGR) [1–3].

Padma Murthi and Cathy Vaillancourt (eds.), *Preeclampsia: Methods and Protocols*, Methods in Molecular Biology, vol. 1710, https://doi.org/10.1007/978-1-4939-7498-6_13,

GATA3 is a well-known regulator of trophoblast-specific gene expression [4], expressed in placental tissues (EVCT and VCT [5, 6]). Recently, it has been shown that TWIST1 is involved in trophoblast syncytialization [7, 8]. As GATA3 and TWST1 are key placental factors, potentially more expressed in mononuclear VCT and ST, respectively, we investigated the possibility that both factors are used as specific nuclear markers of in vitro trophoblast differentiation.

The peroxisome proliferator-activated receptor-γ (PPARγ) is a member of the nuclear receptor superfamily that binds PPRE sequence to regulate, in a ligand-dependent manner, the transcription of target genes. Studies of PPARγ-deficient mice have demonstrated its essential role in placental development [9]. In the human placenta, PPARγ is expressed in VCT and is activated during its differentiation into ST [10, 11]. Altered expression or activation of PPARγ is observed in placental pathologies (PE or IUGR [12, 13]).

To properly assess the use of GATA3 or TWIST1 immunostaining to evaluate the fusion index, (1) we used an agonist (GW1929) and an antagonist (GW9662) of PPARγ so that an increased activity of PPARγ increases the in vitro differentiation of human placental VCT (i.e., higher fusion index as compared to control), while a reduced activity of PPARγ decreases it (i.e., lower fusion index compared to control), and (2) we compared these new fusion index scores to the classical one, based on DAPI/desmoplakin immunostaining [14, 15] (Fig. 1).

2 Materials

2.1 Cell Culture and PPARγ Agonist (GW1929) or Antagonist (GW9662) Treatments

1. Sterile 12-well chamber (removable), cell culture-treated plastic slide.
2. Primary villous cytotrophoblasts (VCT) isolated from human term placental tissues as described in Chapter 17.
3. Cell medium: DMEM medium supplemented with 10% fetal bovine serum (FBS), 1% 100× L-glutamine, 1% 100× penicillin-streptomycin.
4. 10 mM GW1929 in 100% ethanol (EtOH). Aliquot and store at −20 °C.
5. 10 mM GW9662 in 100% EtOH. Aliquot and store at −20 °C.

2.2 Immunofluorescence Staining Components

1. 1× Dulbecco's phosphate-buffered saline (PBS) without calcium and magnesium.
2. Cell fixative solution: 4% paraformaldehyde (PFA) in PBS.
3. Permeabilizing solution: 0.5% Triton X-100 in PBS.
4. PBST: 0.1% Tween-20 in PBS.

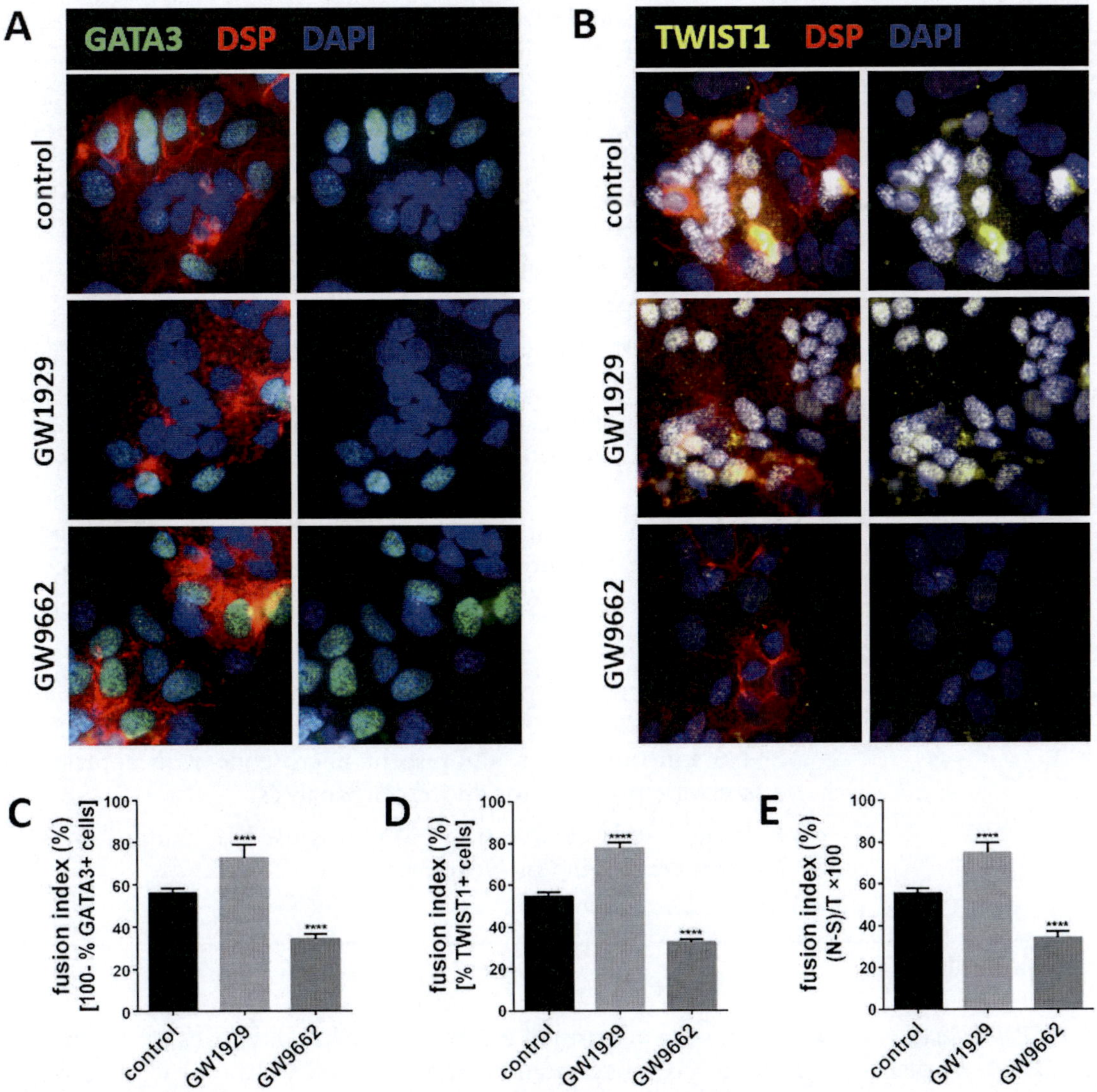

Fig. 1 Immunolocalization of proteins for GATA3 and TWIST1 during in vitro differentiation of human villous cytotrophoblast (VCT). After 24 h of culture, VCT were incubated for the next 48 h with 1 μM of PPARγ agonist (GW1929) or antagonist (GW9662). After 72 h of culture, cells were fixed, and subjected to fusion assays. VCT and ST nuclei were immunostained with either (**a**) anti-GATA3 (*green*) or (**b**) anti-TWIST1 (*yellow*) and anti-desmoplakin (*red*) antibodies, and counterstained with DAPI (*blue*). (**c**–**e**) Nuclei counting was performed manually using the "Cell Counter" plugin of ImageJ. Fusion index was calculated as follows, (**c**) (100 − % (number of GATA3+ nuclei/total number of DAPI nuclei)) or (**d**) % (number of TWIST1+ nuclei/total number of DAPI nuclei), as compared to classical calculation (**e**), i.e. $[(N - S)/T] \times 100$, where N equals the number of nuclei in syncytia, S equals the number of syncytia, and T equals the total number of nuclei counted. The data are expressed as the mean ± SD of the indicated number. Statistical analysis (paired t-test) was performed using the GraphPad Prism 6 software. ****p-Value < 0.001

5. Blocking solution: 5% bovine serum albumin (BSA, IgG-free) in PBST. Filtered in 22 μm filter system and stored at 4 °C.
6. Primary antibodies against GATA3 mouse monoclonal antibody (HG3-31, sc-268 Santa Cruz), TWIST1 mouse monoclonal antibody (ab50887, Abcam), and desmoplakin rabbit polyclonal antibodies (ab71690, Abcam): 2 μg/mL in blocking solution (*see* **Note 1**).
7. VectaFluor™ Excel Amplified DyLight® 488 Anti-Mouse IgG Kit (*see* **Note 2**).
8. Alexa Fluor 555 donkey anti-rabbit IgG: 5 μg/mL in blocking solution.
9. 4′,6-Diamidino-2-phenylindole dihydrochloride (DAPI): 5 mg/mL in deionized water (dH_2O). Aliquoted and stored at −20 °C.
10. Mounting medium: Fluoromount-G or other Fluorescence Mounting Medium.
11. Coverslip for confocal microscopy.
12. Nail polish.
13. Olympus BX60 epifluorescence microscope equipped with a Sony 3CCD DXC.950 color camera, using the VisionStage 1.6 software or any fluorescent microscope with appropriate software program for fluorescent analysis.
14. ImageJ software (version 1.48v was used) including the Cell Counter plugin (*see* **Note 3**).

3 Methods

3.1 Cell Culture and PPARγ Agonist (GW1929) or Antagonist (GW9662) Treatments

All steps are performed under a sterile hood. Gloves are worn at all times to prevent contamination. Use four wells for each treatment.

1. Plate freshly isolated primary VCT at 4 × 10^4 cells/well in a sterile 12-well cell culture-treated plastic slides 1 day prior to treatments in cell medium (maximum volume = 200 μL). Grow cells at 37 °C under 5% CO_2 in a humidified incubator.
2. Prepare treatment solutions: For 1 μM GW1929, dilute 1 μL of 10 mM GW1929 in 10 mL of cell medium. For 1 μM GW9662, dilute 1 μL of 10 mM GW9662 in 10 mL of cell medium. For vehicle control, dilute 1 μL 100% EtOH in 10 mL of cell medium.
3. Wash cells two times with cell medium and incubate cells in 200 μL of 1 μM GW1929 or 1 μM GW9662 or vehicle control solutions, for 48 h at 37 °C and 5% CO_2 in a humidified incubator.

3.2 GATA3, TWIST1, Desmoplakin Immunofluorescence Staining

1. Remove the culture medium from each well of the 12-well slide and rinse cells twice with PBS to remove the broken cell material.
2. Fix the cells with 4% PFA. Add enough PFA to cover the cells (100 μL/well for 12-well slide) and incubate for 20 min at room temperature. Remove PFA and carefully wash the cells with PBS three times, 5 min each.
3. Permeabilize the fixed cells by incubating in 0.5% Triton X-100/PBS for 30 min at room temperature.
4. Remove 0.5% Triton X-100 solution and block nonspecific antibody-binding sites and reduce background by incubating cells in blocking solution (5% BSA/PBST) for 30 min to 1 h at room temperature (*see* **Note 4**).
5. Remove 5% BSA/PBST solution and incubate cells in diluted primary antibodies solution for 1 h at 37 °C or overnight at 4 °C.
6. Remove primary antibodies solution and carefully wash the cells with PBST three times, 5 min each.
7. Remove PBST and proceed to the amplified fluorescent staining as detailed by manufacturer's protocol. Incubate cells for 15 min with Amplifier Antibody solution at room temperature.
8. Remove Amplifier Antibody solution and carefully wash the cells with PBST three times, 5 min each.
9. Remove PBST and incubate cells for 30 min with VectaFluor™ Reagent at room temperature, protected from light as the light can quench the fluorescence. The slide can be placed in a dark box or covered with aluminum foil during the incubation period.
10. Remove VectaFluor™ Reagent and carefully wash the cells with PBST three times, 5 min each.
11. Remove PBST and incubate cells with fluorescent-labeled secondary antibody solution (Alexa Fluor 555 donkey anti-rabbit IgG diluted 1:400 in blocking buffer or PBST) for 1 h at room temperature.
12. Remove secondary antibody solution and carefully wash the cells with PBST three times, 5 min each.
13. DNA counterstain and incubate cells with DAPI solution (1:20,000 in PBST) for 10 min at room temperature.
14. Remove DAPI solution and carefully wash the cells with PBST three times, 5 min each.
15. Remove the 12-well chamber (silicone gasket) by hand or by using tweezers.

16. Wick away excess fluid from the slide and mount the slide with a coverslip 24 mm × 60 mm using Fluoromount-G or other Fluorescent Mounting Medium.
17. Remove any excess mounting medium from around the edges of the coverslip by pipetting or using a wiper, and then seal it with a hardening material such as nail polish to prevent drying and movement under microscope.
18. Store slide on a flat, dry surface protected from light and let stand overnight at 4 °C.
19. Image cells with the 63× oil objective of an epifluorescence microscope (Fig. 1).
20. Analyze/count manually stained nuclei using the "cell counter" tool of ImageJ, (GATA3+/DAPI for mononuclear cytotrophoblast, TWIST1+/DAPI for differentiated syncytiotrophoblast, and DAPI/desmoplakin for classical fusion index calculation).
21. Calculate the fusion index: [100 − % (number of GATA3+ nuclei/total number of DAPI nuclei)] or [% (number of TWIST1+ nuclei/total number of DAPI nuclei)] as compared to classical calculation $[(N - S)/T] \times 100$, where N equals the number of nuclei in syncytia, S equals the number of syncytia, and T equals the total number of nuclei counted.

4 Notes

1. We can also use GATA3 goat polyclonal antibodies (AF2605, R&D) without the amplification staining step.
2. The immunofluorescent staining also works with classical secondary antibodies, but the brightness and contrast of the staining are better with the amplification method. In case for secondary antibodies, GATA3 staining needs Alexa Fluor 488 donkey anti-mouse IgG or Alexa Fluor 488 donkey anti-goat IgG if antibody cited in **Note 1** is used.
3. ImageJ free software, for example, can be downloaded at https://imagej.nih.gov/ij/.
4. Alternatively, blocking can be achieved by incubating the cells with 10% normal donkey serum diluted in PBST.

Acknowledgments

This work was supported by ANSES (PhthalatPreG project).

References

1. Huppertz B, Kingdom JC (2004) Apoptosis in the trophoblast—role of apoptosis in placental morphogenesis. J Soc Gynecol Investig 11(6):353–362. https://doi.org/10.1016/j.jsgi.2004.06.002
2. Longtine MS, Chen B, Odibo AO, Zhong Y, Nelson DM (2012) Villous trophoblast apoptosis is elevated and restricted to cytotrophoblasts in pregnancies complicated by preeclampsia, IUGR, or preeclampsia with IUGR. Placenta 33(5):352–359. https://doi.org/10.1016/j.placenta.2012.01.017
3. Roland CS, Hu J, Ren CE, Chen H, Li J, Varvoutis MS, Leaphart LW, Byck DB, Zhu X, Jiang SW (2016) Morphological changes of placental syncytium and their implications for the pathogenesis of preeclampsia. Cell Mol Life Sci 73(2):365–376. https://doi.org/10.1007/s00018-015-2069-x
4. Ralston A, Cox BJ, Nishioka N, Sasaki H, Chea E, Rugg-Gunn P, Guo G, Robson P, Draper JS, Rossant J (2010) Gata3 regulates trophoblast development downstream of Tead4 and in parallel to Cdx2. Development 137(3):395–403. https://doi.org/10.1242/dev.038828
5. Chiu YH, Chen H (2016) GATA3 inhibits GCM1 activity and trophoblast cell invasion. Sci Rep 6:21630. https://doi.org/10.1038/srep21630
6. Mirkovic J, Elias K, Drapkin R, Barletta JA, Quade B, Hirsch MS (2015) GATA3 expression in gestational trophoblastic tissues and tumours. Histopathology 67(5):636–644. https://doi.org/10.1111/his.12681
7. Lu X, He Y, Zhu C, Wang H, Chen S, Lin HY (2016) Twist1 is involved in trophoblast syncytialization by regulating GCM1. Placenta 39:45–54. https://doi.org/10.1016/j.placenta.2016.01.008
8. Ng YH, Zhu H, Leung PC (2011) Twist regulates cadherin-mediated differentiation and fusion of human trophoblastic cells. J Clin Endocrinol Metab 96(12):3881–3890. https://doi.org/10.1210/jc.2010-2714
9. Barak Y, Nelson MC, Ong ES, Jones YZ, Ruiz-Lozano P, Chien KR, Koder A, Evans RM (1999) PPAR gamma is required for placental, cardiac, and adipose tissue development. Mol Cell 4(4):585–595
10. Schaiff WT, Carlson MG, Smith SD, Levy R, Nelson DM, Sadovsky Y (2000) Peroxisome proliferator-activated receptor-gamma modulates differentiation of human trophoblast in a ligand-specific manner. J Clin Endocrinol Metab 85(10):3874–3881. https://doi.org/10.1210/jcem.85.10.6885
11. Tarrade A, Schoonjans K, Guibourdenche J, Bidart JM, Vidaud M, Auwerx J, Rochette-Egly C, Evain-Brion D (2001) PPAR gamma/RXR alpha heterodimers are involved in human CG beta synthesis and human trophoblast differentiation. Endocrinology 142(10):4504–4514. https://doi.org/10.1210/endo.142.10.8448
12. Fournier T, Guibourdenche J, Handschuh K, Tsatsaris V, Rauwel B, Davrinche C, Evain-Brion D (2011) PPARgamma and human trophoblast differentiation. J Reprod Immunol 90(1):41–49. https://doi.org/10.1016/j.jri.2011.05.003
13. Kadam L, Kohan-Ghadr HR, Drewlo S (2015) The balancing act—PPAR-gamma's roles at the maternal-fetal interface. Syst Biol Reprod Med 61(2):65–71. https://doi.org/10.3109/19396368.2014.991881
14. Degrelle SA, Gerbaud P, Leconte L, Ferreira F, Pidoux G (2017) Annexin-A5 organized in 2D-network at the plasmalemma eases human trophoblast fusion. Sci Rep 7:42173
15. Frendo JL, Cronier L, Bertin G, Guibourdenche J, Vidaud M, Evain-Brion D, Malassine A (2003) Involvement of connexin 43 in human trophoblast cell fusion and differentiation. J Cell Sci 116(Pt 16):3413–3421. https://doi.org/10.1242/jcs.00648

Chapter 14

Ex Vivo Dual Perfusion of the Human Placenta: Disease Simulation, Therapeutic Pharmacokinetics and Analysis of Off-Target Effects

Paul Brownbill, Neil Sebire, Erin V. McGillick, Stacey Ellery, and Padma Murthi

Abstract

In recent years ex vivo dual perfusion of the human placental lobule is seeing an international renaissance in its application to understanding fetal health and development. Here, we discuss the methods and uses of this technique in the evaluation of (1) vascular function, (2) transplacental clearance, (3) hemodynamic and oxygenation changes associated with pregnancy complications on placental structure and function, and (4) placental toxicology and post-perfusion evaluation of tissue architecture.

Key words Placenta, Perfusion, Methods, Pharmacokinetics, Fetoplacental, Vascular resistance, Structural integrity, Preeclampsia, Off-target effects

Overview

Ex vivo dual perfusion of the human placenta lobule is the only experimental model that presents an opportunity to explore human placental pharmacokinetics, pharmacodynamics, and transplacental clearance of xenobiotics, gases, nutrients, and other endogenous substances [1–10]. It also lends itself to studies of endocrine and vesicle release, immunology, and vascular resistance in health and diseased states [11–18]. Although variation exists in its methodology detail internationally, most centers conform to the accepted general principles of established dual circulations; homeostasis of temperature, pH, and colloid osmotic pressures and osmolality of perfusate; flow rates relative to tissue mass; fetoplacental resistance limitations; and transmembrane leakiness thresholds. In this regard, robust evaluation of post-perfusion tissue structure, following perfusion of third trimester placenta, has occurred [19]. More recently studies utilizing this technique have focused on oxygen consumption [20] and on the comparative in vivo and ex vivo clearance of paracellular markers for the human placenta [21]. The unique structural, hemodynamic, and functional nature of the human placenta

Padma Murthi and Cathy Vaillancourt (eds.), *Preeclampsia: Methods and Protocols*, Methods in Molecular Biology, vol. 1710,
https://doi.org/10.1007/978-1-4939-7498-6_14, © Springer Science+Business Media LLC 2018

delineates this ex vivo perfusion model from other in vivo and ex vivo animal placental models. The important human placental factors to consider here are the hemomonochorial type, with a single continuous syncytiotrophoblast epithelium at the capillary exchanger site; villous maternal blood flow engaging in multi-villous exchange; vascularized fetal blood flow, with sinusoidal capillaries and a continuous endothelium; species specific, influx and efflux transporters; and a high collagen content [22–24].

1 Introduction

Ex vivo dual perfusion of the human placenta involves establishing physiological perfusion of buffer through two independent circulatory systems, creating the necessary haemodynamics to facilitate a quantitative understanding of solute transfer, endogenous substance release, and resistance to flow in the fetoplacental circulation. Study themes where the ex vivo placental perfusion model has been employed include (1) transplacental transfer of endogenous substances, oxygen, microbes, parasites, and xenobiotics [2, 6, 25–29], (2) regulation and dysregulation of fetoplacental vascular tone [12, 30–33], (3) placental inflammatory mediation processes [16], (4) endocrine release [26, 34], and (5) syncytiotrophoblast shedding; oxygen transfer and metabolism [20, 35]. This technique has provided a greater understanding of fetoplacental function in pregnancies complicated by (1) preeclampsia [36], (2) fetal growth restriction [31], and (3) gestational diabetes [37].

Fetoplacental flow is established first, within a pair of chorionic plate vessels—one artery and one vein—serving one or more villous trees within an intact lobule of the human placenta. This region is then grossly flow matched on the maternal side, by mimicking spiral artery flow using one or more cannulas, which is/are simply inserted through the decidual plate to irrigate the intervillous space. A physiological salt solution is perfused into each circulatory system that is isotonic with fetal and maternal blood, with a composition that buffers at pH 7.3–7.4 and is therefore permissive of the maintenance of endothelial and trophoblast integrity, is anticoagulatory, ensures a vasodilatory potential, provides some colloid osmotic pressure to prevent intervillous space and capillary fluid loss, and is oxygenated to establish aerobic metabolism necessary to sustain active uptake and efflux transporter systems, modulation of vascular resistance, protein synthesis, and endocrine release.

For successful perfusion experiments, the local arrangements within the clinical research setting should be established, so that midwifery/nursing staff and surgeons understand the need to have the placenta, from recruited cases, handed over for research needs as soon as possible after delivery, ideally within 10–15 min, so that perfusion can be established within the laboratory within 30 min. Once fetal-side ischemia commences, blood begins to clot within the microcirculation, and cell-free hemoglobin has damaging consequences on nitric oxide sequestration and has other irreversible effects through vasoconstriction and inflammation [38]. It is also necessary to perform preparatory work the day before perfusion, and a little more on the day of perfusion, prior to placenta collection, inspection, cannulation, and establishment of homeostasis before experimentation. There are key quality control measures, which must be adhered to in the maintenance of tissue structural integrity and in preventing leakage artifact from the fetal to the maternal circulation. Fetomaternal leakage takes two forms: postpartum breakages in the villous tree structure, which provides a route of least resistance for fetal perfusate escape, along a hydrostatic pressure gradient and into the intervillous space, and the bulk flow of perfusate through existing paracellular routes when this fetomaternal hydrostatic pressure differential exceeds approximately 30 mmHg [12, 39, 40]. The latter phenomenon is associated with elevated fetal-side inflow hydrostatic pressure, which is evoked by prolonged postpartum ischemia, whereby hemostasis leads to platelet activation and irreversible vasoconstriction within the placental microcirculation. Establishing fetal-side perfusion within 30 min, or at least ensuring a fetal-side flush with heparinized perfusate in this time period, would normally ensure a basally relaxed fetoplacental microcirculation, preventing fetomaternal leakage to an acceptable level.

Fetal-side (and sometimes maternal-side) inflow hydrostatic pressure is monitored in real time, to visualize the ease of postischemic blood elution within the first phase of fetal-side perfusion. A steady-state low fetomaternal hydrostatic pressure differential (below 30 mmHg) is preventative of a perfusate fetomaternal "bulk flow" effect and the loss of barrier architectural integrity, whereas a sustained excessive fetal vascular resistance will compromise the tissue structural integrity, by vacuolating the vasculosyncytial membrane, leading to an increased diffusional pathway length. According to Fick's law of diffusion, this would otherwise interfere with nutrient transfer efficacy and the accuracy of interpretation and in vivo of pharmacokinetics. Fetal-side inflow hydrostatic pressure is also directly used in experiments designed to assess the regulation of fetoplacental vascular tone, important in the adequacy of provision of fetal blood flow to and from the placenta, in the supply of nutrients and oxygen, and in the elimination of waste products of metabolism.

Herein, we discuss the methods for ex vivo dual placental perfusion system and uses of this technique to evaluate (1) vascular function, (2) transplacental clearance, (3) hemodynamic and oxygenation changes associated with pregnancy complications on placental structure and function, and (4) placental toxicology and post-perfusion evaluation of tissue architecture.

2 Materials

2.1 Perfusate Composition

Commonly, a modified Earle's bicarbonate buffer (EBB) is employed to each circulation (*see* **Note 1**). The standard EBB composition is 2.4 mM $CaCl_2$, 0.4 mM $MgSO_4$, 117 mM NaCl, 5.3 mM KCl, 1 mM NaH_2PO_4, and 26 mM $NaHCO_3$. Supplementation usually includes 5.6 mM glucose and 5000 IU/mL heparin sodium and may include 0.04 mM L-arginine; 0.1% (w/v) bovine serum albumin (fraction V; *see* **Note 2**), 3.5% (w/v) dextran (*see* **Note 3**) and antibiotics (e.g., 100 mg/L kanamycin).

2.2 Equipment (Fig. 1)

1. Temperature-controlled perfusion cabinet (37 °C at placental mounting height), complete with internal scaffolding, or a benchtop perfusion chamber [41] consisting of an outer water jacket for maintaining temperature at 37 °C and an inner assembly, clamping into position the perfused lobule.
2. Placenta clamping platform, if using perfusion cabinet.
3. Circulating water bath, set to deliver heated water to the benchtop perfusion chamber, equilibrating to 37 °C, if using.
4. Water bath to heat perfusates to 37 °C for open-circuit perfusion.
5. Fetal and maternal peristaltic pumps with appropriate manifold tubing fitted to ensure pumps work within their midrange at 6 mL/min and 14 mL/min, respectively, with scope for fetal-side pumps to operate up to 12 mL/min, if investigating flow-mediated vasodilation (*see* **Note 4**).
6. Hydrostatic pressure transducers, coupled to a pressure logger and computer with software installed for recording, with real-time screen readout.
7. Gas cylinders and regulators to supply required levels of oxygen and carbon dioxide to perfusates.
8. In-line oxygenator system for exchanging oxygen and carbon dioxide to required levels.
9. In-line heat exchanger supplying heated water from a circulating water bath for effective closed circuit perfusion if performing closed-circuit perfusion.
10. A bubble trap for each circuit to prevent non-soluble gases reaching the perfused tissue.
11. A chamber fitted with an oxygen electrode or optode for each circuit to measure oxygen supply to the fetal villous microcirculation and the maternal intervillous space, plus an additional

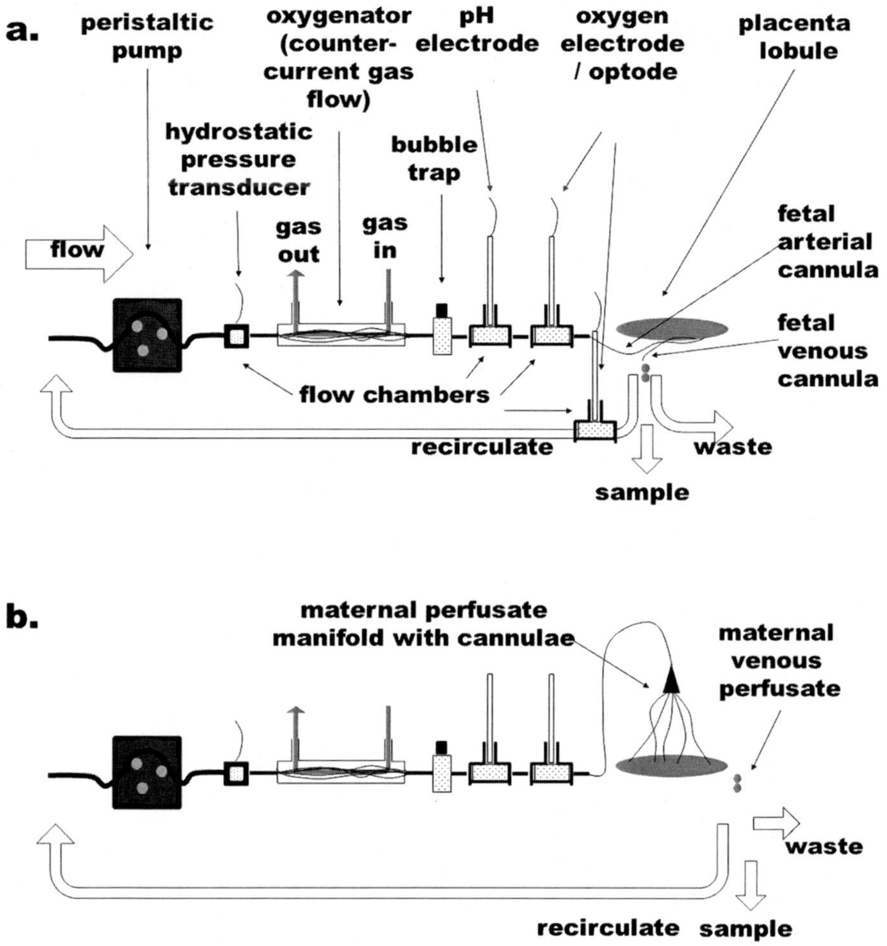

Fig. 1 Schematic of the ex vivo dual perfusion of the human placental lobule. Depicting fetal-side (**a**) and maternal-side (**b**) perfusion, the capacity to measure real-time inflow hydrostatic pressure as a measure of resistance to flow; pH, which is particularly important in closed-circuit perfusion, ppO_2 in the fetal and maternal inflow perfusate and the fetal venous perfusate, permitting a measure of tissue oxygen consumption and transfer. An oxygenator is employed within each circuit, typically supplying 0 mmHg O_2/38 mmHg CO_2 (bal. N2) to the fetal circulation and 712 mmHg O_2/38 mmHg CO_2 to the maternal circulation (superoxic model; [41]) or 150–160 mmHg O_2/38 mmHg CO_2 to the maternal circulation (normoxic model, [47]). An alternative to an oxygenator is through-gassing a perfusate reservoir within a water bath using a sintered gassing tube (for open-circuit perfusion only). Options are available to recirculate perfusate in closed-circuit perfusion with reservoir sampling or send to waste in the open-circuit method with direct sampling. If using the benchtop perfusion system, two perfusate heat exchangers, or equivalent arrangement, one in each circuit, would need to be employed prior to the oxygenator; alternatively, all equipment may be housed within a heated cabinet

arrangement to measure the partial pressure of oxygen in the fetal venous perfusate and gauge aerobic metabolism and transplacental oxygen transfer if relevant to the study.

12. A further needle-type oxygen electrode/optode to assess intervillous space oxygen gradient mapping, sampled using a micromanipulator, if relevant to the study.
13. A chamber fitted with a pH electrode for each circuit to enable pH adjustment if employing closed-circuit perfusion.
14. Watch-makers' forceps and Vannas scissors for chorionic plate arterial cannulation, forceps and fine pointed scissors for chorionic plate venous cannulation, straight fine Spencer-Well forceps for holding sutures, and standard scissors for trimming the placenta when mounted in the ring.
15. Aspiration pump to remove venous waste when performing open-circuit perfusion.

2.3 Consumables

1. Fetal arterial cannula (*see* **Note 5**).
2. Fetal venous cannula (*see* **Note 6**).
3. Sutures: braided silk with a 3/8 curvature is recommended.
4. Maternal arterial cannula (*see* **Note 7**).
5. Gauze swabs.
6. Lab film—folded over and stretch to a wide square over perfused lobule. Additional for covering perfusate reservoirs during top-gassing.
7. 20 mL syringe for pre-flushing fetal circuit with perfusate, if using the cabinet method.
8. Beakers to collect venous waste for disposal (open-circuit perfusion) or reservoirs to collect and recirculate closed-circuit perfusate.

3 Methods

3.1 Prior to Day of Experimentation

1. Prepare perfusates according to individual requirements (*see* Subheading 2.1). Study design may involve the addition of radio-labeled analytes, agonists, cofactors, or inhibitors; alternatively, for labile and expensive substances, such agents may be added on the day, when the preparation is known to have passed QC measures.
2. If holding tubing for long term in 70% ethanol, flush out with distilled H_2O.
3. Check that peristaltic pumps are holding their calibrated flows. Flow settings vary by center, but the range is 4–6 mL/min for the fetal circulation and 12–14 mL/min for the maternal circulation. Fetal-side circuit may increase by integers of 2 mL/min if "flow-ramping" in vascular studies.

4. Check that the hydrostatic pressure transducers are holding their calibration, using a column of water equivalent to 25 mmHg (circa 33.25 cm H_2O). If necessary, recalibrate or perform spreadsheet correction factor on experimental results.
5. In the absence of a placenta, perfuse the tubing in each circulatory system with water, hold the experimental cannula at the experimental height position for the placenta, and record inflow hydrostatic pressures for at least one revolution of the pumps. These data can be later used to correct for total resistance of the tubing with placenta following experimentation, to derive a representation of placental resistance alone.
6. Check gas levels in cylinders and water levels in all baths.
7. Prepare all dissection equipment, sutures, gauze, lab film, and placenta clamping apparatus, so that time can be saved during cannulation and placental assembly on the day of perfusion.
8. Liaise with research midwives/obstetric nurses for the recruitment of patients, as research volunteers, for the donation of their placentas.

3.2 Preparation on Day of Experimentation

1. Switch on perfusate pumps, perfusion cabinet or circulating water bath, reservoir water bath, hydrostatic pressure and O_2 recording equipment, and aspirator pumps.
2. Turn on gas regulators and employ gas to exchangers or through-gas reservoirs within water bath, according to design.
3. If through-gassing is to be employed within a water bath-heated reservoir, for open-circuit perfusion, it is advised that the albumen solution (at 10× or 100× strength) is left out until perfusate O_2/CO_2 saturation has been reached; then the albumen is added, followed by perfusate top-gassing above the meniscus with lab film sealing the top of the perfusate reservoir bottle. Gas exchanger systems are a far superior way of ensuring that the correct partial pressures of O_2 and CO_2 are reached.

3.3 Placenta Collection, Inspection, Cannulation, and Establishment of Homeostasis

1. Record time of birth, and once the placenta has been checked for clinical purposes, transport to the laboratory within 15–20 min.
2. Inspect the decidual surface to identify a lobule devoid of breakages to the villous structure. Placing a gloved hand underneath the placenta, in contact with the chorionic plate, and rotating the placenta during inspection usually reveal fissured breaks in the decidua, which helps in the elucidation of septa damage and also decidual separation at the placenta margins. In all cases of damage, the villous tissue will appear as a rough texture and would incur a leakage from the fetoplacental microcirculation into the intervillous space upon estab-

lishing fetal-side perfusion. Select a lobule that is absent of such postpartum breaks.

3. If a suitable area is identified, prime all perfusion tubing with perfusate, displacing the water with perfusate. For closed-circuit systems that will initially operate in an open-circuit manner, be sure to also prime current closed-circuit dead space.
4. Turn the placenta over, to reveal the chorionic plate, and remembering lobule arrangements and tissue zones to be avoided where there are tears, select a pair of chorionic plate artery and veins, corresponding to the intact lobule and clear the plate of any blood using gauze swabs, in preparation for cannulation.
5. Distinguish arteries from veins within the selected area (*see* **Note 8**).
6. Decide on where the suture point will be for the arterial cannula to capture the zone of perfusion interest. Again, vascular anatomy exploration is key in determining the likelihood of perfusion into the desired and undesired zones.
7. Make a small incision in the artery wall 1–2 cm afferent to the desired suture point.
8. Using a 20 mL syringe, with fetal arterial cannula attached and primed with perfusate, insert the beveled end of the cannula into the lumen, being careful not to include air, and negotiate necessary branches, passing the desired suture point by at least 5 mm. The progression of the cannula through the artery can be aided by flushing the artery a little with the perfusate, which has the effect of expanding the vessel diameter.
9. Suture around the vessel wall, being careful not to encounter villous tissue, or pierce the vessel wall, employing a double knot.
10. Make a small incision in the chorionic plate vein some 2 cm closer to the cord insertion point than the artery; cannulate and suture (as in **steps 8** and **9**; however, flushing during advancement of the venous cannula will not be possible).
11. Flush slowly manually with 20 mL heparinized perfusate and check for leaks on the chorionic plate. The perfusate must run visibly diluted from the venous cannula, and resistance to hand plunging should be low, with the lobule not appearing hard to touch. If the latter two are not achievable, it is most likely that the blood within the microcirculation has started to clot. For bench-mounted perfusion systems, it may be desirable to commence fetal-side perfusion via the peristaltic pump immediately.

12. Mount the placenta within the perfusion clamp system according to individual apparatus design. Generally, lab film is then imposed over the chorionic plate. The amnion/chorion membranes of the villous tissue in neighboring lobules to the one of interest are then spiked within the apparatus to hold the lobule firmly in place and help seal the tissue within a Perspex frame.
13. According to a specific engineering design of the equipment, a second Perspex ring arrangement is passed over the spike, allowing the tissue to be clamped with fly nuts [41]. The chorionic plate cannulas are held together to pass through a break in the circle of the second ring structure arrangement, so that they do not become trapped, and perfusate can flow through without constraint.
14. The double ring clamp, with its sandwiched placenta, is then trimmed of surplus tissue and cord, inverted and placed within the perfusion cabinet, or jacketed water heater system.
15. Turn on the digital acquisition program to record real-time inflow hydrostatic pressure data.
16. Establish fetal-side flow if not already done and start stop clock ($T = 0$).
17. Fetal-side inflow hydrostatic pressure should drop off to a reduced steady-state baseline within a few minutes and should rest at a value below 60 mmHg.
18. Check fetal venous "recovery," expressed as a fraction of inflow. Starting venous flow rates should be 80% required for fetoplacental vascular studies and 100% for clearance studies. Any compromise in the 100% recovery threshold for clearance studies should be evaluated for aberrant nonphysiological transfer.
19. Fetal-side inflow hydrostatic pressure should rest below 60 mmHg to avoid a fetomaternal leak driven by bulk flow.
20. Commence maternal-side perfusion by inserting all cannula below the decidual surface to a depth of circa 1 cm. The cannula should be checked for flow before inserting and should be evenly distributed within the perfused lobule area. Maternal cannulation should be achieved by $T = 15$ min.
21. Continue perfusion to help the tissue reach physiological homeostasis until $T = 30$ min.
22. The preparation is now ready for experimentation. During experimentation fetal and maternal venous perfusates or the reservoirs may be sampled for analyte assay. The use of antibiotics is highly recommended for perfusions exceeding 6 h. Placental ultrastructure analysis is recommended for transfer studies, especially if extended beyond 6 h.

3.4 Applications of the Model

3.4.1 Vascular Function

Studies evaluating fetoplacental resistance might incur the evaluation of potential vasoconstrictors, or vasodilators. Such experiments are best performed in open-circuit perfusion. Vasoconstrictors can be administered from a new reservoir bottle for a set period of time, from a syringe as a bolus or a syringe drive as an extended bolus period. Vasoconstriction responses can be plotted as absolute increases in pressure. For investigations into potential vasodilatory effects of agonists, it is necessary to invoke some tone into the fetoplacental circulation, since the vasculature is quite basally relaxed. This is best achieved either through the prior and continuous administration of U46619 (usually 1–2 pM), a thromboxane A2 mimetic, into the fetal-side perfusion line from a 100× stock concentration within a syringe drive or by switching the fetal perfusate reservoir to a composition where sodium chloride is substituted for potassium chloride to a value of circa 11 mM. In either case an elevated baseline inflow hydrostatic pressure must be established. Other agonists may have desensitizing response and so do not hold resistance in a steady manner. Single boluses of the vasodilatory test agonist are administered in turn, with sufficient recovery time to see the fetal-side inflow hydrostatic pressure level return to its prior resting state. Data is expressed as a percentage change in fetal-side inflow hydrostatic pressure at the trough compared to the previous steady state. This representation tends to standardize the data between preparations, where the starting resistance will vary in each lobule.

In all cases vehicle control boluses should be employed in the design. Recovery time must be sufficient to permit a return to baseline pressure before a new dose is administered. Desensitization effects of the experimental agonist may be investigated in a separate series of perfusions, where the same dose is administered repeatedly and responses observed. It helps to perform pilot investigations to determine the longevity of agonist-evoked effects and recovery periods before designing the definitive experiment, with timelines for experimental interventions. Injections from syringes and drives must occur afferent to the peristaltic pump, via a silicone port, to prevent shear stress surges through the fetoplacental vasculature, which would evoke a competing paracrine vasodilation signal. The lability of agonist should be considered in designing the administration route. Syringe drives holding the agonist at ambient temperature at a stock concentration are preferable, where the rate of administration into the fetal perfusate inflow line can be factored against flow rate of the syringe driver, to achieve a steady-state working concentration upon reaching the fetoplacental microcirculation. Syringe driver flow rates will require calibrating when factoring against fetal-side perfusion flow rates.

3.4.2 Transplacental Clearance Studies

Understanding the pharmacokinetics of human placental transfer is of key importance to appreciating fetal exposure in the human. Substances may be transferred across the placenta in a variety of processes, including (1) simple diffusion, either through plasma membrane, if lipophilic or gaseous, or via paracellular routes if hydrophilic and of a suitable molecular radius, (2) bulk flow, (3) facilitated and active transfer processes, and (4) endocytosis and exocytosis, and have been extensively reviewed [42]. There is species specificity in influx and efflux process, as well as in placental architecture [43, 44]. These factors make the ex vivo dual perfusion of the human placenta a particularly attractive model to utilize, not least by the pharmaceutical industry, who realize that human placental transfer data will assist in more accurate "dosage margin setting" for maternal medications, in conjunction with other data on "no- and lowest observed-adverse-effect levels" (NOAELs/LOAELs) obtained from animal testing [45].

Frequently closed-circuit perfusion is employed in both circulations. A xenobiotic or nutrient is added to the maternal reservoir, along with a standardization marker such as antipyrine. The fetal and maternal reservoirs (circa 200 mL) are sampled periodically for the assay of analyte and antipyrine levels. These levels are expressed temporally in absolute terms and the equilibration time, relative to antipyrine informs on the rate of transfer. Equilibration time is a useful tool in the evaluation of transporter processes, where specific inhibitors might be employed. Expressing the clearance data as a "fetal to maternal ratio" permits a comparison with other studies, where absolute analyte concentrations may vary, but does not account for variation in reservoir volumes or mean perfused tissue mass between studies.

An alternative approach is to study clearance of substances in dual open-circuit perfusion. Bi-directionality can be explored in separate experiments, which could reveal differences in transfer symmetry and processes. In such studies, the donor side concentration (constant in open circuit) is sampled, along with periodic sampling of the acceptor side venous perfusate. Unidirectional clearance (K) is calculated as below:

$$K = \left(\left[\text{acceptorside}\right].Q\right) / \left(\left[\text{donorside}\right].W\right)\left(\text{L} / \text{min per gramplacenta}\right)$$

where "Q" is the measured flow rate in the acceptor circulation and "W" is the wet weight of the perfused cotyledon [46].

For standardization, it is common to include inert paracellular markers such as creatinine, or FITC-inulin, which can be assayed. Clearance can be expressed against time for analytes and markers. A steady-state clearance is usually reached within 30 min, so collection of venous perfusate continues for at least 40 min, at 5 min intervals, to establish that steady state has indeed occurred. When clearance is plotted against time, there is normally a convex curve on the approach to steady state.

3.4.3 Ex Vivo Placental Perfusion as a Model of Trophoblast Shedding

The release of particulate and soluble materials from the placenta into the maternal blood space is the focus of study in understanding dysregulation of peripheral maternal systemic microvasculature in the disease of preeclampsia. The ex vivo human placental perfusion model has been adapted in several ways to emulate hemodynamic and oxygenation changes thought to occur in the placenta of such pregnancies, and furthermore, placental lobules from preeclamptic pregnancies have been directly perfused, to examine the release of syncytiotrophoblast vesicles and endogenous substances. Using placental lobules from normal pregnancy, turbulent flow of blood anticipated to occur around the placental villous trees in preeclampsia, when spiral arteries fail to transform, has been mimicked by increasing intervillous space perfusate flow [35]. In this study, maternal flow was increased to 45 mL/min via five cannulas in a single lobule, which revealed elevated release of lactate dehydrogenase, alkaline phosphatase, human chorionic gonadotropin, and the chemokines GROα and RANTES, expressed as rate of release per unit tissue mass, compared to normal flow rates of 14 mL/min. In a different adaptation, the intervillous space of a single lobule was perfused at normal flow rates of 14 mL/min with hypoxic levels of physiological buffer, distributed via 22, instead of five maternal cannulas [47]. A relative hypoxic environment caused increases in the release of macrophage inflammatory protein-1α, and the cytokines and oxidative stress markers, IL-6, IL-8, TNF-α, IFN-γ, and endothelin-1, compared to normoxic perfusion with the same number of cannulas [13, 47]. In further studies, placentas from preeclamptic pregnancies were perfused directly to evaluate the qualities of syncytiotrophoblast microvesicles and also the quantity of soluble angiogenic growth factors [17, 35].

Many of these studies involve the use of metabolomics. In collecting venous perfusates for metabolomics, it is essential to process the venous perfusates as quickly as possible, by centrifuging (1500 × *g* for 10 min at 4 °C), holding the collection tubes on ice if necessary, prior to processing. Supernatants should be aliquoted and snap frozen at −80 °C after spinning. Open-circuit perfusion is preferable if metabolomics is to be employed, as recirculation in closed circuit at 37 °C will permit metabolite breakdown of released substances, making the interpretation of timed analyte accrual difficult. For cytokines and the release of other substances requiring a genomic upregulation following an experimental intervention, it is expected that a perfusion duration of 5–6 h would be needed to see such changes in the perfusate. However, other substances may be stored within cells, perhaps as precursor molecules, and their release might report quickly within the experimental time period.

3.4.4 Placental Toxicology and Post-perfusion Evaluation of Tissue Architecture

Recent OECD recommendation on changes to reproductive toxicology testing within the chemical industry requires an assessment of "internal dose" in hazard assessments, with a heightened requirement for toxicokinetic analysis, including regulatory triggers to study endocrine disruption [48]. The ex vivo human placental perfusion model offers the opportunity to study the effects of xenobiotics on placental endocrinology and metabolism, with the added advantage over other human placental models of illustrating changes in the polarity of release endocrine signals and xenobiotic metabolites into the fetal and maternal venous perfusates [26]. In this regard it is useful to assess human chorionic gonadotropin release as a potential marker of endocrine disruption. A new focus is now being directed to consider other endocrine outputs, such as aromatase activity and retinoic acids [49, 50]. Lactate dehydrogenase is normally detectable in the maternal venous perfusate, but increases may indicate a change in trophoblast function [35]. Placental alkaline phosphatase is also found in the maternal venous perfusate, but an increased release would indicate damage to the microvillous membrane of the syncytiotrophoblast [35]. Such experiments would be designed to include a control perfusion phase, in which the clearance of paracellular markers might be included along with steady-state endocrine and metabolite release, as well as an intervention phase with the xenobiotic, monitoring similar outcomes. Temporal vehicle controls are also essential as separate experiments.

The evaluation of post-perfusion barrier and vascular architecture is an essential process, since xenobiotics might evoke cellular mechanisms that lead to changes in barrier properties and perfusion efficacy, which, experimentally, could be linked to observations of altered placental transfer of paracellular and lipophilic markers. It is therefore valuable to couple physiological transfer and pharmacokinetic data with a qualitative histological assessment on the preservation of the placental barrier. Figure 2 shows the term normal villous architecture from placentas that had been fixed immediately postpartum (Fig. 2a, b), compared to similar tissue that had undergone a 4 h ex vivo dual perfusion with a modified Earle's bicarbonate buffer (Fig. 2c, d). Numerous terminal villi and stem villi are scattered throughout each micrograph. It can be seen that ex vivo perfusion did not affect the trophoblast layer structure, in so far as the epithelium is without vacuolation and remained thin and continuous, except for prepartum denudation events (Fig. 2) [2]; the endothelial layer within each vessel type is also intact, and the length of pathway between the maternal-side intervillous space and the fetal vascular is qualitatively unaffected at the terminal villi. It should be noted that in the freshly fixed tissue, maternal red blood cells are present within the intervillous space and fetal red blood cells within many of the villous vessels. Following ex vivo perfusion, the main changes that occur are the washing out of blood cells from both the fetal circulation and the maternal intervillous space, accounting for the difference in overall appearances between the perfused and non-perfused groups. Furthermore, with perfusion there is apparent separation of the

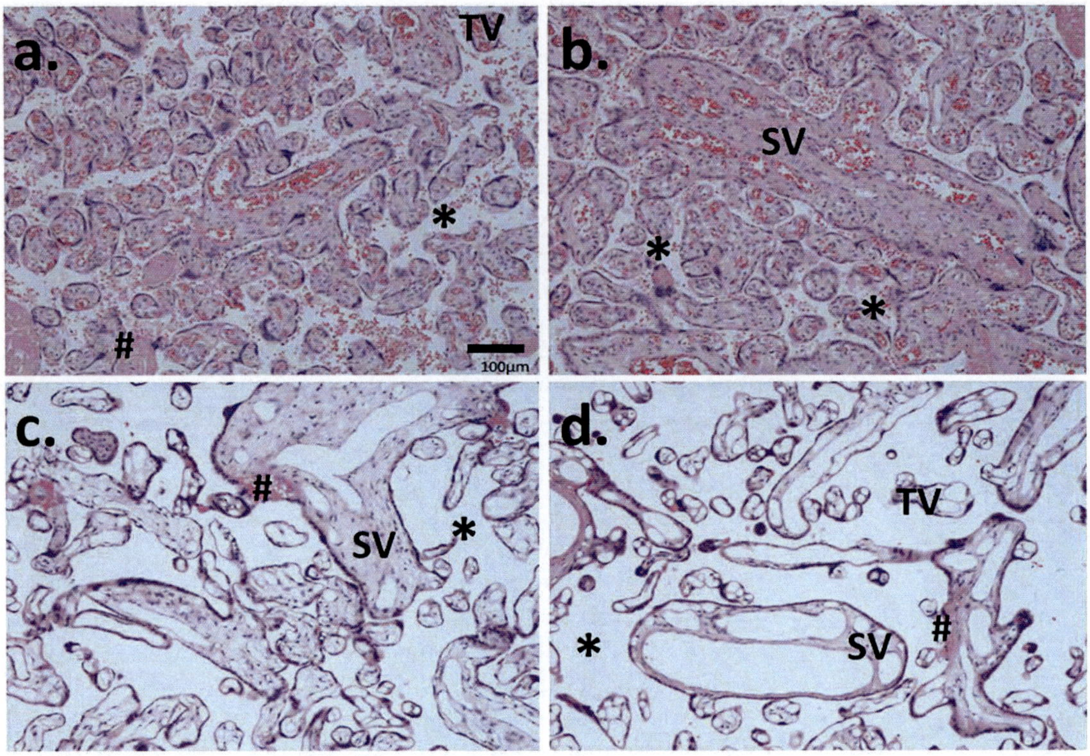

Fig. 2 Hematoxylin and eosin-stained sections of the human ex vivo perfused placenta. Freshly fixed normal term placenta (**a**, **b**) and a normal placenta that had been perfused ex vivo for 4 h and then perfusion fixed from the maternal circulation, during physiological perfusion of the fetal vasculature (**c**, **d**). Features depicted are the intervillous space (*), prepartum denuded trophoblast (#), stem villi (SV), and terminal villi (TV). Scale bar = 100 μm

chorionic villi and also an increase in villous vascular diameter, due to the continued inflation of the vascular lumen and intervillous space compartment during perfusion fixation, while the fetal vessels continued to be perfused with buffer. These factors should be taken into account when assessing specimens of this type.

4 Notes

1. Perfusate composition may vary between laboratories and modified according to specific research questions.
2. In pharmacokinetic investigations, where the analyte binds to albumen, transfer rates may beheavily influenced by the albumen concentration and species from which the albumen is derived; consideration might be given to the use of human serum albumen [51].
3. Clinical grade; 40 or 70 kDa (i.e., a guaranteed molecular weight, rather than a range of dextrans with different molecular

weights); fetal-side concentrations are enhanced on the fetal side in some laboratories where perfused tissue mass is low and fetomaternal HP differential is high, to discourage bulk flow.

4. Tubing type should be considered with respect to gas permeability and also tubing binding potential. Where oxygenators are employed prior to the fetal and maternal cannula, this is not important; otherwise Tygon is the material of choice. To prevent tubing binding of agonists, platinum-coated tubing should be considered.
5. The fetal arterial cannula use may vary, for example, for cabinet method with placenta platform, 15 cm of transparent polythene tubing (i.d., 1.0 mm; o.d., 1.6 mm), with beveled cut end and attached to a tubing adapter.
6. The fetal venous cannula may vary, for example, for cabinet method with placenta platform 15 cm of transparent vinyl tubing (i.d., 2 mm; o.d., 3 mm). The i.d. should not be less than this, ensuring that undue pressure is not imposed on the upstream microcirculation.
7. The maternal arterial cannula may vary in material and number, for example, 10 cm length of polythene tubing × 5, with beveled cut ends (i.d., 0.58 mm; o.d., 0.96 mm) diverging from a manifold of 1–5 ports for superoxic maternal perfusate or 5–25 ports for an adapted approach to perfusing the maternal side with normoxic levels of soluble gas, deriving a median partial pressure of >35 mmHg.
8. Arteries usually cross over the veins, but if uncertain explore the full arterial network.

References

1. Berveiller P, Gil S, Vialard F (2017) Placental perfusion: interest and limits. J Matern Fetal Neonatal Med 30:1347–1348
2. Brownbill P et al (2000) Denudations as paracellular routes for alphafetoprotein and creatinine across the human syncytiotrophoblast. Am J Physiol Regul Integr Comp Physiol 278(3):R677–R683
3. Eisenmann CJ, Miller RK (1994) The placental transfer and toxicity of selenite relative to cadmium in the human term perfused placenta. Placenta 15(8):883–895
4. Kummu M et al (2015) Organic anion transporter 4 (OAT 4) modifies placental transfer of perfluorinated alkyl acids PFOS and PFOA in human placental ex vivo perfusion system. Placenta 36(10):1185–1191
5. Abumaree MH et al (2014) IFPA Meeting 2013 Workshop Report III: maternal placental immunological interactions, novel determinants of trophoblast cell fate, dual ex vivo perfusion of the human placenta. Placenta 35:S15–S19
6. May K et al (2011) Perfusion of human placenta with hemoglobin introduces preeclampsia-like injuries that are prevented by alpha1-microglobulin. Placenta 32(4):323–332
7. Mathiesen L et al (2010) Quality assessment of a placental perfusion protocol. Reprod Toxicol 30(1):138–146
8. Nanovskaya T et al (2012) Transplacental transfer of vancomycin and telavancin. Am J Obstet Gynecol 207(4):331.e1–331.e6
9. Perazzolo S et al (2017) The influence of placental metabolism on fatty acid transfer to the fetus. J Lipid Res 58(2):443–454
10. Lees CC et al (2015) 2 year neurodevelopmental and intermediate perinatal outcomes in

infants with very preterm fetal growth restriction (TRUFFLE): a randomised trial. Lancet 385(9983):2162–2172
11. Brownbill P et al (2003) Neurokinin B is a paracrine vasodilator in the human fetal placental circulation. J Clin Endocrinol Metab 88(5): 2164–2170
12. Brownbill P, Sibley CP (2006) Regulation of transplacental water transfer: the role of fetoplacental venous tone. Placenta 27:560–567
13. Jain A et al (2014) Hypoxic treatment of human dual placental perfusion induces a preeclampsia-like inflammatory response. Lab Invest 94(8): 873–880
14. Leach L, Firth JA (1992) Fine structure of the paracellular junctions of terminal villous capillaries in the perfused human placenta. Cell Tissue Res 268(3):447–452
15. Malek A et al (1995) Continuous measurement of ATP by 31P-NMR in term human dually perfused placenta in vitro: response to ischemia. J Appl Physiol 78(5):1778–1786
16. Schamberger S et al (2013) Establishment of a one-sided ex vivo human placenta perfusion model to assess adhesion and invasion behavior of T cell leukemia cell lines. Leuk Lymphoma 54(8):1811–1813
17. Tannetta DS et al (2015) Syncytiotrophoblast extracellular vesicles from pre-eclampsia placentas differentially affect platelet function. PLoS One 10(11):e0142538
18. Gordon Z et al (2016) Ex vivo human placental perfusion model for analysis of fetal circulation in the chorionic plate. J Ultrasound Med 35(3):553–560
19. Illsley NP et al (1985) Human placental ultrastructure after in vitro dual perfusion. Placenta 6(1):23–32
20. Schneider H (2000) Placental oxygen consumption. Part II: in vitro studies - a review. Placenta 21(Suppl A):S38–S44
21. Brownbill P et al (2016) An international network (PlaNet) to evaluate a human placental testing platform for chemicals safety testing in pregnancy. Reprod Toxicol 64:191–202
22. Leach L, Firth JA (1997) Structure and permeability of human placental microvasculature. Microsc Res Tech 38(1-2):137–144
23. Chernyavsky IL et al (2011) Transport in the placenta: homogenizing haemodynamics in a disordered medium. Philos Trans A Math Phys Eng Sci 369(1954):4162–4182
24. Walker N et al (2017) Placental transporter localization and expression in the human: the importance of species, sex and gestational age differences1. Biol Reprod 96:733
25. Miller RK et al (2003) Marginal transfer of ReoPro (Abciximab) compared with immunoglobulin G (F105), inulin and water in the perfused human placenta in vitro. Placenta 24(7):727–738
26. Cleal JK et al (2007) Modification of fetal plasma amino acid composition by placental amino acid exchangers in vitro. J Physiol Lond 582(2):871–882
27. Myllynen P, Vahakangas K (2013) Placental transfer and metabolism: an overview of the experimental models utilizing human placental tissue. Toxicol In Vitro 27(1):507–512
28. Pehrson C et al (2016) Adhesion of Plasmodium falciparum infected erythrocytes in ex vivo perfused placental tissue: a novel model of placental malaria. Malar J 15(1):292
29. Porter C et al (2016) Certolizumab pegol does not bind the neonatal Fc receptor (FcRn): consequences for FcRn-mediated in vitro transcytosis and ex vivo human placental transfer. J Reprod Immunol 116:7–12
30. Glance DG et al (1984) The effects of the components of the renin-angiotensin system on the isolated perfused human placental cotyledon. Am J Obstet Gynecol 149(4):450–454
31. Jones S et al (2015) Dysregulated flow-mediated vasodilatation in the human placenta in fetal growth restriction. J Physiol 593(14): 3077–3092
32. Gude NM (1988) An investigation into the mechanisms controlling vascular tone of the fetal vessels of the human isolated perfused placenta. PhD thesis. Monash University, Clayton VIC
33. Cindrova-Davies T et al (2013) Reduced cystathionine γ-lyase and increased miR-21 expression are associated with increased vascular resistance in growth-restricted pregnancies: hydrogen sulfide as a placental vasodilator. Am J Pathol 182(4):1448–1458
34. Mortimer RH et al (2012) Secretion and transfer of the thyroid hormone binding protein transthyretin by human placenta. Placenta 33(4):252–256
35. Hutchinson ES et al (2009) Assessment of the link between spiral artery diameters, intervillous flow and pre-eclampsia pathogenesis using the in vitro dually perfused human placenta. Reprod Sci 16(3):173A
36. Balan A et al (2017) The effects of pravastatin on the normal human placenta: lessons from ex-vivo models. PLoS One 12(2):e0172174
37. Osmond D et al (2000) Effects of gestational diabetes on human placental glucose uptake, transfer, and utilisation. Diabetologia 43(5): 576–582

38. Brook A et al (2013) Free fetal haemoglobin elevates vascular tone in the fetoplacental circulation. Placenta 34:A40
39. Kertschanska S, Kosanke G, Kaufmann P (1997) Pressure dependence of so-called transtrophoblastic channels during fetal perfusion of human placental villi. Microsc Res Tech 38: 52–62
40. Sebire NJ, Talbert D (2004) The dynamic placenta: II. Hypothetical model of a fetus driven transplacental water balance mechanism producing low apparent permeability in a highly permeable placenta. Med Hypotheses 62(4):520–528
41. Schneider H, Huch A (1985) Dual in vitro perfusion of an isolated lobe of human placenta: method and instrumentation. Contrib Gynecol Obstet 13:40–47
42. Dilworth MR, Sibley CP (2013) Review: transport across the placenta of mice and women. Placenta 34(Suppl):S34–S39
43. Ceckova-Novotna M, Pavek P, Staud F (2006) P-glycoprotein in the placenta: expression, localization, regulation and function. Reprod Toxicol 22(3):400–410
44. Carter A (1993) In: Hanson M, Spencer J, Rodeck C (eds) Fetal placental circulation, in fetus and neonate physiology and clinical applications. Cambridge University Press, Cambridge, pp 116–136
45. Guittina P, Elefant E, Saint-Salvi B (2000) Hierarchization of animal teratology findings for improving the human risk evaluation of drugs. Reprod Toxicol 14(4):369–375
46. Sibley CP, Boyd RD (1988) Control of transfer across the mature placenta. Oxf Rev Reprod Biol 10:382–435
47. Soydemir F et al (2011) Adapting in vitro dual perfusion of the human placenta to soluble oxygen tensions associated with normal and pre-eclamptic pregnancy. Lab Invest 91(2):181–189
48. OECD (2015) Test No. 421: reproduction/developmental toxicity screening test. OECD Publishing, Paris
49. Nakanishi T et al (2005) Trialkyltin compounds bind retinoid X receptor to alter human placental endocrine functions. Mol Endocrinol 19(10):2502–2516
50. Sato BL et al (2015) Validation of murine and human placental explant cultures for use in sex steroid and phase II conjugation toxicology studies. Toxicol In Vitro 29(1):103–112
51. Nanovskaya TN et al (2008) Effect of albumin on transplacental transfer and distribution of rosiglitazone and glyburide. J Matern Fetal Neonatal Med 21(3):197–207

Chapter 15

Immunohistological Techniques

Evangelina Capobianco and Nora Martinez

Abstract

Preeclampsia is associated with histological alterations in the placenta. These alterations can be described by means of histological techniques. More specifically, immunohistochemistry could be used to detect proteins, and these in turn may be used to identify a specific cell type, to differentiate it from other cell types and to detect the expression of some markers deregulated in preeclampsia.

This chapter focuses on the detection of specific cellular and molecular markers that evidence the alterations in the human placenta in preeclampsia.

Key words Immunohistochemistry, Placental molecular markers, Preeclampsia, Syncytiotrophoblast, Cytotrophoblast

1 Introduction

The placenta is a highly specialized organ that ensures the exchange of nutrients and waste products between the mother and the fetus that supports the normal growth and development of the fetus. The human placenta is composed of different functional units: the chorionic villi next to the intervillous space filled with maternal blood, the chorionic plate (fetal component), and the basal plate (maternal component). The different tissues that form the placenta are the villous trophoblast (the epithelial cover of the villous tree), the villous stroma with mesenchymal cells, fetal vessels, and free connective tissue cells such as macrophages (Hofbauer cells), mast cells, and plasma cells. Fetal blood enters the placenta via the two umbilical arteries and leaves the placenta via the umbilical vein. Another tissue derived from the trophoblast is the extravillous trophoblast, which invades maternal tissues, finally reaching the walls of spiral arteries as deep as the inner third of the myometrium. Table 1 summarizes molecular markers of the different cell types of the human placenta.

The placenta plays a critical role in the physiopathogeny of preeclampsia. This gestational disorder is characterized by abnormal

Padma Murthi and Cathy Vaillancourt (eds.), *Preeclampsia: Methods and Protocols*, Methods in Molecular Biology, vol. 1710, https://doi.org/10.1007/978-1-4939-7498-6_15,

Table 1
Molecular cell markers for human placenta

Placental cell type	Marker
1. Villous trophoblast	Cytokeratin [7] Syncytin [8] PLAP [9] CD133 [10] PIGF[11]
(a) Syncytiotrophoblast	hCG [12] PP13 [13] Endoglin [14] PPARγ [15] hPL [7] GCM-1 [16]
(b) Cytotrophoblast	E-cadherin [17]
2. Villous stromal cells	CD9 [7] CD45 [7] Vimentin [7]
(a) Mesenchymal cells	Vimentin [18]
(b) Fibroblasts	Vimentin [18] Desmin [19]
(c) Endothelial cells	VEGF [20] Caveolin 1 and 2 [21] von Willebrand factor [22] CD34 [23]
(d) Macrophages (Hofbauer cells)	CD68 [24]

Adapted from *Molecular Markers for human placental investigation* by Berthold Huppertz [1]

PALP placental alkaline phosphatase, *PIGF* placenta growth factor, *CD* cluster of differentiation number, *hCG* human choriogonadotropin, *PP13* = *galectin 13* placental protein 13, *PPARγ* peroxisome proliferator-activated receptor γ, *hPL* human placental lactogen, *GCM-1* glial cell missing 1, *VEGF* vascular endothelial growth factor

differentiation of trophoblasts, producing a defective maternal-fetal interface [2]. Abnormal development of placental villi may induce a deficient trophoblast invasion which is associated with a defective placental implantation [3].

Histological alterations in the placenta include a decreased number of syncytial microvilli and necrotic villous tissues; extensive endothelial injury; inflammatory changes such as vasculitis, chronic villitis, and hemorrhagic endovasculitis; fibrinoid deposition and inflammatory reaction; increased deposition of collagen and laminin; a thin and discontinuous syncytium; and an increased number of syncytial knots (i.e., aggregated syncytiotrophoblastic nuclei at the surface of terminal villi) [4–6].

The morphological and molecular placental alterations in preeclampsia can be evidenced by different histochemical and immunohistochemical techniques. There is a full range of histochemical techniques used to detect the presence of carbohydrates, lipids, proteins, and nucleotides in a tissue section. The techniques of enzymatic histochemistry highlight an enzymatic reaction with specific substrates whose color changes at the site of the enzyme activity (peroxidases, phosphatases, dehydrogenases, diaphorases, acetylcholinesterases, etc.).

This chapter focuses on basic protocols for the identification of proteins in the placental tissue by immunohistochemistry. This technique can be used to determine the cellular source of proteins, identify a specific cell type, and differentiate it from others. Table 2 summarizes the specific placental markers for preeclampsia. Several immunohistochemical techniques use the presence of the peroxidase enzyme directly bound to an antibody or to another molecule that is bound to an antibody, which indicates the place where the primary antibody, used to detect the antigen of interest, is located. This chapter focuses on the description of one of these techniques, the avidin-biotin complex, which uses the high affinity of avidin to biotin and the formation of a stable complex bound to peroxidase. This is a very good method due to its great amplification of the immunostain, which makes it a very sensitive methodology, easy to develop in most laboratories.

Table 2
Molecular specific markers for preeclampsia found in human placenta

Marker	Alteration	Reference
VEGF	↑↓	[25–27]
PIGF	↑	[25]
PP13	↑	[28]
Connexin-43	↑	[29]
E-cadherin	↑	[30]
GCM-1	↓	[31]
Syncytin-1	↓	[32–34]
Syncytin-2	↓	[34]
Nitrotyrosine residues	↑	[35]

Alterations in human placental molecular markers evidenced in preeclampsia
↑ = increased; ↓ = decreased in comparison to normal placental tissues
VEGF vascular endothelial growth factor, *PIGF* placental growth factor, *PP13* placental protein 13, *GCM-1* glial cell missing-1
Note: there are controversial reports about the expression of VEGF in preeclamptic placentas. Some authors have reported a decrease of this factor, whereas others have found an increase

2 Materials

2.1 Tissue Preparation

1. A cool bag and a container to transport the placenta.
2. Sterile scalpels, scissors, and forceps.
3. Petri dishes.
4. Saline solution (9% NaCl in deionized water).

2.2 Fixation, Embedding, and Sectioning of Paraffin Tissue Blocks

1. 4% neutrally buffered formalin solution (100 mL 37% formaldehyde solution in 900 mL phosphate buffered saline (PBS), pH 7.0).
2. Embedding cassettes and molds.
3. Alcohol series: 70% ethanol, 80% ethanol, 96% ethanol, 100% ethanol, 50–50% ethanol-benzene, benzene.
4. Incubator adjusted to 56 °C.
5. Purified paraffin with melting temperature between 56 and 58 °C.
6. Heating plate adjusted to 56 °C.
7. Forceps.
8. Microtome.
9. Glass slides (coated slides are better).
10. Brush.
11. Water bath at 40–45 °C.

2.3 General Histology

1. Glass coplin staining jar with glass cover.
2. Deparaffinization and rehydration: xylene, 100% ethanol, 90% ethanol, 80% ethanol, 70% ethanol, deionized water.

2.4 Standard Immunohistochemistry

1. PBS and PBS-Tween: 10× PBS (80 g NaCl, 2 g KCl, 14.4 g $Na_2HPO_4 \cdot 2H_2O$, 2.4 g KH_2PO_4; bring to 800 mL, adjust the pH to 7.4, and correct the volume with distilled water to reach 1000 mL); 1× PBS (dilute 100 mL of 10× PBS in 900 mL distilled water); and PBS-T (0.5 mL Tween 20 in 1000 mL of 1× PBS). Store these solutions at 4 °C.
2. Blocking endogenous peroxidase activity: 0.3% H_2O_2. Dilute the H_2O_2 30 volume one hundredth with PBS just prior use.
3. For antigen retrieval in citrate buffer (10 mM citric acid, 0.05% Tween 20, pH 6.0): Dissolve 1.92 g of citric acid (anhydrous) in 1000 mL of distilled water. Adjust pH to 6.0 with 1 N NaOH and then add 0.5 mL of Tween 20. Mix well. Store this solution at room temperature for 3 months or at 4 °C for longer storage.
4. Microwave oven or water bath at 97 °C.
5. Hydrophobic pen.

6. Blocking solutions: 150 μL normal serum in 10 mL PBS, 2% bovine serum albumin (BSA) in 0.2% PBS-T (2 g BSA, bring to 100 mL with distilled water and add 200 μL of PBS-T), and 5% nonfat milk in 0.2% PBS-T BSA (5 g nonfat milk, bring to 100 mL with distilled water and add 200 μL of PBS-T).
7. Primary antibody solution. Dilute the primary antibody in PBS-T containing 1% BSA. Tables 1 and 2 summarize the molecular markers for the human placenta and specific markers for preeclampsia.
8. Vectastain Elite ABC Kit (Vector Laboratories) (*see* **Note 1**) provides blocking serum (normal serum) prepared as described in point 6; secondary antibody biotinylated, affinity-purified anti-immunoglobulin (diluted 1:200: add 150 μL of normal blocking serum stock to 10 mL PBS-T (diluted 1:66) in a mixing tube, and then add 50 μL of the antibody stock); and VECTASTAIN Elite ABC reagent (diluted 1:100: to prepare 30 min before use).
9. Chromogenic substrate; 3,3′ diaminobenzidine (DAB); 20 mg DAB, 50 mL of 0.05 M Tris buffer (pH 7.6), 40 μL H_2O_2.
10. Mounting medium for microscopy.
11. Coverslips.

3 Methods

3.1 Tissue Preparation

1. Shortly after delivery, put the placenta into a plastic bag and place the bag on ice in an isolated container to transfer the placenta to the laboratory (*see* **Note 2**).
2. Place the placenta on a tray, cut the tissue needed for your experiments, and place the pieces into petri dishes in saline solution. The size of the pieces should be approximately 0.5 mm × 1–3 cm (*see* **Note 3**).
3. There is no universal fixative, so the most appropriate fixative should be tested for some antibodies. This chapter focuses on formalin-fixed paraffin sections because they are mostly used in pathology with good results. As there is a great controversy about paraffin versus frozen sections, a summary of their advantages and disadvantages is described in Table 3.

3.2 Treatment for Paraffin Tissue Blocks

3.2.1 Fixation

1. Pour the 4% formalin solution into a 50 mL bottle and place the placental tissue. The fixative volume should be 5–10 times of tissue volume (*see* **Note 5**).
2. Close the bottle and fix the tissue for 24 h at room temperature (*see* **Note 6**).
3. Place the tissue into another 50 mL bottle filled with 70% ethanol. The tissues could be stored in this medium at 4 °C or at room temperature.

Table 3
Paraffin versus frozen sections

	Paraffin sections	Frozen sections
Advantages	Easy to store: samples can be stored at room temperature for long periods of time Easy to cut using a microtome without the need for cooling	Faster to prepare: no dewaxing, rehydration or antigen retrieval (the activity and epitope of target antigens can be well preserved) (*see* **Note 4**) Used to detect the substances lost in paraffin
Disadvantages	Pretreatment to unmask cross-linked antigen is often essential Does not provide a sufficient hard matrix for cutting thinner slices (typically 80–100 nm thick)	The technical quality of the section is low (controversial) The section slides might only be stored at low temperature (−80 °C)
Mostly used when:	The antigen survives fixation and processing at 60 °C	The antigen does not survive chemical fixation and/or heating at 60 °C The antigen is soluble in the clearing agent (e.g., lipids) Confocal and electronic microscopy is used

Advantages and disadvantages of choosing each

3.2.2 Embedding

1. Trim the fixed tissues into appropriate size and shape, and place in embedding cassettes.
2. Dehydrate the samples before embedding into paraffin. Pour the alcohol series into 250 mL bottles as follows: 70% ethanol for 20 min, 80% ethanol twice for 20 min, 96% ethanol three times for 20 min, 100% ethanol three times for 15 min, 50–50% ethanol-benzene twice for 10 min, and benzene twice for 5 min (*see* **Note 7**).
3. Place the samples into prewarmed paraffin (56–58 °C) and leave it overnight.
4. Finally, pour prewarmed paraffin into the embedding molds (on a heating plate at 56 °C), and place the embedded tissues inside the paraffin molds.
5. Place the molds at room temperature until the paraffin is hard and remove the paraffin blocks.

3.2.3 Sectioning

1. Trim paraffin blocks to an optimal surface and include the sample with a small paraffin frame.
2. Cut 5 μm slices. A cutting angle of 15 °C is optimal.

3. Use a brush to place the slice in a 40–45 °C water bath (it will expand and wrinkles will vanish).
4. Fish out swimming paraffin section using glass slides and the brush to position the section.
5. Allow the sections to dry overnight at room temperature.

3.3 General Histology

1. Place the slides in appropriate coplins.
2. Deparaffinize the sections in xylene, twice for 20 min.
3. Rehydrate the sections in an alcohol series as follows: 100% ethanol twice for 10 min, 90% alcohol for 10 min, 80% alcohol for 10 min, 70% alcohol for 10 min, and distilled water for 5 min.
4. For general histology and evaluation of the tissue morphology, the slides can be stained with hematoxylin/eosin. Otherwise continue with the immunohistochemistry procedure for the determination of specific markers of the tissue.

3.4 Standard Immuno-histochemistry

1. Transfer the slides into the 0.3% H_2O_2 solution for 20 min to block endogenous peroxidase activity (*see* **Note 8**).
2. Wash the slides twice with PBS and once with PBS-T for 5 min each (*see* **Note 9**).
3. If required, include an antigen retrieval step to enhance the immunostaining using a water bath or microwave treatment with citric buffer at 97 °C.
4. Wash once in distilled water.

The following incubation steps are performed in a humidified chamber at room temperature.

5. Outline sections with a hydrophobic pen.
6. Block the tissue for unspecific binding sites, incubating the slides with a solution of 10% normal blocking serum prepared from the species in which the secondary antibody has been raised (*see* **Note 10**).
7. Blot the excess blocking solution from sections.
8. Incubate sections overnight with the primary antibody at 4 °C (50 μL each section) (*see* **Note 11**). Positive controls: incubate a section with well-known antibodies for the tissue tested. Negative controls: incubate a section with 10% normal serum.
9. Wash the slides twice in PBS and once in PBS-T for 5 min each.
10. Incubate sections for 60 min with secondary antibody at room temperature.
11. Prepare the avidin-biotin complex (ABC) dilution 30 min before the end of the incubation.

12. Wash the slides twice with PBS and once with PBS-T for 5 min each.
13. Incubate sections for 60 min with Vectastain Elite ABC reagent (or the system you choose) at room temperature.
14. Wash the slides twice with PBS and once with PBS-T for 5 min each.
15. Place the slides into the coplin and incubate them with peroxidase substrate solution and the chromogenic substrate DAB solution until desired stain intensity develops (*see* **Note 12**).
16. Stop the reaction with water.
17. Counterstain with hematoxylin (if the antibody location is not nuclear) for 1 min. Then wash with running water for 5 min.
18. Dehydrate the slides through a graded series of alcohols as follows: 70% alcohol for 10 min, 80% alcohol for 10 min, 90% alcohol for 10 min, 100% ethanol twice for 10 min, and xylene solvent twice for 20 min.
19. Mount in the synthetic mounting medium using a coverslip.

4 Notes

1. A variety of systems of detection are used for immunohistochemistry. A representative detection kit used in our laboratory is presented.
2. If there is at least a 10–30 min gap between the delivery room and laboratory, a term placenta can be kept on ice (without contact) without additional solutions.
3. When cutting pieces of the placenta, hold it with forceps at the edge without compressing the fragile villous tissue.
4. Way of mounting for freezing: the O.C.T. (optimal cutting temperature) compound is a matrix for cryostat sectioning at temperatures of −10 °C and below. The dissected tissue can be frozen between −20 °C and −80 °C.
5. Fixation in formalin solution requires a minimal diffusion distance of the fixative. Therefore, samples obtained from the placenta should have a maximal width of 5 mm. Other sizes may be chosen, but keep in mind that fixation of the samples is performed with embedding cassettes. This will restrict the size of the samples to about 3 × 1–2 × 0.5 mm.
6. The fixation time of all the tissues in a same experiment should be the same.
7. The time for the alcohol series has to be adapted depending on the volume of the samples.

8. Incubation with a 3% H_2O_2 solution is also possible and requires only 5–10 min. The H_2O_2 solution should always be prepared and used fresh.
9. PBS and PBS-T buffers are used in all steps, but other buffers such as Tris buffer solution (TBS) and Tris buffer solution-Tween (TBS-T) may be used.
10. Otherwise, use another blocking solution: 2% BSA in 0.2% PBS-T or 5% nonfat milk in 0.2% PBS-T if the host of the secondary antibody is goat.
11. These are the conditions for the antibodies used in our lab. However, for some primary antibodies, an incubation time of 60 min at room temperature is sufficient to result in a clear staining with low background. Changes of the times and temperature may be necessary depending on the antibody.
12. Two chromogens are classically used in immunohistochemistry: aminoethyl carbazole (AEC) and DAB. However, other substrates or fluorochromes can be used. AEC produces an insoluble product that is red, whereas DAB produces a brown water-insoluble end product.

Acknowledgments

This work was partly supported by the Agencia Nacional de Promoción Científica y Tecnológica de Argentina (PICT 2014-0411).

References

1. Huppertz B (2006) Molecular markers for human placental investigation. In: Soares MHJ (ed) Placenta and trophoblast. Methods and protocols. Human Press, Totowa, NJ, pp 337–350
2. Cross JC (2000) Genetic insights into trophoblast differentiation and placental morphogenesis. Semin Cell Dev Biol 11(2):105–113
3. Newhouse SM, Davidge ST, Winkler-Lowen B, Demianczuk N, Guilbert LJ (2007) In vitro differentiation of villous trophoblasts from pregnancies complicated by intrauterine growth restriction with and without preeclampsia. Placenta 28(10):999–1003
4. Soma H, Yoshida K, Mukaida T, Tabuchi Y (1982) Morphologic changes in the hypertensive placenta. Contrib Gynecol Obstet 9:58–75
5. Ishihara N, Matsuo H, Murakoshi H, Laoag-Fernandez JB, Samoto T, Maruo T (2002) Increased apoptosis in the syncytiotrophoblast in human term placentas complicated by either preeclampsia or intrauterine growth retardation. Am J Obstet Gynecol 186(1):158–166
6. Burton GJ, Jones CJ (2009) Syncytial knots, sprouts, apoptosis, and trophoblast deportation from the human placenta. Taiwan J Obstet Gynecol 48(1):28–37
7. Frank HG, Morrish DW, Potgens A, Genbacev O, Kumpel B, Caniggia I (2001) Cell culture models of human trophoblast: primary culture of trophoblast--a workshop report. Placenta 22(Suppl A):S107–S109. https://doi.org/10.1053/plac.2001.0644
8. Mi S, Lee X, Li X, Veldman GM, Finnerty H, Racie L, LaVallie E, Tang XY, Edouard P, Howes S, Keith JC Jr, McCoy JM (2000) Syncytin is a captive retroviral envelope protein involved in human placental morphogenesis. Nature 403(6771):785–789
9. Leitner K, Szlauer R, Ellinger I, Ellinger A, Zimmer KP, Fuchs R (2001) Placental alkaline

phosphatase expression at the apical and basal plasma membrane in term villous trophoblasts. J Histochem Cytochem 49(9):1155–1164

10. Potgens AJ, Bolte M, Huppertz B, Kaufmann P, Frank HG (2001) Human trophoblast contains an intracellular protein reactive with an antibody against CD133--a novel marker for trophoblast. Placenta 22(7):639–645. https://doi.org/10.1053/plac.2001.0701
11. Vuorela P, Hatva E, Lymboussaki A, Kaipainen A, Joukov V, Persico MG, Alitalo K, Halmesmaki E (1997) Expression of vascular endothelial growth factor and placenta growth factor in human placenta. Biol Reprod 56(2): 489–494
12. Peleg D, Peleg A, Shalev E (2000) Immunodetection of living trophoblast. Isr Med Assoc J 2(11):821–822
13. Than NG, Romero R, Goodman M, Weckle A, Xing J, Dong Z, Xu Y, Tarquini F, Szilagyi A, Gal P, Hou Z, Tarca AL, Kim CJ, Kim JS, Haidarian S, Uddin M, Bohn H, Benirschke K, Santolaya-Forgas J, Grossman LI, Erez O, Hassan SS, Zavodszky P, Papp Z, Wildman DE (2009) A primate subfamily of galectins expressed at the maternal-fetal interface that promote immune cell death. Proc Natl Acad Sci U S A 106(24):9731–9736. https://doi.org/10.1073/pnas.0903568106
14. Potgens AJ, Kataoka H, Ferstl S, Frank HG, Kaufmann P (2003) A positive immunoselection method to isolate villous cytotrophoblast cells from first trimester and term placenta to high purity. Placenta 24(4):412–423
15. Tarrade A, Schoonjans K, Guibourdenche J, Bidart JM, Vidaud M, Auwerx J, Rochette-Egly C, Evain-Brion D (2001) PPAR gamma/RXR alpha heterodimers are involved in human CG beta synthesis and human trophoblast differentiation. Endocrinology 142(10): 4504–4514
16. Baczyk D, Drewlo S, Proctor L, Dunk C, Lye S, Kingdom J (2009) Glial cell missing-1 transcription factor is required for the differentiation of the human trophoblast. Cell Death Differ 16(5):719–727. https://doi.org/10.1038/cdd.2009.1
17. MacCalman CD, Furth EE, Omigbodun A, Bronner M, Coutifaris C, Strauss JF III (1996) Regulated expression of cadherin-11 in human epithelial cells: a role for cadherin-11 in trophoblast-endometrium interactions? Dev Dyn 206(2):201–211
18. Kohnen G, Kertschanska S, Demir R, Kaufmann P (1996) Placental villous stroma as a model system for myofibroblast differentiation. Histochem Cell Biol 105(6):415–429
19. Kohnen G, Castellucci M, Hsi BL, Yeh CJ, Kaufmann P (1995) The monoclonal antibody GB 42--a useful marker for the differentiation of myofibroblasts. Cell Tissue Res 281(2): 231–242
20. Demir R, Kayisli UA, Seval Y, Celik-Ozenci C, Korgun ET, Demir-Weusten AY, Huppertz B (2004) Sequential expression of VEGF and its receptors in human placental villi during very early pregnancy: differences between placental vasculogenesis and angiogenesis. Placenta 25(6):560–572. https://doi.org/10.1016/j.placenta.2003.11.011
21. Lyden TW, Anderson CL, Robinson JM (2002) The endothelium but not the syncytiotrophoblast of human placenta expresses caveolae. Placenta 23(8-9):640–652
22. Lang I, Pabst MA, Hiden U, Blaschitz A, Dohr G, Hahn T, Desoye G (2003) Heterogeneity of microvascular endothelial cells isolated from human term placenta and macrovascular umbilical vein endothelial cells. Eur J Cell Biol 82(4):163–173
23. Fina L, Molgaard HV, Robertson D, Bradley NJ, Monaghan P, Delia D, Sutherland DR, Baker MA, Greaves MF (1990) Expression of the CD34 gene in vascular endothelial cells. Blood 75(12):2417–2426
24. Wetzka B, Clark DE, Charnock-Jones DS, Zahradnik HP, Smith SK (1997) Isolation of macrophages (Hofbauer cells) from human term placenta and their prostaglandin E2 and thromboxane production. Hum Reprod 12(4): 847–852
25. Kurtoglu E, Altunkaynak BZ, Aydin I, Ozdemir AZ, Altun G, Kokcu A, Kaplan S (2015) Role of vascular endothelial growth factor and placental growth factor expression on placenta structure in pre-eclamptic pregnancy. J Obstet Gynaecol Res 41(10):1533–1540
26. Lyall F, Young A, Boswell F, Kingdom JC, Greer IA (1997) Placental expression of vascular endothelial growth factor in placentae from pregnancies complicated by pre-eclampsia and intrauterine growth restriction does not support placental hypoxia at delivery. Placenta 18(4):269–276
27. Akercan F, Cirpan T, Terek MC, Ozcakir HT, Giray G, Sagol S, Karadadas N (2008) The immunohistochemical evaluation of VEGF in placenta biopsies of pregnancies complicated by preeclampsia. Arch Gynecol Obstet 277(2):109–114
28. Than NG, Balogh A, Romero R, Karpati E, Erez O, Szilagyi A, Kovalszky I, Sammar M, Gizurarson S, Matko J, Zavodszky P, Papp Z, Meiri H (2014) Placental protein 13 (PP13) - a placental immunoregulatory galectin protecting pregnancy. Front Immunol 5:348
29. Otto T, Gellhaus A, Luschen N, Scheidler J, Bendix I, Dunk C, Wolf N, Lennartz K,

Koninger A, Schmidt M, Kimmig R, Fandrey J, Winterhager E (2015) Oxygen sensitivity of placental trophoblast connexins 43 and 46: a role in preeclampsia? J Cell Biochem 116(12):2924–2937

30. Li HW, Cheung AN, Tsao SW, Cheung AL, WS O (2003) Expression of e-cadherin and beta-catenin in trophoblastic tissue in normal and pathological pregnancies. Int J Gynecol Pathol 22(1):63–70
31. Chen CP, Chen CY, Yang YC, TH S, Chen H (2004) Decreased placental GCM1 (glial cells missing) gene expression in pre-eclampsia. Placenta 25(5):413–421
32. Zhuang XW, Li J, Brost BC, Xia XY, Chen HB, Wang CX, Jiang SW (2014) Decreased expression and altered methylation of syncytin-1 gene in human placentas associated with preeclampsia. Curr Pharm Des 20(11):1796–1802
33. Roland CS, Hu J, Ren CE, Chen H, Li J, Varvoutis MS, Leaphart LW, Byck DB, Zhu X, Jiang SW (2016) Morphological changes of placental syncytium and their implications for the pathogenesis of preeclampsia. Cell Mol Life Sci 73(2):365–376
34. Vargas A, Toufaily C, LeBellego F, Rassart E, Lafond J, Barbeau B (2011) Reduced expression of both syncytin 1 and syncytin 2 correlates with severity of preeclampsia. Reprod Sci 18(11):1085–1091
35. Myatt L, Rosenfield RB, Eis AL, Brockman DE, Greer I, Lyall F (1996) Nitrotyrosine residues in placenta. Evidence of peroxynitrite formation and action. Hypertension 28(3):488–493

Chapter 16

Using a Next-Generation Sequencing Approach to Profile MicroRNAs from Human Origin

Dominic Guanzon, Juvita Delancy Iljas, Gregory E. Rice, and Carlos Salomon

Abstract

Next-generation sequencing is a powerful method to interrogate the nucleotide composition for millions of DNA strands simultaneously. This technology can be utilized to profile microRNAs from multiple origins, such as tissues, cells, and body fluids. Next-generation sequencing is increasingly becoming a common and readily available technique for all laboratories. However, the bottleneck for next-generation sequencing is not within the laboratory but with the bioinformatics and data analysis of next-generation sequencing data. This chapter briefly describes the methods used to prepare samples for next-generation sequencing within the laboratory, before a deeper description of the methods used for data analysis.

Key words Next-generation sequencing, MicroRNA, Bioinformatics, Data analysis

1 Introduction

Within the past 10 years, there has been a steady increase in the development and utilization of next-generation sequencing (NGS) technologies within the laboratory [1]. In 2005, NGS was introduced into the market, which allowed researchers to economically, rapidly, and efficiently sequence whole genomes and transcriptomes [2]. There are two main competitors in the NGS field: Life Technologies which uses semiconductor technology and Illumina with their sequencing-by-synthesis chemistry using fluorescently labeled nucleotides [3, 4]. This chapter utilizes Illumina sequencing technology, which is based on the detection of fluorescently labeled nucleotides during DNA strand synthesis [3]. The labeled nucleotides also contain a reversible terminator which does not allow the next nucleotide to bind until the terminator is removed. Subsequently, the detection of the fluorescent signal which is unique for each A, T, C, and G nucleotide is performed, before terminator removal that allows the next nucleotide to be incorporated [3]. The specific Illumina sequencing platform we

Padma Murthi and Cathy Vaillancourt (eds.), *Preeclampsia: Methods and Protocols*, Methods in Molecular Biology, vol. 1710, https://doi.org/10.1007/978-1-4939-7498-6_16,

utilized is the NextSeq 500 coupled with the high-output flow cell (75 cycles), which has the capacity to generate up to 400 million single end reads [3].

This chapter will focus on the application of NGS technology to profile microRNAs (miRNAs), which falls under the term of small RNA sequencing. MiRNAs are small noncoding RNAs (approximately 22 nucleotides in length) that epigenetically regulate gene expression at the translational level [5]. It is hypothesized that miRNAs play a role in the pathology of preeclampsia [6, 7]. Furthermore, miRNAs are of particular interest as circulating biomarkers, due to their high stability in body fluids [8]. Therefore, identification of miRNAs and understanding its involvement in pathology can be valuable for diagnostic and therapeutic approaches. NGS can be used as a powerful tool to profile and identify candidate miRNAs in these pathologies [9, 10]. Furthermore, NGS is readily becoming an easily accessible and common technique within the laboratory. However, NGS generates large amounts of data which biomedical researchers struggle to analyze and interpret, becoming a bottleneck for biomedical research [11]. Therefore, this chapter will describe the methods used to analyze small RNA NGS data, with particular emphasis on miRNAs.

2 Materials

2.1 Reagents and Equipment Required for NGS

1. TruSeq small RNA library preparation kit.
2. NextSeq 500 high-output kit.
3. T4 RNA Ligase 2, Deletion Mutant (200 U/μL) (Epicentre).
4. SuperScript II Reverse Transcriptase.
5. 5× Novex TBE running Buffer.
6. Novex TBE Gels, 6%, 10 well.
7. 5× Novex Hi-Density TBE Sample Buffer.
8. SYBR® Gold Nucleic Acid Gel Stain (10,000× Concentrate in DMSO).
9. Illumina NextSeq 500 NGS platform.
10. Thermal cycler.

2.2 Software Required

1. TagCleaner program (version 0.16).
2. FASTX-Toolkit program (version 0.0.13).
3. miRDeep2 program (version 2.0.0.7).
4. R software (version 3.2.2).
5. DESeq2 package (version 1.10.1).
6. gplots package (version 2.17.0).

7. Cytoscape (version 3.4.0).
8. CyTargetLinker (version 3.0.1).
9. BiNGO (version 3.0.2).

3 Methods

3.1 Library Preparation for Next-Generation Sequencing

The Illumina NextSeq 500 NGS platform was utilized to profile miRNAs within our RNA samples. A library must first be generated in order to sequence a sample. This is achieved using the TruSeq small RNA library preparation kit from Illumina. Small RNA libraries were prepared following the manufacturer's protocol for this kit. This protocol and slight modifications will be briefly mentioned below:

1. Dilute RNA libraries to 1 μg/5 μL (for total RNA) or 50 ng/5 μL (for purified small RNA) in nuclease free water (*see* **Note 1**).
2. Ligate the 3′ and 5′ adaptors, and then perform reverse transcription according to the manufacturer's kit protocol.
3. Amplify the complimentary DNA (cDNA) using PCR. For this reaction, make a master solution with ultrapure water and RP1 (RNA PCR Primer) only (*see* **Note 2**). Pipette this master solution into each cDNA sample tube, followed by the PML (PCR mix) solution (25 μL), and finally the index adaptors into each cDNA sample tube (*see* **Note 3**). This PCR amplified product is now referred to as the small RNA library.
4. Pool small RNA libraries together (total volume = 50 μL) and mix with 10 μL of Novex® Hi-Density TBE Sample Buffer (*see* **Note 4**). Load this mixture into two lanes of a Novex 6% TBE 10-well gel, flanked by CRL (custom RNA ladder) and HRL (high-resolution ladder) DNA ladders. Run this gel at 145 V for 60 min at 4 °C, until the blue dye exits the gel.
5. Stain this gel with SYBR gold solution (1× concentration in 50 mL TBE running buffer). Visualize this gel using a UV trans-illuminator, and excise small RNAs using a razor blade (Fig. 1).
6. Fragment the gel pieces using a gel breaker tube into a 2 mL tube. Add 200 μL of ultrapure water to this tube, and elute the pooled small RNA library overnight with shaking.
7. Separate the liquid (containing the pooled small RNA library) from the gel pieces using a 5 μm filter tube.
8. Dilute the pooled small RNA library, and load onto a high-output flow cell (75 cycles) following the manufacturer's protocol specified in the NextSeq 500 high-output kit.
9. Sequence small RNA library using the Illumina NextSeq 500 platform, according to the manufacturer's protocol.

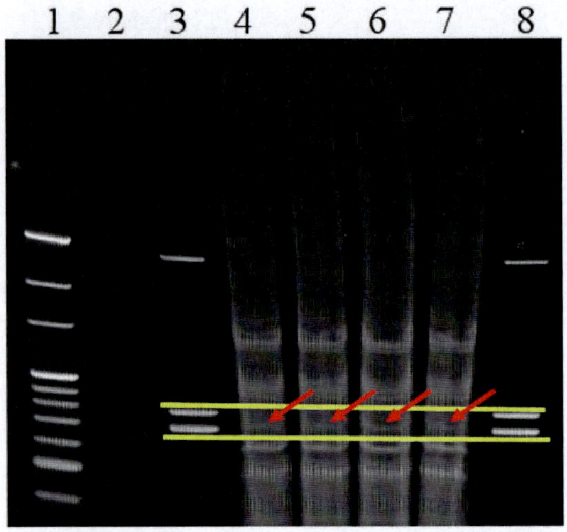

Fig. 1 Gel electrophoresis of pooled small RNA libraries. Gel electrophoresis of pooled small RNA libraries were stained with SYBR gold and visualized using the Bio-Rad gel doc system under UV. Typically, only two lanes (25 μL each) of pooled small RNA libraries are flanked by the CRL, instead of the four lanes showed in this gel. The *red arrows* indicate the band containing miRNAs. The *yellow lines* indicate where we cut the gel, and the region between these lines excised. This region was trimmed to remove excess gel that did not stain for DNA, before further downstream processing. *Lane 1* = HRL (high-resolution ladder), *Lane 2* = empty, *Lane 3* = CRL (custom RNA ladder), *Lane 4–7* = pooled small RNA libraries, and *Lane 8* = CRL

3.2 Pre-processing FASTQ Data Files

After sequencing, a FASTQ file is generated. This file has to be further processed to remove index and adaptor sequences (Fig. 2) and trimmed to 28 nucleotides. This can be achieved using the programs TagCleaner and FASTX-Toolkit, respectively [12]. If a FASTQ file is not properly processed, these artificial sequences will interfere with further downstream miRNA identification.

1. Download and install the TagCleaner program (version 0.16) (http://tagcleaner.sourceforge.net/index.html).
2. Remove adaptors using the TagCleaner program. Removal of adaptor sequences would typically result in a read distribution as seen in Fig. 3. An example of the command we ran to remove adaptors from our sequences is shown below (*see* **Note 5**):

```
tagcleaner -verbose -64 -fastq Input_file.fastq
-info -tag3
TGGAATTCTCGGGTGCCAAGG -trim_within 76 -mm3 3
-cont -log Processing.log -out Output_file.
fastq
```

3. Download and install the FASTX-Toolkit program (version 0.0.13) (http://hannonlab.cshl.edu/fastx_toolkit/index.html).

@NS500334:80:HKMG3BGXY:1:11101:21990:1056 1:N:0:TGACCA

CCACGNTCCCGTGG**<u>TGGAATTCTCGGGTGCCAAGGAACTCCAGTCACTGACCAATCTCGTATGCCGTCTTCTGCTT</u>**

+

AAAAA#EEEEEEEEEEEEEEEEEEEEEEEEEEEEEEEEEEEEEEEEEEEEEEEAEEEEEEEEEEEEEEEEEEEEEE

Fig. 2 Layout of a FASTQ file. A FASTQ is a text file format which has four repeating lines. The first line is a sequence identifier with an optional description, the second line is the raw sequence, the third line is for additional information (optional), and the fourth line is the quality score for each nucleotide in the raw sequence. The *bold* and *underlined* region is the artificial sequence (adaptors), while the text in *red* is the unique index for the sample

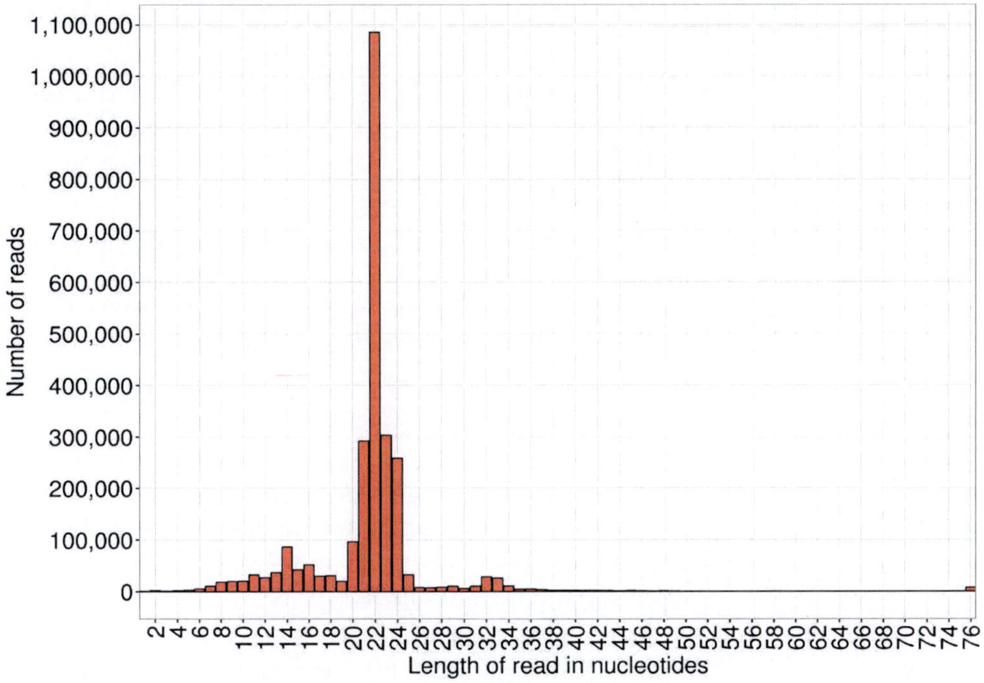

Fig. 3 Read distribution after removal of adaptor sequences. An example of the read distribution after removal of adaptor sequences. The largest peak is at 22 nucleotides, which is normally distributed between 19 and 25 nucleotides. This region contains miRNAs, which are approximately 22 nucleotides in length

4. Trim sequences to 28 nucleotides using the FASTX-Toolkit. An example of the command we ran to achieve this is shown below (*see* **Note 6**):

```
fastx_trimmer -Q33 -v -f 1 -l 28 -i Input_file.
fastq -o Output_file.fastq
```

3.3 Identification of miRNAs

Subsequently, the processed file from Subheading 3.2 is analyzed to identify miRNAs using the program miRDeep2 [13]. A more detailed and useful tutorial can be found here [14]. This section will explain how we use miRDeep2:

1. Download and install the miRDeep2 program (version 2.0.0.7) (https://www.mdc-berlin.de/8551903/en/).

2. Download the databases required from the following sources:

The human genome (hg19) indexed by Bowtie: (http://bowtie-bio.sourceforge.net/index.shtml).

miRNA databases "hairpin.fa" and "mature.fa": (http://www.mirbase.org/index.shtml).

3. Extract human mature and hairpin miRNAs (from mature.fa and hairpin.fa databases) using miRDeep2 and the following commands:

```
extract_miRNAs.pl mature.fa hsa mature > ma-
ture_hsa.fa
extract_miRNAs.pl hairpin.fa hsa > hairpin_
hsa.fa
```

4. Use the mapper module in miRDeep2 to align our sequences to the human genome, using the following command (*see* **Note 7**):

```
mapper.pl Input_file.fastq -e -h -l 16 -m -p
hg19 -q -s reads_file.fa -t reads_genome.arf
```

5. Quantify miRNAs using quantifier module in miRDeep2, using the following command (*see* **Note 8**):

```
quantifier.pl -m mature_hsa.fa -p hairpin_hsa.
fa -t hsa -y now -r reads_file.fa
```

6. The quantifier module generates an expression HTML file which can be opened with your internet browser. This file contains a summary of miRNAs and their counts identified for each sample. Clicking on the miRNA link will open a PDF file, an example shown in Fig. 4.
7. Extract raw counts and corresponding miRNAs from the miRBase.mrd data file for each sample. This file is located in the expression_analyses folder generated by miRDeep2. We use a custom in house python script to do this.

3.4 Normalization, Differential Expression, and Statistical Analysis

The miRNA and corresponding raw counts from Subheading 3.3 can be further analyzed using the package DESeq2 [15]. This package will normalize the counts, perform differential expression between control and treatment groups, and perform statistical analysis on these differences to determine statistical significance. A detailed tutorial for DESeq2 is available at the Bioconductor website shown below:

(https://bioconductor.org/packages/release/bioc/html/DESeq2.html)

1. Download and install the R software (version 3.2.2), the DESeq2 package (version 1.10.1), and the gplots package (version 2.17.0).

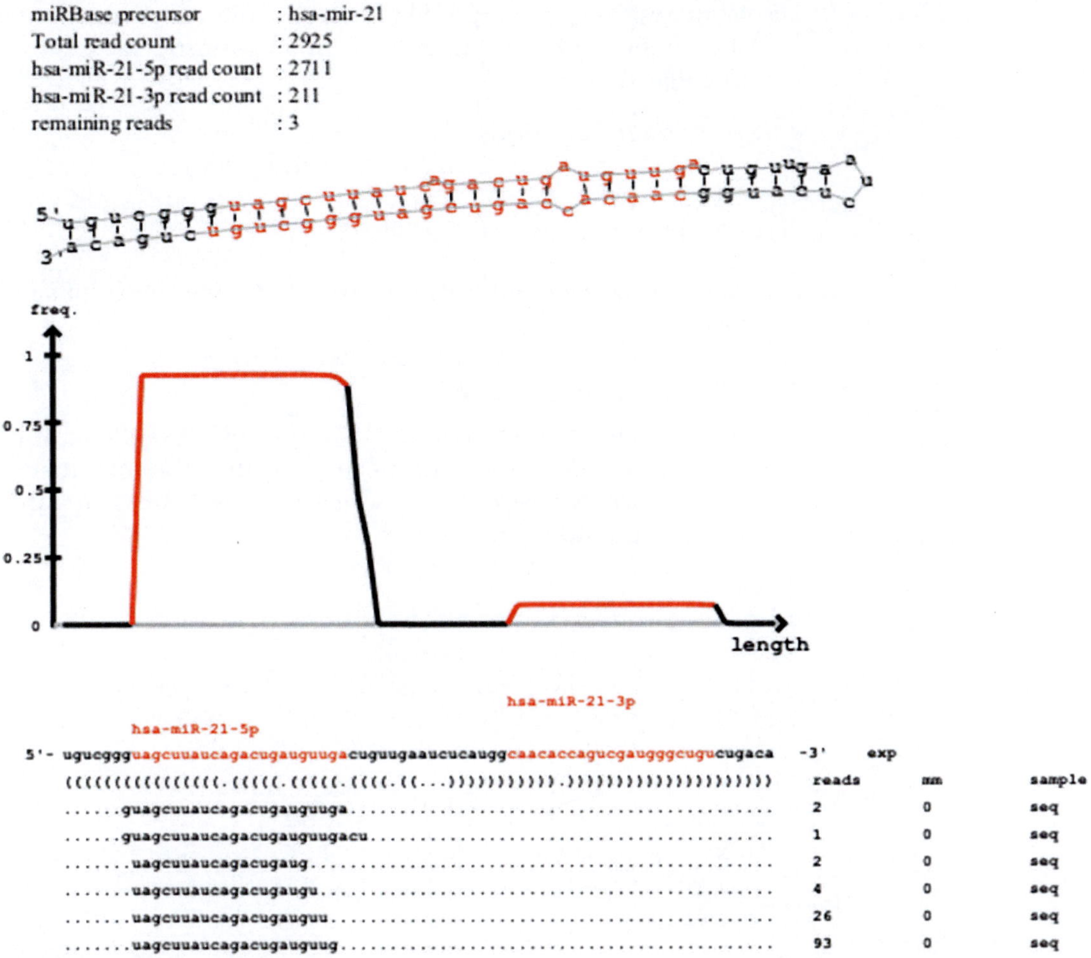

Fig. 4 Example of the PDF output for hsa-miR-21, produced by miRDeep2. This PDF generated by the quantifier module shows the sequences which align to the 5′ and 3′ end of the precursor miRNA for hsa-miR-21. A density plot and the counts for hsa-miR-21-5p and hsa-miR-21-3p are also shown within the PDF

2. Load the library and import Input.csv and Design.csv files, using the commands below (*see* **Note 9**):

```
library(DESeq2)
countData <- read.csv("Input.csv", header = TRUE,
row.names = 1)
colData <- read.csv("Design.csv", header = TRUE,
row.names = 1)
```

3. Construct a DESeqDataSet, using the commands below:

```
dds <- DESeqDataSetFromMatrix(countData =
countData, colData = colData, design = ~ con-
dition)
```

4. Perform normalization, differential expression, and statistics, using the command below:

```
dds <- DESeq(dds)
```

5. Write results to an output file sorted by adjusted *p*-value, using the commands below. An example output statistics file is shown in Table 1:

```
res <- results(dds)
res_for_output <- res[order(res$padj),]
write.csv(as.data.frame(res_for_output),
file="Output_statistics.csv")
```

6. The normalized counts can be exported using the commands below:

```
write.csv((counts(dds, normalized = TRUE)),
file="Count_data.csv")
```

7. A heatmap can be created using miRNAs selected by increasing statistical significance, using the commands below (*see* **Note 10**). This heatmap will be generated using the gplots package:

```
library(gplots)
rld <- rlogTransformation(dds, blind = TRUE)
select2 <- order(res$padj)[1:6]
png("P_value_log.png", width = 8.3, height =
11.7, units = "in", res = 300)
heatmap.2(assay(rld)[select2,],
col=rev(redgreen(75)), trace="none",
margin=c(45,20), scale = "none",
dendrogram="both", cexCol= (1), cexRow= (1),
density.info="none", lhei = c(0.1, 0.8))
dev.off()
```

Table 1
The layout for the Output_statistics.csv file

	baseMean	log2FoldChange	lfcSE	stat	*p*-value	padj
hsa-miR-100-3p	5.196513	1.253012	0.646877	1.937019	0.052743	0.131858
hsa-miR-100-5p	3487.186	1.120397	0.533381	2.100558	0.03568	0.131858
hsa-miR-1-1-3p	9.540297	−0.23907	0.556833	−0.42933	0.667682	0.834602
hsa-miR-1-2-3p	10.05194	−0.258	0.552325	−0.46711	0.640423	0.834602
hsa-miR-101-1-3p	2189.641	0.011113	0.486653	0.022835	0.981782	0.981782
hsa-miR-1-1-5p	0	NA	NA	NA	NA	NA

The layout of the results file produced by DESeq2. The column baseMean is the average of miRNA-normalized counts across all samples. The column log2FoldChange is the log 2 fold change observed, using the "control" as reference and comparing to the "treatment" condition (within the Design.csv file). The lfcSE is the standard error of log 2 fold change, while stat is the calculated Wald statistic. The columns *p*-value and padj are *p*-value and adjusted *p*-value, respectively

3.5 Identifying miRNA-Regulated Genes and Gene Ontology Pathway Analysis

Candidate miRNAs can subsequently be analyzed to identify their target genes and associated gene ontology pathways. For the purposes of this tutorial, hsa-miR-21-5p, hsa-miR-126-3p, and hsa-miR-20a-5p will be analyzed, which are miRNAs involved in preeclampsia [16]. Identifying genes regulated by these miRNAs can be achieved using the CyTargetLinker application in Cytoscape [17]. Furthermore, gene ontology analysis can be performed on these target genes, using the Cytoscape application BiNGO [18]. A detailed tutorial for using both CyTargetLinker and BiNGO can be found below:(http://apps.cytoscape.org/apps/cytargetlinker) (http://apps.cytoscape.org/apps/bingo)

1. Download and install Cytoscape (version 3.4.0) and the applications CyTargetLinker (version 3.0.1) and BiNGO (version 3.0.2).
2. Download the databases for CyTargetLinker from the following sources:

   RegINs database: (http://projects.bigcat.unimaas.nl/cytargetlinker/regins/)
3. Download the databases for BiNGO from the following sources:

   Gene annotation: (http://geneontology.org/page/download-annotations)

   Gene ontology: (http://geneontology.org/page/download-ontology)
4. Import the input file containing miRNAs using the instructions below (*see* **Note 11**):

   Go to File → Import → Network → File; Select microRNA as the source node and press Ok.
5. Create the microRNA regulatory gene network using the instructions below. An example of this regulatory gene network can be seen in Fig. 5:

   Go to Apps → CyTargetLinker → Extend Network; In the Directory containing RegINs option, click the browse button, and select the directory with previously downloaded RegIN databases; In the Settings option, select "Add targets" and press Ok; In the pop-up window, select the RegIN databases microcosm, mirtarbase, and targetscan, then press Ok.
6. Genes regulated by candidate miRNAs can be narrowed down, by selecting for genes shared between two or more databases. This can be achieved using the instructions below:

   Go to CyTargetLinker tab in the Control Panel; Change the Overlap threshold, which means the number of databases for which a gene should be shared.
7. A gene ontology network can be constructed on identified genes, using the BiNGO application. An example of this regulatory network can be seen in Fig. 6. Follow the instructions below to create this network:

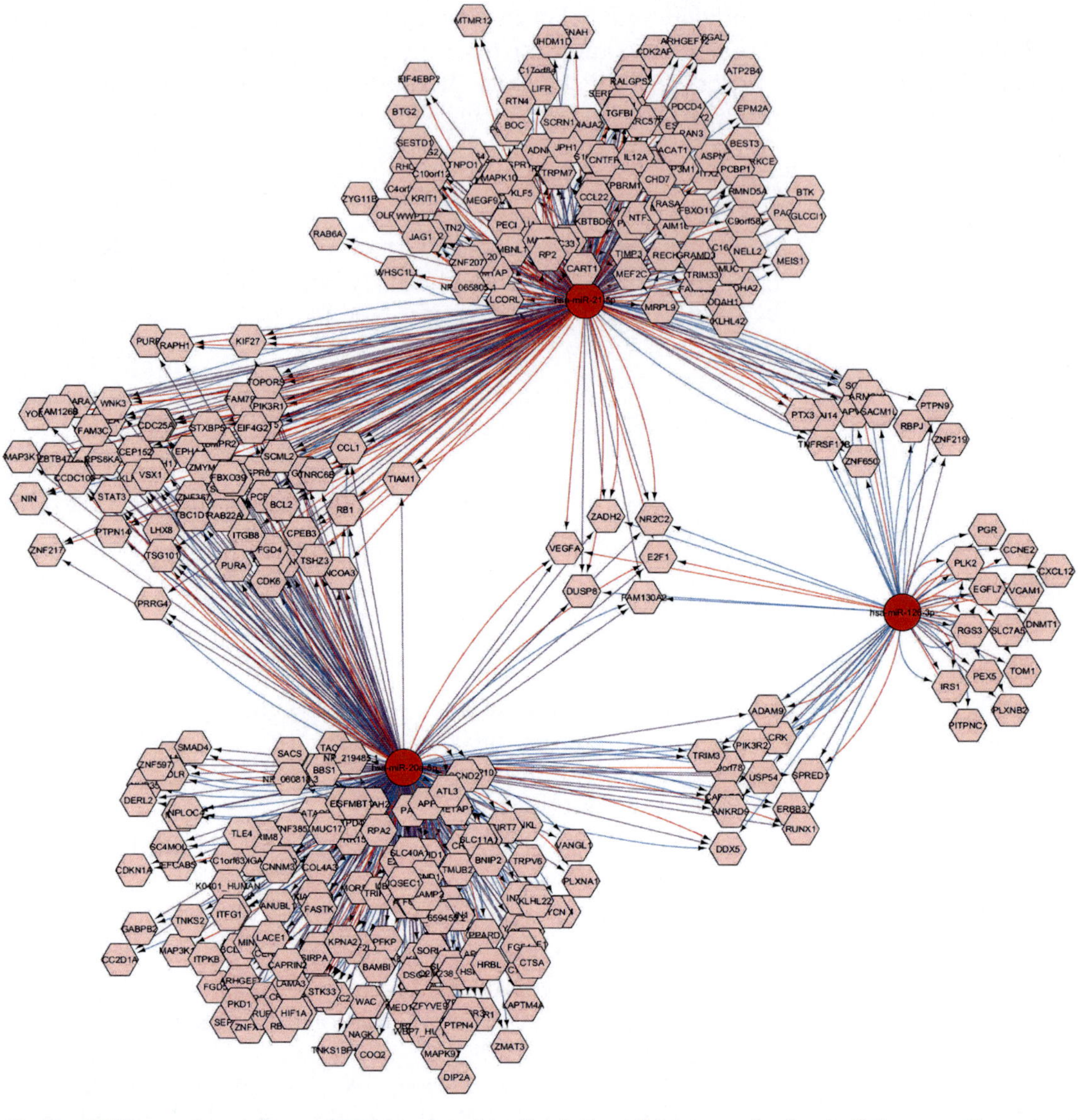

Fig. 5 miRNA-gene regulatory network produced by the CyTargetLinker application in Cytoscape. Example of a miRNA-gene regulatory network produced by the Cytoscape application CyTargetLinker. This network is for three miRNAs, where genes are shared by at least two or more databases. The *circles in red* are miRNAs, the pink hexagons are gene targets, and the number of *arrows* to the gene indicates the number of databases that share the gene

Select the genes by holding the control button and placing a box over all the genes in the network produced by CyTargetLinker; Go to Apps → BiNGO; In the new window, type a name for the Cluster name option; For the Select ontology file option, press the drop-down arrow and go to Custom. Navigate to the gene ontology file that was previously downloaded,

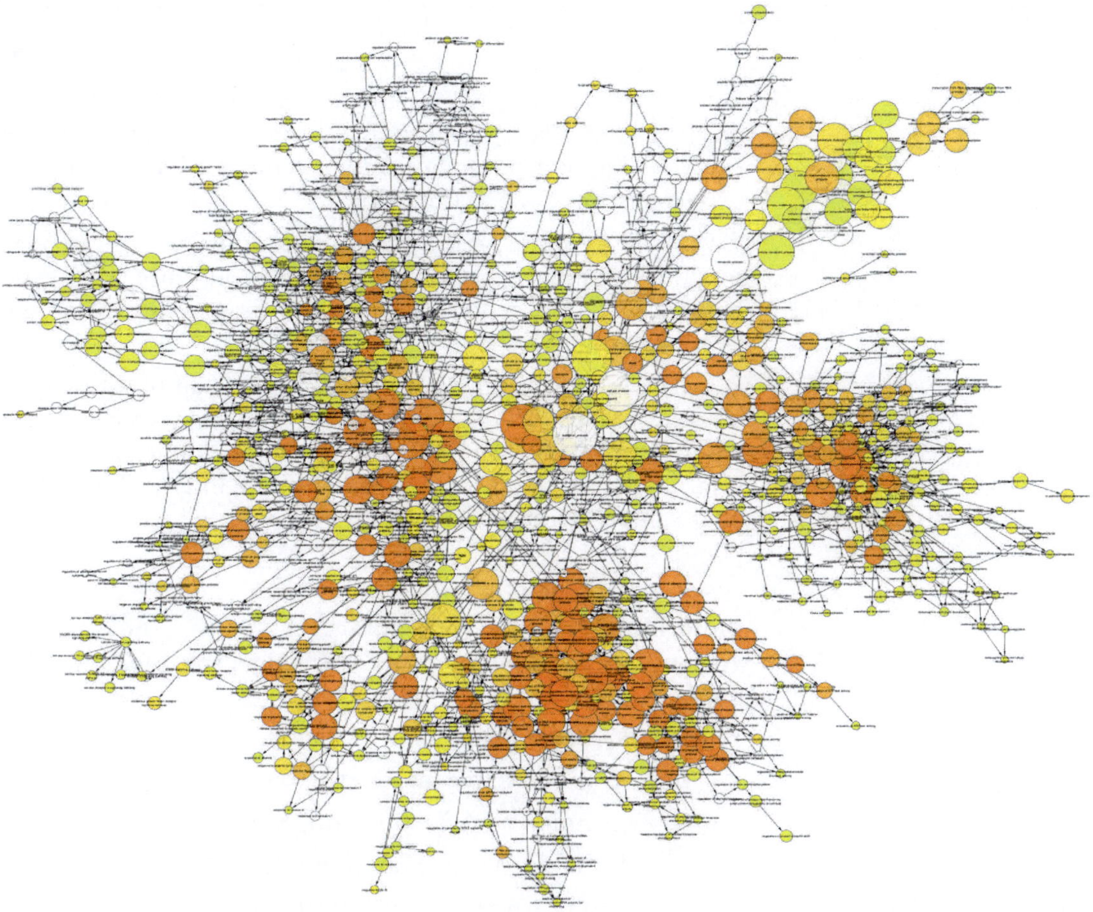

Fig. 6 Gene ontology network produced by the BiNGO application in Cytoscape. Example of the gene ontology network produced by BiNGO, using the genes identified by the CyTargetLinker application in Cytoscape. Each circle represents a gene ontology term, while an increase in the circle size is proportional to the number of genes associated with the gene ontology term. The increase in color from yellow to orange is proportional to increasing significance (*p*-adjusted value <0.05)

select the file, and press Open; For the Select organism/annotation option, press the drop-down arrow and go to Custom. Navigate to the annotation file that was previously download, select the file and press open; Select the box Check box for saving Data, and click on the button named Save BiNGO Data file in. Navigate to the folder you want to save the data, and press Save; Click on the button named Start BiNGO.

8. Gene targets from CyTargetLinker and gene ontology terms from BiNGO can be exported as a table for further analysis. Furthermore, the output file (.bgo) produced by BiNGO can be opened by Excel, which will display additional information about the gene ontology network.

4 Notes

1. We extracted total RNA using the miRNeasy mini kit, while purified small RNA was extracted using the PureLink miRNA isolation kit. We have successfully sequenced RNA samples extracted from both of these kits.
2. The PML (PCR mix) is the limiting solution within the TruSeq small RNA library preparation kit. Do not use 10% extra reagent as the kit recommends for preparing multiple libraries, as you will not have enough PML solution.
3. A single TruSeq small RNA kit can process up to 24 samples but only comes with 12 unique indexes (each index has 10 μL, enough for five reactions). There are 48 unique indexes in total. Make sure you have enough unique indexes for each of your samples (for pooling) before preparing your small RNA libraries.
4. We have pooled up to 24 libraries and successfully sequenced these libraries using the Illumina NextSeq 500 platform. When pooling libraries, make sure they each have a unique index.
5. The options in the command are as follows:
   - verbose (print status messages).
   - 64 (if running a 64-bit operating system).
   - fastq Input_file.fastq (fastq input file).
   - info (additional trimming/splitting information).
   - tag3 TGGAATTCTCGGGTGCCAAGG (trim from three prime end up to and including this sequence region). This adaptor is the sequence used for reverse transcription during library preparation.
   - trim_within 76 (search for the tag3 sequence within the first 76 nucleotides of the three prime end).
   - mm3 3 (allows up to three mismatches when aligning the tag3 sequence to the target sequence).
   - cont (continuously removes tag sequence repeats).
   - log Processing.log (name of the log file).
   - out Output_file.fastq (name of the output file).
6. The reason for trimming to 28 nucleotides is because this is the maximum miRNA length within our database. The options for the command are below:
   - Q33 (tells program to use Sanger encoded quality scores)
   - v (reports number of sequences)
   - -f 1 (keeps the first base)

- l 28 (keeps the 28th base)
- i Input_file.fastq (name of input file which was processed by TagCleaner)
- o Output_file.fastq (name of output file)

7. The options for the command are below:
   - Input_file.fastq (the processed FASTQ file from Subheading 3.2).
   - e (specified the input file is in the FASTQ format).
   - -l 16 (discards the reads shorter than 16 nucleotides). The length of 16 nucleotides was chosen because it is the smallest miRNA length within our database.
   - m (collapses the reads).
   - p hg19 (maps to the reference genome, where the prefix of the file name is hg19).
   - q (maps sequences allowing one mismatch).
   - s reads_file.fa (writes processed reads to this file name).
   - t reads_genome.arf (writes read mappings to this file name).
8. The options for the command are below:
   - m mature_hsa.fa (name of the mature miRBase database file)
   - p hairpin_hsa.fa (name of the hairpin miRBase database file)
   - t hsa (looks for human identifier in the UCSC browser)
   - y now (time stamp for output files)
   - r reads_file.fa (input file with the processed reads created by the miRDeep2 mapper module)
9. Example of Input.csv and Design.csv files is shown in Tables 2 and 3, respectively. Make sure that the order of the samples in the horizontal direction (for Input.csv file) and samples in the vertical direction (for Design.csv file) is the same.
10. For selecting the number of miRNAs displayed on the heatmap, modify the command below:

```
select2 <- order(res$padj)[1:6]; # For 6 miRNAs
select2 <- order(res$padj)[1:3]; # For 3 miRNAs
select2 <- order(res$padj)[1:100]; # For 100
miRNAs etc.
```

Furthermore, the parameters such as margins and text size will have to be adjusted, to make the heatmap presentable. You can modify these parameters in the command below:

```
heatmap.2(assay(rld)[select2,],
col=rev(redgreen(75)), trace="none",
margin=c(45,20), scale = "none",
```

Table 2
Input.csv file layout

MicroRNA	Sample 1	Sample 2	Sample 3	Sample A	Sample B	Sample C
hsa-miR-1-1-3p	4	4	12	12	13	27
hsa-miR-1-1-5p	0	0	0	0	0	0
hsa-miR-1-2-3p	4	5	12	12	13	30
hsa-miR-100-3p	1	0	3	28	8	11
hsa-miR-100-5p	654	1797	476	7363	8285	13640
hsa-miR-101-1-3p	1118	1056	1473	6736	1791	4351

This is the input file used for the DESeq2 package. These miRNA counts were extracted from the miRBase.mrd file produced by the miRDeep2 program

Table 3
Design.csv file layout

	Condition
Sample 1	Control
Sample 2	Control
Sample 3	Control
Sample A	Treatment
Sample B	Treatment
Sample C	Treatment

This is a design file used for the DESeq2 package. This DESeq2 analysis will compare between two groups, a control group and a treatment group

Table 4
Input file used for CyTargetLinker in Cytoscape

MicroRNA
hsa-miR-21-5p
hsa-miR-126-3p
hsa-miR-20a-5p

```
dendrogram="both", cexCol= (1), cexRow= (1),
density.info="none", lhei = c(0.1, 0.8))
```

11. Example of the input file is shown in Table 4. Make sure that the nomenclature for your miRNAs is correct, or the databases will not recognize the miRNAs.

Acknowledgment

CS was in receipt of a Lions Medical Research Foundation Fellowship. This study was supported by the Lions Medical Research Foundation, UQ ECR Award, Royal Brisbane and Women's Foundation, Diabetes Australia, and UQ-Ochsner Seed Grant. The ISO17025 accredited research facility was supported by grants from the Therapeutics Innovation Australia and the National Collaborative Research Infrastructure Strategy.

This review is supported partly by funding from the Lions Medical Research Foundation (LMRF), The University of Queensland, and Fondo Nacional de Desarrollo Científico y Tecnológico (FONDECYT 1170809), Chile.

References

1. Morozova O, Marra MA (2008) Applications of next-generation sequencing technologies in functional genomics. Genomics 92:255–264
2. Cullum R, Alder O, Hoodless PA (2011) The next generation: using new sequencing technologies to analyse gene regulation. Respirology 16:210–222
3. Goodwin S, McPherson JD, McCombie WR (2016) Coming of age: ten years of next-generation sequencing technologies. Nat Rev Genet 17:333–351
4. Pareek CS, Smoczynski R, Tretyn A (2011) Sequencing technologies and genome sequencing. J Appl Genet 52:413–435
5. Moss EG (2002) MicroRNAs: hidden in the genome. Curr Biol 12:R138–R140
6. Murphy MS, Tayade C, Smith GN (2017) Maternal circulating microRNAs and pre-eclampsia: challenges for diagnostic potential. Mol Diagno Ther 21:23
7. Pillar N et al (2015) The possible involvement of microRNAs in preeclampsia and gestational diabetes mellitus. Best Practice and Research. Clin Obstet Gynaecol 29:176–182
8. Brase JC et al (2010) Serum microRNAs as non-invasive biomarkers for cancer. Mol Cancer 9:306
9. Seashols-Williams S et al (2016) High-throughput miRNA sequencing and identification of biomarkers for forensically relevant biological fluids. In: Electrophoresis
10. Gao L, Jiang F (2016) MicroRNA (miRNA) Profiling. Methods Mol Biol 1381:151–161
11. Marx V (2013) Biology: the big challenges of big data. Nature 498:255–260
12. Schmieder R et al (2010) TagCleaner: identification and removal of tag sequences from genomic and metagenomic datasets. BMC Bioinformatics 11:341
13. Friedlander MR et al (2008) Discovering microRNAs from deep sequencing data using miRDeep. Nat Biotechnol 26:407–415
14. Mackowiak SD (2011), Identification of novel and known miRNAs in deep-sequencing data with miRDeep2. Curr Protoc Bioinformatics. Chapter 12: Unit 12.10.
15. Love MI, Huber W, Anders S (2014) Moderated estimation of fold change and dispersion for RNA-seq data with DESeq2. Genome Biol 15:550
16. Escudero CA et al (2016) Role of extracellular vesicles and microRNAs on dysfunctional angiogenesis during preeclamptic pregnancies. Front Physiol 7:98
17. Kutmon M et al (2013) CyTargetLinker: a cytoscape app to integrate regulatory interactions in network analysis. PLoS One 8:e82160
18. Maere S, Heymans K, Kuiper M (2005) BiNGO: a Cytoscape plugin to assess overrepresentation of gene ontology categories in biological networks. Bioinformatics 21:3448–3449

Chapter 17

Isolation and Purification of Villous Cytotrophoblast Cells from Term Human Placenta

Hélène Clabault, Laetitia Laurent, J. Thomas Sanderson, and Cathy Vaillancourt

Abstract

The placenta is a key element during pregnancy for the health of the fetus and the mother, which justifies why placental studies are so important. One of the best models for placental studies is the primary cell culture of cytotrophoblast cells from human term placentas. In this chapter, we will detail firstly the isolation of cytotrophoblast cells, with tissue preparation, digestion, Percoll gradient, and cell freezing, and secondly the cell immunopurification and seeding.

Key words Immunopurification, Percoll gradient, Syncytiotrophoblast, Placenta, Primary cell culture

1 Introduction

There are several models to study the development and functioning of the placenta. Each model, which will be described quickly here, allows studying part of the mechanisms involved. Nevertheless, since the placenta is a very complex organ, none of the below-mentioned models can exactly reflect all the functions of the human placental tissue in vivo. First of all, placental tissues from human or animal models can be fast frozen and then used to evaluate the level of expression of different targets under physiological conditions or also following some treatment or diseases. Unfortunately, this model cannot allow studying the behavior of the cytotrophoblast cells, which is essential for the understanding of the placental functions. Villous explants containing the whole villous structure and cell types are often used to study placental physiology. This model has the advantages of closely matching human placental physiology but is limited for intensive biochemistry and molecular

Hélène Clabault and Laetitia Laurent contributed equally to this work.

Padma Murthi and Cathy Vaillancourt (eds.), *Preeclampsia: Methods and Protocols*, Methods in Molecular Biology, vol. 1710, https://doi.org/10.1007/978-1-4939-7498-6_17,

biology studies. There are also a few trophoblastic cell lines, all derivate from choriocarcinoma, which are commercially available such as BeWo, Jeg-3, and JAR (the latter are derivate from the former), and are commonly used to study human placental functions [1–3]. An inconvenient of these cell lines is the necessity of chemical induction for achieving a differentiation. BeWo cells, which are the most used model, can biochemically and morphologically differentiate following an induction (*e.g.*, forskolin stimulation), which make them good differentiation and fusion models. They have also the ability to form confluent monolayer on permeable support, which allows studying the transplacental transport of drugs [4]. Caution should be used, however, as these lines unlikely reflect in vivo trophoblast function. A recent study showed a very weak correlation between gene expression in human cytotrophoblasts and BeWo cells [5].

Finally, the other way to study the cytotrophoblastic function is to establish a primary cell culture from placenta. The advantage of using placenta is that it represents a large reservoir of materials for isolation of trophoblast cells compared to biopsies, the usual way to obtain human live tissue. Moreover, primary cells are able to syncytialize spontaneously and, as such, allow studying human trophoblast cell fusion, syncytiotrophoblast formation, and regeneration. Taking this into account, we believe that human primary trophoblast culture remains a suitable and robust model for studying placenta.

Concretely, for this manipulation, it is important to consider that it is a relatively long experiment, with significant handling costs. Indeed, it takes approximately 8 h of continuous manipulation after obtaining the placenta and then 3 h for trophoblasts purification. We estimate that the isolation of cytotrophoblast cells from a term human placenta costs about 400 USD (for double preparation) of consumable products such as chemicals and small disposable materials. The most expensive consumables are DNase type IV (130 USD), trypsin (100 USD), and DMEM high glucose (40 USD). For the thawing and the immunomagnetic purification, we estimate 130 USD. The isolation technique requires little work space, ideally a double bench. The necessary equipment is fairly basic (centrifuge, sterile hood). The immunopurification, however, requires an autoMACS® magnetic separator.

In this chapter, we describe the procedure to isolate and purify the cytotrophoblast cells from human term placenta. The procedures, adapted from Kliman et al., are based on enzymatic dissociation of villous placental tissue, followed by gradient centrifugation and immunomagnetic bead purification [6]. All steps are summarized in Table 1; a video is also available on JoVE [7].

Table 1
Summary of isolation, purification, and purity analysis of villous cytotrophoblasts (vCTB) by step

Steps	Proceedings	Succinct descriptions
Isolation		
1	Transportation	– Quick transportation of placenta (≤1 h)
2	Tissue preparation	– Remove fetal and maternal membranes – Mince 30–35 g of tissue after having remove blood vessels
3	Digestion	– Four digestions for 30 min at 37 °C in shaking water bath with HBSS + $CaCl_2$ + $MgSO_4$ + digestive enzymes: trypsin I and DNAse I type IV ± P/S
4	Centrifugation	– Keep supernatant from digestions 2 to 4, put it on FCS – Centrifugation (1250 × *g*, 15 min at RT) – Pellets rinsing with DMEM-P/S
5	Percoll	– Deposit cells on Percoll gradients – Centrifugation without brake (507 × *g*, 30 min, at RT)
6	Centrifugation	– Keep vCTB which are between 1.048 and 1.060 densities – Wash cells in DMEM-P/S – Centrifugation (1250 × *g*, 10 min, at RT)
7	Count	– Pellet resuspension in FBS – Count and cell viability determination
8	Cryofreezing	– Cryofreezing in FBS and 10% DMSO
Purification		
9	Thawing	– Quick thawing frozen cells – Resuspension with autoMACS® running buffer + P/S
10	Count	– Cells count with trypan blue
11	Labeling	– Incubation 30 min with running buffer + anti-HLA-ABC Ab – Wash
12	Immunopurification	– Cells resuspension with magnet microbeads MACS® – vCTB immunopurification
13	Count	– Cells count with trypan blue
14	Seeding	– vCTB seeding after resuspension in culture media (DMEM + HEPES + FBS + P/S)
15	Changing medium	– 4 h after incubation at 37 °C, wash (×2) with medium culture

HBSS Hank's balanced salt solution, *$CaCl_2$* calcium chloride, *$MgSO_4$* magnesium sulfate, *DNAse* deoxyribonuclease, *P/S* penicillin/streptomycin, *FCS* fetal calf serum, *RT* room temperature, *DMEM* Dulbecco's modified eagle medium, *FBS* fetal bovine serum, *DMSO* dimethyl sulfoxide, *Ab* antibody, *HEPES* 2-[4-(2-hydroxyethyl)-1-piperazinyl]ethanesulfonic acid
Adapted from [10] according to the protocol used in our laboratory [7]

2 Materials

2.1 Equipment

The quantities for a double preparation are given in brackets. Note that all surgical equipment should be sterile.

1. autoMACS® columns.
2. autoMACS® magnetic separator.
3. Büchner funnel.
4. Cell strainers 100 μm nylon.
5. Fine-toothed forceps [2].
6. Gauze sponge.
7. 50 mL corex tube [2].
8. Metzenbaum [2] and pointed scissors [2].
9. Peristaltic pump.
10. Pyrex flat (21 × 30 cm).
11. 250 mL sterile trypsinizing flasks [2].
12. Watch glass [2].

2.2 Chemical Products

1. Anti-human HLA ABC purified clone W6/32.
2. Anti-mouse IgG microbeads.
3. autoMACS® running buffer.
4. autoMACS® rinsing solution.
5. 100 mM calcium chloride (store at 4 °C).
6. Culture medium: Dulbecco's modified eagle medium (DMEM) high glucose with 25 mM HEPES, 10% of fetal bovine serum (FBS) (store at 4 °C).
7. Deoxyribonuclease (DNase) type IV.
8. Fetal calf serum (FCS).
9. 10× Hank's buffered salt solution (HBSS) without calcium and magnesium.
10. 800 mM magnesium sulfate (store at 4 °C).
11. Modified HBSS: 1 vial (9.25 g) 1× HBSS without calcium and magnesium, 25 mL 1 M HEPES, pH = 7.4 (store at 4 °C).
12. Penicillin/streptomycin (P/S; 10,000 units/mL penicillin G, 100 mg/mL streptomycin sulfate).
13. Percoll.
14. Saline (NaCl) solution (10 L; 0.9%).
15. Trypsin type I.

3 Methods

3.1 Cell Isolation

3.1.1 Eve or the Day of the Manipulation

1. Weigh the different quantities of trypsin (Table 2), twice for a double preparation, in a plastic weight boat. Label, cover with paraffin, and store them at 4 °C until use.
2. Reconstitute DNase by dissolving 1 vial (100 mg) in 1 mL of modified HBSS. Keep at 4 °C until use.
3. Prepare a 90% Percoll solution: mixing 36 mL of Percoll with 4 mL of 10× HBSS. Prepare Percoll solutions in disposable culture tubes, as written in Table 3 (*see* **Note 1**). Keep at 4 °C until use.
4. Add 4 mL of P/S in 200 mL of DMEM. Keep at 4 °C until use.

3.1.2 Isolation of Trophoblast Cells

Be aware that during the whole process, the placenta and its pieces must be kept in saline buffer.

1. In a water bath at 37 °C, warm two aliquots of 1 mL P/S, eight bottles of modified HBSS for digestions (digestion 1, 2 × 150 mL; digestion 2, 2 × 100 mL; digestion 3, 2 × 75 mL; and digestion 4, 2 × 75 mL), 200 mL of DMEM-P/S, and 50 mL of FCS. For FCS, as soon as thawed, put it at room temperature for acquiring the right density.
2. Following the delivery of the baby, bring the placenta to the laboratory as quickly as possible (≤1 h) in a cold saline buffer (*see* **Note 2**).
3. Dispose of the placental blood in a liquid trash. Weigh the placenta in a pre-weighed flat plastic pot.

Table 2
Quantities for digestion solutions

	Digestion 1	Digestion 2	Digestion 3	Digestion 4
Modified HBSS (mL)	150	100	75	75
$MgSO_4$ (μL)	150	100	75	75
$CaCl_2$ (μL)	150	100	75	75
Trypsine (U)	1,824,000	1,200,000	960,000	960,000
DNase IV (μL) (0.1 mg/μL)	300	200	150	150
P/S (mL)	1	/	/	/

For a double digestion, all solutions have to be prepared twice
HBSS Hank's buffered salt solution, *$MgSO_4$* magnesium sulfate, *$CaCl_2$* calcium chloride, *DNase* deoxyribonuclease, *P/S* penicillin and streptomycin

Table 3
Quantities for Percoll solution

Concentration (%)	70	65	60	55	50	45	40	35	30	25	20	15	10	5
90% Percoll (mL)	2.33	2.17	2.00	1.83	1.67	1.50	1.33	1.17	1.00	0.83	0.67	0.50	0.33	0.17
Modified HBSS (mL)	0.67	0.83	1.00	1.17	1.33	1.50	1.67	1.83	2.00	2.17	2.33	2.50	2.67	2.83

4. Cover the placenta with saline solution.
5. Take note of the following: umbilical cord length, implantation (central or not), placental length, width and form (oval, discoid), membranes color, cotyledons (entire or not), and pathologies.
6. Cut the umbilical cord, by doing a 1 cm diameter circle in the placental cord base. Keep it in formalin if required by the histopathology hospital department.
7. Remove the amnion (thin membrane covering the fetus) and the outer 2 cm of the placenta (this part is too thin and does not contain many trophoblasts).
8. Cut the entire placenta in 5 × 5 cm pieces. Rinse several times (~four times) in saline buffer to remove blood cells. After this step, the liquid should be limpid.
9. Remove fetal (amnion and chorion) and maternal membranes. In a watch glass, mince tissue to remove blood vessels and calcifications using forceps and the back of a Metzenbaum scissors. When a piece of placenta is completely minced, put it in a Büchner funnel under a beaker (*see* **Note 3**). Shed the saline buffer, rinse again, and place it in a weighing boat on ice. Repeat until having 60–70 g of minced tissue for a double preparation (30–35 g for a single preparation).
10. Equally divide the 60–70 g of minced placental tissue in the two trypsinization flasks.
11. Prepare the first digestion solutions with heated modified HBSS, $MgSO_4$, $CaCl_2$, trypsine, DNase and P/S, according to Table 2. Transfer these solutions in the trypsinization flasks.
12. Vigorously mix, before putting the flasks in a shaking water bath for 30 min (50 cycles/min). Mix flasks every 5 min to provide a homogenous digestion (*see* **Note 4**).
13. At the end of the first digestion, remove the flasks from the water bath and put them on a bench at a 45° angle. Decant for about 1 min.
14. With the help of a 10 mL sterile pipette, discard 80 mL of liquid, avoiding any tissue.
15. Prepare the second digestion solution as described in Table 2, put the solution in trypsinization flasks, mix, and incubate 30 min in a water bath, mixing every 5 min (as in **step 12**).
16. At the end of the second digestion, remove the flasks from the water bath and put them on a bench at a 45° angle. Decant for about 1 min. With the help of a 10 mL sterile pipette, withdraw 80 mL of liquid and put it gently on a cell strainer (100 μm nylon) placed on top of a 50 mL tube.

17. Aliquot 13.5 mL of the second digestion collected liquid in 15 mL tubes. With a glass Pasteur pipette, very gently and slowly, add 1.5 mL of FCS at the bottom of tubes. The two liquids must not mix. Centrifuge all tubes at 1250 × *g* without brake at room temperature during 20 min.
18. After the centrifugation, pellets with four layers should be formed from top to bottom: digestion solution, FCS with DNase and trypsin, trophoblast cells, and blood cells. With a vacuum pump, aspirate supernatants, taking care to avoid withdrawing the trophoblasts layer. It is very important to remove the whitish precipitate at the FCS interface, by aspirating along the tube's wall (Fig. 1).
19. Resuspend each pellet with 1 mL of warm DMEM-P/S (flick each tube four or five times). Collect all resuspended cells in two tubes with a Pasteur pipette. Let the tubes stand by at room temperature.
20. Begin layering the Percoll gradient. Take two 50 mL corex tubes, and fix the outflow tubing of the peristaltic pump on each tube. The liquid should flow along the tube wall without forming droplets.

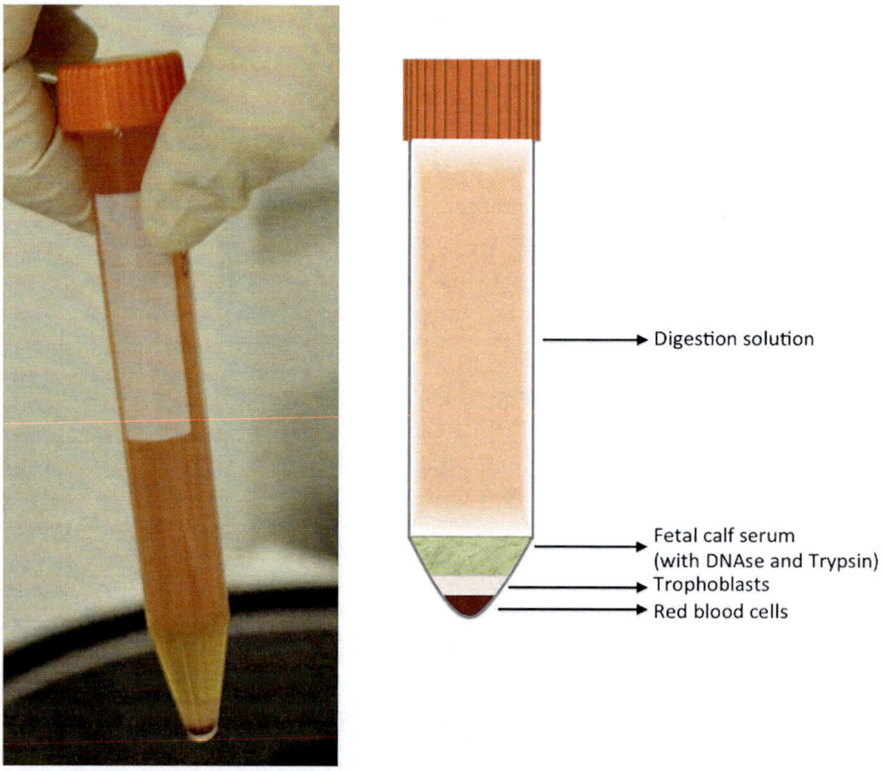

Fig. 1 Digestion tube. After the centrifugation, pellets with four layers should be formed from top to bottom: digestion solution, FCS with DNase and trypsin, trophoblast cells, and blood cells

21. Take the different Percoll solutions previously prepared (as described in Table 3). Layer each Percoll solution, in a decreasing fashion (70–5% concentrations), with a slow peristaltic pump (1 mL/min) (*see* **Note 5**). Vortex each Percoll solution before layering it. Keep at room temperature.
22. At the end of the third and fourth digestions, perform again **steps 16–19**. For the last digestion, collect as much supernatant as possible.
23. Once all digestions are completed, there will be eight tubes with trophoblasts. Fill them to 15 mL with warm DMEM--P/S. Centrifuge at 1250 × *g* with brake, during 10 min at room temperature. Remove the supernatant with the vacuum pump, taking care to avoid aspirating the white pellets.
24. Resuspend each pellet with 1 mL of warm DMEM-P/S by flicking all tubes four or five times each. Collect all liquids in two 15 mL tubes (*see* **Note 6**). It is very important to rinse tubes well, to avoid losing cells. Fill with warm DMEM-P/S, to have two tubes of 8 mL.
25. With a Pasteur pipette, very gently and slowly, take support on the wall of the tube and apply cell suspensions in Percoll gradients. Centrifuge without brake at 507 × *g* during 30 min at room temperature. It is important that the centrifuge is perfectly balanced. Handle the tubes very gently to avoid mixing the gradients.
26. At the end of the centrifugation, move the tubes near the vacuum pump. Place a lamp behind to visualize the bands well. Trophoblasts cells are located between 40% and 50% Percoll concentrations (*see* **Note 7**). With the vacuum pump, take support on the tube wall and remove the top layer up to the trophoblast cells (>50% Percoll concentration). With a Pasteur pipette, take the cells of interest and put them in a 50 mL tube (*see* **Note 8**).
27. Fill the tube to 50 mL with warm DMEM-P/S. Centrifuge with brake at 1250 × *g* during 10 min at room temperature (*see* **Note 9**).

From this step on, work under sterile conditions.

28. Resuspend the pellet with 20 mL of FBS. Keep on ice.
29. Count the cells and determine their viability using trypan blue dye.
30. Add 2.22 mL of sterile DMSO. Mix gently by flicking. Aliquot 1.5 mL of cell suspension into cryogenic vials. Put in freezing container and store at −80 °C for 12–24 h, before putting the vials in a liquid nitrogen tank.

3.2 Cell Purification

3.2.1 Preparation Steps

1. Prepare the autoMACS® by installing the autoMACS® rinsing solution, the autoMACS® running buffer, and a new autoMACS® column in the negative port. Solutions need to be at room temperature for the purification of cells.
2. Perform the "clean program" of the autoMACS®.
3. Clean up the ports, then place three 50 mL tubes identified negative 1, positive 1, and positive 2 under respective ports.
4. Prepare a sterile aliquot of cold running buffer: 50 mL is necessary for 50 million cells. Add 1 mL of P/S in 50 mL of running buffer. Keep solutions on ice.
5. Add 1% of P/S in the culture medium and keep it at 37 °C.

3.2.2 Cell Purification Steps

1. If starting from a frozen stock of villous mononuclear cells, thaw cells quickly in a 37 °C water bath. Transfer the cells into a 50 mL tube and resuspend gently in about 20 mL cold running buffer containing P/S.
2. Centrifuge at 450 × *g* for 5 min at 4 °C.
3. Remove gently the supernatant, then resuspend in 20 mL cold running buffer. Keeping the cells on ice, count the cells and determine their viability using trypan blue dye.
4. Centrifuge again at 450 × *g* for 5 min at 4 °C. Carefully remove the supernatant and then resuspend in 1 mL cold running buffer. Add 10 μL of mouse anti-HLA-ABC.
5. The cell suspension will be viscous; mix well by flicking the tube several times and incubate for 30 min at 4 °C. Mix gently the cells every 5 min.
6. After the incubation, add 6 mL of cold running buffer and centrifuge at 450 × *g* for 5 min at 4 °C.
7. Remove gently and discard the supernatant, resuspend in 6 mL of cold running buffer, and repeat the centrifugation at 450 × *g* for 5 min at 4 °C.
8. After discarding the supernatant, resuspend cells in 900 μL of cold running buffer. Label cells by adding 100 μL anti-mouse IgG microbeads. Incubate for 15 min at 4 °C. Mix gently the cells every 5 min.
9. Following the incubation, wash cells by adding 6 mL of cold running buffer and centrifuge at 450 × *g* for 5 min at 4 °C.
10. Discard the supernatant, then resuspend in 5 mL of cold running buffer.
11. Place the cell suspension under the uptake port and perform the separation program on the autoMACS.
12. Keep the negative fraction, which contains villous trophoblasts, and add 20 mL of cold running buffer. Centrifuge the purified cells at 450 × *g* for 5 min at 4 °C.

13. Remove gently the supernatant, then resuspend in 20 mL of warm culture medium. Keeping the cells at room temperature, count the cells and determine their viability using trypan blue dye (*see* **Note 10**).
14. Seed cells in the warm culture medium:
    (a) 96 wells plate: 150,000 cells/well
    (b) 24 wells plate: 1.6 million cells/well
    (c) 6 wells plate or 35-mm petri dish: 4.5 million cells/well.
15. Incubate at 37 °C and 5% CO_2 for at least 4–6 h, which allows cells to attach to the surface of the plate and then rinse twice with pre-warmed culture medium to remove nonattached cells. Refresh the medium every 24 h.

4 Notes

1. Two layers of Percoll solution can be used. Put 20 mL of 60% Percoll at the bottom of the tube and then, with the peristaltic pump, add 20 mL of 25% Percoll. After centrifugation, trophoblast cells will be at the interface between both layers of the Percoll.
2. Transport buffer (~500 mL/placenta) can be used instead of saline. This buffer is composed of DMEM medium (26.74 g) completed with HEPES (11.916 g), sodium bicarbonate (7.4 g), penicillin (4 mg), gentamicin (100 mg), and amphotericin (10 mg). Dissolve all powders in 2 L of milliQ water, adjust pH at 7, and filter (0.2 μm).
3. Instead of a Büchner funnel to rinse minced placenta with saline solution, it is possible to use gauze sponge or sieve with an appropriate pore size.
4. For a uniform heat transfer, the bath water level should exceed the liquid level in the trypsinization flask.
5. If there is no peristaltic pump in your laboratory, you can flow the Percoll very gently with Pasteur pipettes.
6. It is possible to discard the fourth digestion if the white pellet is very small.
7. Given that trophoblasts cells localization is approximate in the gradient Percoll, it can vary in each experiment.
8. It is possible that it will be difficult to take only trophoblast cells because blood cells are often too close by. If there are blood cells mixed with your trophoblasts, keep going with the experiment. Blood cells will be eliminated during the immunopurification and centrifugation steps realized to wash the cells after freezing. If blood cells are still present even after all these

steps, it is nevertheless possible to seed them and then wash cells carefully several times with warm culture medium at each change of medium.

9. At this point, it is possible not to freeze the trophoblast cells and directly perform the purification. For that, replace the medium by cold running buffer (under sterile conditions), then continue to Subheading 3.2.2 below.
10. To verify cell purity using flow cytometry, keep one million cells (2 × 500,000 cells in two microtubes). Briefly, wash the cells twice with HBSS and then block nonspecific antigen sites with HBSS containing FBS during 30 min at room temperature. Wash once and then stain the positive tube cells with anti-cytokeratin-7 antibody (1.25 μg/million cells) or add HBSS-BSA in the negative tube. After 45 min of incubation at room temperature, wash the cells and proceed with the flow cytometry analysis [8, 9]. A cell preparation is considered to be pure when there is a minimum of 96% of positive cells staining with the anti-cytokeratin-7 antibody.

Acknowledgments

This work was financially supported by the March of Dimes Foundation Social and Behavioral Sciences Research grant (#12-FY12-179; C.V. and J.T.S.) as well as by scholarship awards to H.C. from the "Réseau Québécois en Reproduction-NSERC-CREATE" and the "Fondation Universitaire Armand-Frappier INRS."

References

1. Pattillo RA, Gey GO (1968) The establishment of a cell line of human hormone-synthesizing trophoblastic cells in vitro. Cancer Res 28:1231–1236
2. Kohler PO, Bridson WE (1971) Isolation of hormone-producing clonal lines of human choriocarcinoma. J Clin Endocrinol Metab 32:683–687
3. Hochberg A, Rachmilewitz J, Eldar-Geva T, Salant T, Schneider T, de Groot N (1992) Differentiation of choriocarcinoma cell line (JAr). Cancer Res 52:3713–3717
4. Prouillac C, Lecoeur S (2010) The role of the placenta in fetal exposure to xenobiotics: importance of membrane transporters and human models for transfer studies. Drug Metab Dispos 38:1623–1635
5. Bilban M, Tauber S, Haslinger P, Pollheimer J, Saleh L, Pehamberger H, Wagner O, Knofler M (2010) Trophoblast invasion: assessment of cellular models using gene expression signatures. Placenta 31:989–996
6. Kliman HJ, Nestler JE, Sermasi E, Sanger JM, Strauss JF III (1986) Purification, characterization, and in vitro differentiation of cytotrophoblasts from human term placentae. Endocrinology 118:1567–1582
7. Sagrillo-Fagundes L, Clabault H, Laurent L, Hudon-Thibeault AA, Salustiano EM, Fortier M, Bienvenue-Pariseault J, Wong Yen P, Sanderson JT, Vaillancourt C (2016) Human primary trophoblast cell culture model to study the protective effects of melatonin against hypoxia/reoxygenation-induced disruption. J Vis Exp (113). https://doi.org/10.3791/54228

8. Campbell FM, Bush PG, Veerkamp JH, Dutta-Roy AK (1998) Detection and cellular localization of plasma membrane-associated and cytoplasmic fatty acid-binding proteins in human placenta. Placenta 19:409–415
9. Moreau R, Daoud G, Bernatchez R, Simoneau L, Masse A, Lafond J (2002) Calcium uptake and calcium transporter expression by trophoblast cells from human term placenta. Biochim Biophys Acta 1564:325–332
10. Cervar-Zirkovic M, Stern C (2011) Trophoblast isolation and culture. In: Kay HH, Nelson DM, Wang Y (eds) The placenta: from development to disease. Wiley-Blackwell, London, pp 155–162

Chapter 18

Analyzing Trophoblast Function Using Cell-Based Assays

Katie L. Powell and Anthony W. Ashton

Abstract

Functional cell-based assays are useful for comparing the effect of a treatment, drug, or condition on cells in culture. Cell lines are a commonly used model to replicate a normal biological process or a pathological condition. Trophoblasts within the placenta are required to perform a variety of functions, which include proliferation, differentiation, migration, and invasion for efficient placentation to occur. These functions are impaired in trophoblasts from preeclamptic pregnancies, and therefore functional cell-based assays can be utilized to measure differences and dissect molecular regulatory pathways.

Key words Trophoblasts, Cell lines, Proliferation, Apoptosis, Migration, Invasion, Adhesion

1 Introduction

The healthy growth and development of a fetus is largely attributed to the placenta. Efficient placental development is reliant on trophoblasts, which incorporate undifferentiated cytotrophoblasts and differentiated syncytiotrophoblast performing a number of key functions simultaneously. Cytotrophoblasts are a highly invasive and proliferative cell type that are responsible for anchoring the placenta to the uterus and invading the decidua to remodel maternal spiral arteries to increase blood flow to the placenta. They also fuse to form a large multinucleated layer called the syncytium (syncytiotrophoblast) in floating villi that acts as a barrier between the maternal and fetal circulations. The syncytiotrophoblast is bathed in maternal blood and thereby facilitates the transport of nutrients and oxygen to the placenta and the removal of waste products [1–3].

Preeclampsia is a serious complication of pregnancy that is associated with abnormal placentation [3–5]. It is widely accepted that trophoblast invasion is perturbed in preeclamptic placentae. These trophoblasts only invade the superficial decidua, which limits the remodeling of maternal spiral arteries. The maintenance of high resistance vessels subsequently prevents adequate

Padma Murthi and Cathy Vaillancourt (eds.), *Preeclampsia: Methods and Protocols*, Methods in Molecular Biology, vol. 1710,
https://doi.org/10.1007/978-1-4939-7498-6_18,

uteroplacental perfusion [6, 7]. Studies have also found that preeclamptic placentae have reduced intramural extravillous cytotrophoblasts in myometrial vessels, increased rates of apoptosis, abnormal expression of adhesion molecules by invasive cytotrophoblasts, and increased production of antiangiogenic factors including sFlt-1 and sEng [7–11].

The key processes of trophoblasts (including proliferation, apoptosis, migration, invasion, and adhesion) can all be assessed in vitro using cell culture models. Cell lines including the choriocarcinoma cells BeWo, JEG-3, JAR [12], and HTR-8/SVneo (immortalized first trimester chorionic villus explant) [13] are commonly used for such assays. There are numerous methodologies that can be used to analyze each of these cellular functions. In this chapter, robustly tested and published techniques for analyzing trophoblast function will be described.

2 Materials

2.1 Cell Lines and Culture Conditions

There are many cell lines that are commonly used to study specific aspects of trophoblast biology. Established cell lines are often used in preference to primary trophoblasts as they will continue to proliferate in culture, which is necessary for long-term observational studies and if genetic modification is required for studying the effects of altered gene expression [13, 14]. The choice of cell line is however largely dependent on the cell line's phenotype corresponding to the cellular function that is requiring investigation. A few commonly used cell lines will be briefly described in this section, which may act as a guide as to the type/s of assays they are best suited to.

There are two main categories that the cell lines originate from, being those derived from a cancer (gestational choriocarcinoma), for example, BeWo, JEG-3, and JAR cell lines, and those derived from primary placental tissue, for example, HTR-8 and HTR-8/SVneo. The BeWo, JEG-3, and JAR cell lines were derived from human choriocarcinoma tissue that has undergone repeated rounds of growth within the cheek pouch of hamsters and clonal selection in culture, over many years [15–17]. The HTR-8 cell line was originally derived from first trimester placental tissue collected during pregnancy termination. These cells were subsequently immortalized by transfection with the SV40 (simian virus 40) large T antigen, now referred to as HTR-8/SVneo [13].

Ensuring the cells are cultured under optimal conditions in the appropriate medium is paramount for measuring changes in normal cellular function. According to the American Type Culture Collection (ATCC) and the European Collection of Authenticated Cell Cultures (ECACC), the recommended culture medium is:

1. BeWo—Ham's F-12 medium modified to contain 2 mM L-glutamine and 10% (v/v) fetal bovine serum (FBS) or F-12K (Kaighn's modification of Ham's F-12) medium containing 2 mM L-glutamine and 1500 mg/L sodium bicarbonate and modified to contain 10% (v/v) FBS.
2. JEG-3—Eagle's minimal essential medium (EMEM) modified to contain Earle's balanced salt solution, 1% (v/v) nonessential amino acids, 2 mM L-glutamine, 1 mM sodium pyruvate, 1500 mg/L sodium bicarbonate, and 10% (v/v) FBS.
3. JAR—RPMI-1640 medium modified to contain 2 mM L-glutamine, 10 mM HEPES, 1 mM sodium pyruvate, 4500 mg/L glucose, 1500 mg/L sodium bicarbonate, and 10% (v/v) FBS.
4. HTR-8/SVneo—RPMI-1640 medium modified to contain 2 mM L-glutamine, 10 mM HEPES, 1 mM sodium pyruvate, 4500 mg/L glucose, 1500 mg/L sodium bicarbonate, and 10% (v/v) FBS.

In addition, BeWo cells can be successfully cultured in DMEM and RPMI medium and JEG-3 cells in RPMI medium. Culture medium is also routinely supplemented with antibiotics (10–50 mg/mL streptomycin and 10–50 IU/mL penicillin), and the concentration of FBS varies between 5 and 10% (v/v) [14, 18–20].

Differences in expression of trophoblast markers, cell adhesion molecules, receptors, cytokines, and proteases between the cell lines contribute to their phenotype and hence their utility in specific functional assays. BeWo cells are a good model for studying the villous trophoblast as they can fuse to form a syncytium, which is ideal for use in syncytialization assays, which is described in detail in Chapter 13. BeWo cells are most commonly used for assessing the effects of syncytialization as there are very few other cell lines with this capability [18, 19, 21]. They do however have limited ability to migrate in vitro [19]. JEG-3, JAR, and HTR-8/SVneo cell lines exhibit characteristics of the extravillous cytotrophoblast and are ideal for assessing migration, invasion, and adhesion [19, 22]. Some researchers prefer using the HTR-8/SVneo cell line over choriocarcinoma cells due to their non-cancerous origin, but despite this, no one single cell line is suitable for assessing all cellular functions. Therefore, careful consideration must be taken when selecting a cell line for use in specific functional assays.

For all functional assays, cell lines are cultured in the relevant culture medium as described above, on tissue culture treated plastic ware (*see* **Note 1**). Prepare all solutions using analytical grade reagents diluted in ultrapure water, which comprises deionized water purified to a sensitivity of 18.2 MΩ cm. Store solutions at room temperature unless otherwise stated.

2.2 General

1. Phosphate-buffered saline (PBS): 10× stock prepared by weighing 80 g NaCl, 2 g KCl, 14.4 g of Na_2HPO_4, and 2.4 g of KH_2PO_4. Make the solution up to 1 L using water and ensure the pH is 7.4. To make a 1× solution, transfer 100 mL of 10× stock into a 1 L glass bottle containing 900 mL of water. Autoclave to sterilize.
2. 0.4% (w/v) trypan blue: Weigh 0.4 g trypan blue dye and add to 100 mL 1× PBS. Mix to dissolve and filter the solution through a 0.22 μm filter to remove any undissolved dye.
3. Hemocytometer.

2.3 Proliferation

Proliferation assays are used to compare the growth of cells over a defined period of time. A number of assays are used for testing cell proliferation. Some assays measure metabolic activity, for example, MTT and XTT assays, which are not necessarily reflective of proliferative state especially as some drugs or culture conditions may interfere with mitochondrial activity. The most accurate proliferation assays are the ones that either measure DNA replication or intact cells. Methylene blue dye is routinely used to rapidly and reproducibly count live cells cultured in multi-well culture plates [19, 23].

1. 10% (v/v) neutral buffered formalin.
2. 0.01 M borate buffer: Weigh 0.62 g boric acid and add to 900 mL of water. Adjust the pH to 8.5 using 1 M NaOH and make the final volume up to 1 L using water.
3. 0.1% (w/v) methylene blue solution: Weigh 1 g methylene blue and transfer into a 100 mL glass bottle containing 100 mL of 0.01 M borate buffer. Mix using gentle agitation on a rotating platform. Ensure the pH of the solution is 8.5 and filter the solution through a 0.22 μm filter into a clean 100 mL glass bottle to remove undissolved dye material.
4. Developing buffer (1:1 ethanol absolute, 0.1 M HCl): Measure 50 mL of 0.1 M HCl and pour into a 100 mL glass bottle. Measure 50 mL of ethanol (absolute), pour into the glass bottle, and stir gently.
5. 96-well plate.
6. Spectrophotometer.

2.4 Apoptosis

Apoptosis assays are performed in conjunction with proliferation assays to measure the health of the cells. As cells undergo apoptosis, their nuclear compartment, as well as their cytoplasm, eventually undergoes fragmentation generating "apoptotic bodies" (small membrane-surrounded vesicles). The processing of the nucleus to states less than diploid ($2n$) is a regular feature. The small size and lower DNA content of an apoptotic nucleus can be assessed by flow cytometry after staining with a dye capable of binding the DNA (such as propidium iodide), which is the basis of the apoptosis assay described in this chapter [19, 24].

1. TrypLE Express (*see* **Note 2**).
2. 10 mg/mL propidium iodide solution: Weigh 50 mg of propidium iodide into a 10 mL tube. Add 5 mL of water and invert to mix to generate a 10 mg/mL stock solution. Filter the stock through a 0.22 μm filter and store at 4 °C.
3. RNase A (stock concentration of 10 mg/mL).
4. Solution I: Weigh 58.4 mg NaCl, 100 mg sodium citrate dihydrate, and 30 μL NP-40 and transfer into a 100 mL glass bottle containing 100 mL of water. Filter the solution through a 0.22 μm filter into a clean 100 mL glass bottle. Store the solution at 4 °C. Immediately prior to use, add 2.5 μL of propidium iodide (from the 10 mg/mL stock) and 1 μL of RNase A (from a 10 mg/mL stock) per 1 mL of solution I.
5. Solution II: Weigh 1.5 g citric acid and 8.55 g sucrose and transfer into a glass bottle containing 100 mL of water. Filter the solution through a 0.22 μm filter into a clean 100 mL glass bottle. Store the solution at 4 °C. Immediately prior to use, add 2.5 μL of propidium iodide (from the 10 mg/mL stock) and 1 μL of RNase A (from a 10 mg/mL stock) per 1 mL of solution II.
6. Flow cytometry tubes with inbuilt 70 μm nylon mesh.
7. Flow cytometer and associated analysis software (*see* **Note 3**).

2.5 Migration

Motility is a requirement for all cells to invade, escape the vascular tree, and colonize a surface. Random migration across a 2D surface (chemokinesis) does not rely on the response to a directional stimulus (chemotaxis) but occurs in response to cues such as planar cell polarity and chemorepulsive signals from intercellular junctions [25]. The most cost-effective chemokinesis assay is the scratch assay, which is performed in culture plates, meaning it can be easily adapted for large-scale analyses [19, 24].

1. P200 pipette tip.
2. Cell culture medium: The formulation is dependent on the cell line being cultured for the experiment.
3. Inverted microscope and camera.

2.6 Invasion

The cellular process of invasion is similar to that of migration; however, invasion requires the movement through a 3D matrix. This process incorporates the movement of cells due to environmental stimuli (migration) as well as adhesion and degradation of the surrounding extracellular matrix [25].

1. The reagents specified in Subheading 2.5.
2. Matrigel: Pipette 3 mL of Matrigel (stock solution 10 mg/mL; *see* **Note 4**) into a 10 mL tube containing 7 mL of serum-free culture medium to make a 3 mg/mL working solution (*see* **Notes 5** and **6**).

2.7 Adhesion

Adhesion is a cellular process by which all adherent cell lines interact with the extracellular matrix of their tissues, which provides structural and biochemical cues to modulate cell behavior. Adhesion is closely linked with migration and invasion and is mediated by integrins (dimers of α and β subunits), cellular adhesion molecules, and proteoglycan receptors. Integrin engagement promotes focal adhesion formation with activation of focal adhesion kinase and recruitment of vinculin to the cytoplasmic tail of the β integrin [26]. Signaling cues and deformations of the actin cytoskeleton produced by new focal adhesion formation direct planar cell polarity and ultimately the directionality of migration. One method for assessing adhesion is to examine binding capacity of cells to a variety of extracellular matrix proteins in culture [19].

1. Extracellular matrix proteins: Fibrillary proteins (collagen I, collagen IV, gelatin), glycoproteins (elastin, vitronectin, and fibronectin), and proteoglycans (heparin, chondroitin, and dermatan sulfates) should be examined. A final concentration of 10 μg/mL (except for vitronectin at 5 μg/mL) in autoclaved water is sufficient for most cell lines.
2. 24-well plate.
3. Cell dissociation solution.

3 Methods

3.1 Proliferation

1. Detach the cells from the culture plate by pipetting 1 mL of TrypLE Express into each well and incubating at 37 °C in a humidified cell culture incubator for 5 min or until the cells start to detach. Inhibit TrypLE Express by adding an equal volume of growth media and recover cells by centrifugation at 400 × *g* for 5 min. Aspirate media and suspend cells in 2 mL of 1× PBS. Take 50 μL of the cell suspension and mix with 450 μL of trypan blue. Trypan blue will differentiate live cells (clear) that can excrete the dye from dead cells (blue). Place diluted cells in trypan blue into a hemocytometer and count the clear cells in each of the four corner chambers. To calculate cell number, multiply the average count from the four chambers by 10^4 (as each chamber constitutes only 1/10,000th of a mL) and then by 10 for the dilution factor.

2. Based on the cell count, plate cells in 12-well plates (*see* **Note 1**) at low enough concentration such that they will still be subconfluent at the end of the growth period (25–50,000/well depending upon the cell type). Plate sufficient number of replicates (normally two to three) that will provide reliable data at each time point.
3. Plate a standard curve of cells as well to allow for extrapolation of the results. A suitable standard curve should be empirically determined for each cell line but should be from low confluence (5–10,000 cells per well) to 100% confluence. This should be harvested on day 0 and left in fixative until the assay is stained.
4. Grow cells overnight. The next day harvest a time point of each to provide a background reading (time 0 h) that accounts for errors in pipetting and initial cell counts.
5. To determine cell counts, first remove medium from cells and wash each well with 500 μL of 1× PBS making sure not to disturb the monolayer of cells you are trying to count. Discard the wash solution, and fix the cells by pipetting 500 μL of 10% (v/v) neutral buffered formalin into each well. Incubate the cells in fixative for 10 min at room temperature (*see* **Note 7**). After incubation discard the fixative solution.
6. Stain the cells by pipetting 500 μL of 0.1% (w/v) methylene blue solution into each well and incubating for 30 min. Again, take care not to disturb the monolayer of cells you are trying to count.
7. Discard the methylene blue solution and carefully wash each well four times with 1 mL of 0.01 M borate buffer, discarding the buffer after each wash (*see* **Note 8**). Remove all borate buffer and allow the wells to dry by turning the plate upside down on the bench for a minimum of 1 h (*see* **Note 9**).
8. Elute the dye by pipetting 500 μL of developing buffer into each well and placing the plate on a rotating platform shaker for 1 min to ensure the cells have lysed and released the methylene blue stain. Remove 100 μL of solution per well and transfer into 1 well of a 96-well plate. Read the absorbance of the samples at 650 nm (*see* **Note 10**). Comparison of the optical densities from the test wells against the standard curve of cells will provide a means to determine absolute cell number rather than changes in relative absorbance.

3.2 Apoptosis

1. Grow cells in 6-well plates until 70% confluence is reached (*see* **Note 1**) and treat with vehicle or apoptosis-inducing/inhibiting agents for the appropriate length of time. Apoptotic cells detach into the culture media. To estimate apoptosis remove media from cells and set aside.

2. Detach the cells from the culture plate by pipetting 1 mL of TrypLE Express into each well and incubating at 37 °C in a humidified cell culture incubator for 5 min or until the cells start to detach. Add the detached cells to the reserved media from **step 1**. Pellet the cells by centrifuging at 400 × *g* for 5 min. Discard the culture supernatant and gently suspend the cell pellet in 2 mL of 1× PBS. Repeat the centrifugation step and remove all supernatant from the cell pellet.
3. Gently suspend each cell pellet in 1 mL of solution I (*see* **Note 11**) and incubate the cells for 1 h at room temperature.
4. Pipette 1 mL of solution II into each tube containing nuclei in solution I and gently pipette up and down to mix (*see* **Note 11**).
5. Pellet the nuclei by centrifuging at 1000 × *g* for 5 min, and remove all but 1 mL of solution from each tube (*see* **Note 12**). Suspend the pelleted nuclei in the remaining 1 mL of solution and pass through a 70 μm nylon mesh into a flow cytometry tube to remove clumps (*see* **Note 13**).
6. Set up the flow cytometer for analysis using the FL2 channel. Propidium iodide has a maximum excitation wavelength of 535 nm and a maximum emission wavelength of 617 nm when bound to nucleic acids. *Do not* gate the "debris" out of the flow analysis as much of it will represent your apoptotic populations. Analyze the samples for the presence of hypodiploid peaks using the FL2 area data. Examples of the analysis are below (Fig. 1). Normal cell populations segregate into peaks for G_0/G_1 (arrested cells) and G_2/M (dividing cells) that have twice the DNA content and twice the nuclear size as G_0/G_1 cells. S-phase cells are between. Apoptotic cells (*filled with blue*) are present in low levels in normal BeWo cells (Fig. 1a) but increase upon serum starvation (Fig. 1b). As such, this assay can also be used in conjunction with proliferation assays to examine cell cycle blockade.

3.3 Migration

1. Grow cells in 6-well plates until all wells have simultaneously established a confluent monolayer (*see* **Note 1**). The level of confluence is crucial and needs to be the same in all wells.

   Remove all culture medium from the wells. Using a P200 pipette tip, make two horizontal and one vertical wound to the monolayer (Fig. 2a).
2. Carefully wash the wells with 1 mL of culture medium to remove the detached cells. Make sure not to affect the integrity of the cell monolayer as it is important for the success of the assay. Replace the culture medium in each well (3 mL per well) (*see* **Note 14**).
3. Photograph at least two points in each well where the horizontal and vertical wounds intersect as shown by the dotted lines

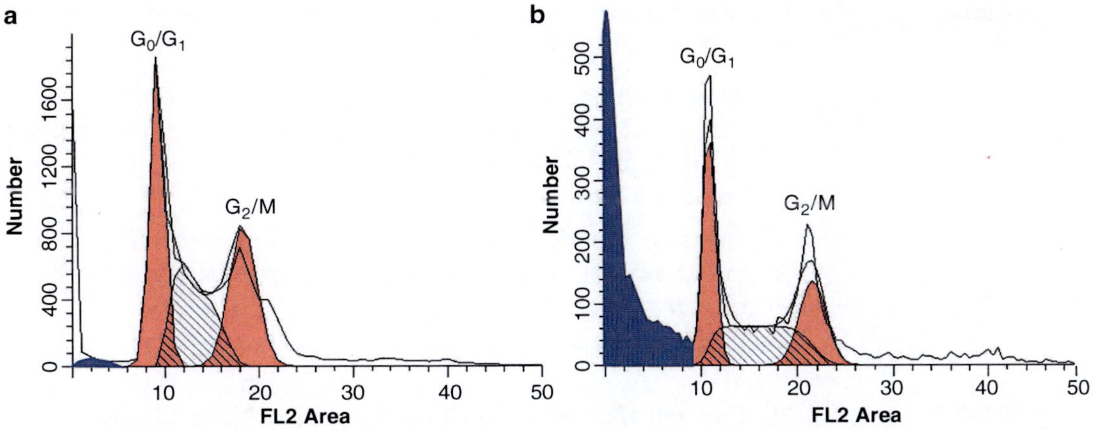

Fig. 1 Analysis of DNA content for apoptosis using flow cytometry. Cells were stained with propidium iodide as described and run on a flow cytometer to analyze DNA content (FL2 area). Normal cells show peaks for G_0/G_1 and G_2/M (*filled with red*) with an intervening S-phase (*filled with lines*). The apoptotic cells appear as a population to the left of the G_0/G_1 population (*filled with blue*). BeWo cells grown in full culture medium (**a**) and under serum starvation conditions (**b**)

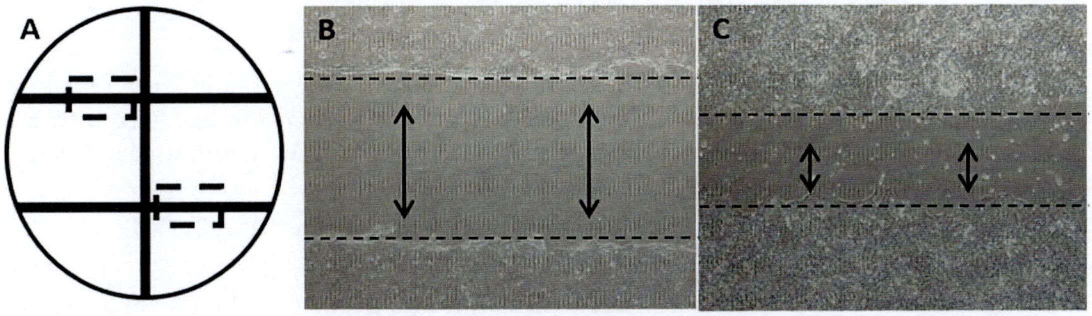

Fig. 2 Schematic of the chemokinesis (scratch) assay. (**a**) Pattern of scratches made in the monolayer at the beginning of the assay. The *dotted boxes* indicate the areas of the wound that are photographed. Wounding the assay at time 0 h (**b**) creates a deficit in the monolayer of JEG-3 cells. Cells migrate into and recolonize the wound over 48 h (**c**). *Dotted lines* in (**b**) and (**c**) denote the migrating front of cells in the monolayer

in Fig. 2a (*see* **Note 15**) using a camera mounted onto an inverted microscope. Photograph the wounds immediately after creating them to establish a 0 h time point and again in the same position 24 h and 48 h post wounding. Photographing exactly the same field at 0 h and at the end of the assay is imperative to the success of the assay.

4. Analyze the distance the cells migrated using TScratch software by subtracting the area of the wound after 48 h (Fig. 2c) from the initial 0 h wound (Fig. 2b).

3.4 Invasion

The experimental setup for this assay is similar to the migration assay. Follow **steps 1** and **2** as outlined in Subheading 3.3.

1. After washing, pipette 1.5 mL of Matrigel into each well so that a layer of 1–2 mm deep is covering the cell monolayer. Incubate the plate for 1 h in a 37 °C humidified 5% CO_2 incubator (*see* **Note 4**).
2. Carefully pipette 3 mL of culture medium into each well taking care not to damage the Matrigel that you have just overlaid the cells with.
3. Follow **steps 3** and **4** as outlined in Subheading 3.3.

3.5 Adhesion

1. Pre-coat the wells of a 24-well plate (*see* **Note 1**) with 250 μL of diluted extracellular matrix proteins or water (control) for a minimum of 1 h at 37 °C in a humidified cell culture incubator (*see* **Note 16**).
2. Detach the cells from the culture plate using 2 mL of cell dissociation solution (*see* **Note 17**) and incubate at 37 °C in a humidified cell culture incubator for 5 min or until the cells start to detach. Pipette solution over the monolayer to detach cells and add an equal volume of growth media. Recover cells by centrifugation at 400 × *g* for 5 min.
3. Aspirate the solution and suspend the pellet in 2 mL of culture media. Take 50 μL of the cell suspension and mix with and 450 μL of trypan blue. Perform a cell count as described in Subheading 3.1.
4. Adjust the cell concentration to 2.5×10^5 cells/mL.
5. Remove the coating solutions from the 24-well plates and wash the wells once with 500 μL of 1× PBS. Aspirate the PBS and repeat the wash with another 500 μL of PBS/well. Take care to prevent the wells from drying. Aspirate this second wash just prior to seeding cells.
6. Seed 400 μL (1×10^5 cells in full culture medium) in each well. Incubate the cells for 30 min in a humidified cell culture incubator (*see* **Note 18**).
7. Remove the culture medium. Wash the wells carefully three times with 1 mL of 1× PBS to remove any non-adherent cells, removing the solution after each wash step (*see* **Note 19**).
8. Fix the cells by gently pipetting 500 μL of 10% (v/v) neutral buffered formalin into each well and incubating for 10 min at room temperature as described in Subheading 3.1.
9. Determine the number of cells that adhered to each extracellular matrix protein by staining with methylene blue as described in Subheading 3.1.

4 Notes

1. It is suggested that proliferation assays are performed in 12-well tissue cultured-treated plates, apoptosis, migration, and invasion in 6-well plates and adhesion assays in 24-well plates. The volume of culture medium specified is specific to the size of the tissue culture plates. Adjust the volumes accordingly if alternatively sized wells are used.
2. Various cell dissociation regents can be used instead of TrypLE Express including trypsin or EDTA at a recommended starting concentration of 0.2% (w/v), depending on the cell type undergoing detachment.
3. A BD FACSCalibur flow cytometer with ModFit LT software was used to analyze the apoptosis data described herein; however, alternative flow cytometers and analysis software (CellQuest Pro and FlowJo) can be used. A description of flow cytometry setup and methods is described in Chapter 7.
4. Matrigel will transform from a solution into a gel when incubated at 37 °C. All Matrigel solutions must be kept at 4 °C at all times. Matrigel may be placed in a fridge overnight to facilitate thawing. Before preparing the working solution, pre-chill pipette tips and tubes to 4 °C. Always keep Matrigel on ice while preparing solutions and use only cold, serum-free medium (4 °C), corresponding to the regular culture medium specific to the cell type being analyzed, for diluting Matrigel.
5. The minimum recommended Matrigel concentration to form a gel is 3 mg/mL, but the range of 1.5–5 mg/mL has been reported. Optimization may be required as individual cell lines may have a different response to the stiffness of the gel and have different abilities to produce matrix-degrading enzymes.
6. Collagen I can be used as an alternative matrix to test invasion and also requires preparation at 4 °C. The collagen I gel is prepared by mixing seven volumes of collagen I with one volume of 10× serum-free medium (specific to the cell type in use), one volume of 10 mg/mL sodium bicarbonate, and up to one volume of 0.1 M NaOH to adjust the pH of the solution to 7.4 or water to achieve ten volumes. Collagen I will form a gel best in a 37 °C incubator without 5% CO_2.
7. The neutral buffered formalin can remain on the cells for up to 72 h if required depending on the length of time proliferation is being measured to allow for combined processing once all time points have been completed. Store the tissue culture plates at 4 °C.
8. Washing with borate buffer removes the excess methylene blue solution. This process may require four to six washes

before the buffer can no longer remove excess methylene blue. The borate buffer should be nearly colorless before the remaining steps can be performed. Pay special attention to remove any methylene blue solution from the walls of each well, which may otherwise contaminate the final eluate and introduce errors into the assay.

9. All liquid must be removed from the wells before the elution step can be performed, which may take several hours or overnight if required. The plates can be stored at this step at room temperature until all time points have been collected to allow for batch processing of the remaining steps.
10. Samples should be tested in duplicate or triplicate. If the absorbance reading of any sample exceeded 2.0, the samples will require an additional dilution step. A starting dilution of 1:5 can be tested.
11. Cell pellets containing $1–2 \times 10^6$ cells can be resuspended in 1 mL of solution I, which is the approximate number of cells harvested from 1 well of a 6-well plate at 70% confluence. The number of harvested cells is dependent on the cell line being utilized. If more or less cells need to be assessed, adjust the volume of solution I and II accordingly. This protocol requires equal volumes of solution I and II to be used on the same sample. The addition of solution II results in the destruction of cell membranes leaving only nuclei.
12. After staining with solution II and centrifuging the sample, the pellet should appear a bright pink color.
13. The samples can be stored at 4 °C for 2–3 days prior to analysis via flow cytometry if required.
14. The medium can be supplemented to contain chemokinetic agents to enhance (such as the growth factors FGF-2 and HGF) or inhibit (colchicine and vinblastine) motility.
15. Photographs do not have to be taken at the exact points indicated in Fig. 2a but can be taken at any of the points where the horizontal and vertical wounds intersect. However, the same fields should be photographed at each time point to ensure quantitation is accurate.
16. The 24-well plate can be coated and incubated with extracellular matrix proteins for a minimum of 1 h but can be prepared 24 h prior to commencement of the assay.
17. The attachment assays are assessed over a short time period. As such, cells do not have time to replace adhesive proteins (such as integrins) if lost during harvesting. For this reason, enzyme-based methods of detachment (TrypLE Express, trypsin, etc.) must be avoided and nonenzymatic methods used.

18. Timing is essential. Too little time and not enough cells will be firmly attached. Too long an incubation and you risk assessing a mixture of adhesion and spreading. Normally 30–45 min is sufficient, but this should be determined empirically for each cell line by observing the behavior of the cells.
19. Any cells that do not adhere to the extracellular matrix proteins will be removed by carefully running 1 mL of 1× PBS down the wall of the well and gently tilting the plate so as not to dislodge the loosely adherent cells.

Acknowledgment

This work was supported by project grants (571329, 512154) from the National Health and Medical Research Council of Australia and Heart Research Australia (AWA: 2014-02).

References

1. Cross JC, Werb Z, Fisher SJ (1994) Implantation and the placenta: key pieces of the development puzzle. Science 266(5190):1508–1518
2. Fisher SJ, Damsky CH (1993) Human cytotrophoblast invasion. Semin Cell Biol 4(3):183–188
3. Goldman-Wohl D, Yagel S (2002) Regulation of trophoblast invasion: from normal implantation to pre-eclampsia. Mol Cell Endocrinol 187(1–2):233–238
4. Redman CW, Sargent IL (2005) Latest advances in understanding preeclampsia. Science 308(5728):1592
5. Huppertz B (2008) Placental origins of preeclampsia: challenging the current hypothesis. Hypertension 51(4):970–975
6. Kaufmann P, Black S, Huppertz B (2003) Endovascular trophoblast invasion: implications for the pathogenesis of intrauterine growth retardation and preeclampsia. Biol Reprod 69(1):1–7
7. Zhou Y et al (1993) Preeclampsia is associated with abnormal expression of adhesion molecules by invasive cytotrophoblasts. J Clin Invest 91(3):950–960
8. Lyall F, Robson SC, Bulmer JN (2013) Spiral artery remodeling and trophoblast invasion in preeclampsia and fetal growth restriction: relationship to clinical outcome. Hypertension 62(6):1046–1054
9. Allaire AD et al (2000) Placental apoptosis in preeclampsia. Obstet Gynecol 96(2):271–276
10. Ishihara N et al (2002) Increased apoptosis in the syncytiotrophoblast in human term placentas complicated by either preeclampsia or intrauterine growth retardation. Am J Obstet Gynecol 186(1):158–166
11. Powe CE, Levine RJ, Karumanchi SA (2011) Preeclampsia, a disease of the maternal endothelium: the role of antiangiogenic factors and implications for later cardiovascular disease. Circulation 123(24):2856–2869
12. Orendi K et al (2011) Placental and trophoblastic in vitro models to study preventive and therapeutic agents for preeclampsia. Placenta 32(Suppl):S49–S54
13. Graham CH et al (1993) Establishment and characterization of first trimester human trophoblast cells with extended lifespan. Exp Cell Res 206(2):204–211
14. Bilban M et al (2010) Trophoblast invasion: assessment of cellular models using gene expression signatures. Placenta 31(11):989–996
15. Pattillo RA, Gey GO (1968) The establishment of a cell line of human hormone-synthesizing trophoblastic cells in vitro. Cancer Res 28(7):1231–1236
16. Pattillo RA et al (1971) The hormone-synthesizing trophoblastic cell in vitro: a model for cancer research and placental hormone synthesis. Ann N Y Acad Sci 172(10):288–298
17. Kohler PO et al (1971) Clonal lines of human choriocarcinoma cells in culture. Acta Endocrinol Suppl 153:137–153

18. Pathirage NA et al (2013) Homeobox gene transforming growth factor beta-induced factor-1 (TGIF-1) is a regulator of villous trophoblast differentiation and its expression is increased in human idiopathic fetal growth restriction. Mol Hum Reprod 19(10):665–675
19. Powell KL et al (2016) Role for the thromboxane A2 receptor beta-isoform in the pathogenesis of intrauterine growth restriction. Sci Rep 6:28811
20. Yang Y et al (1993) Molecular, biochemical, and functional characteristics of tumor necrosis factor-alpha produced by human placental cytotrophoblastic cells. J Immunol 150(12):5614–5624
21. Hannan NJ et al (2010) Models for study of human embryo implantation: choice of cell lines? Biol Reprod 82(2):235–245
22. Zygmunt M et al (1998) Invasion of cytotrophoblastic JEG-3 cells is stimulated by hCG in vitro. Placenta 19(8):587–593
23. Oliver MH et al (1989) A rapid and convenient assay for counting cells cultured in microwell plates: application for assessment of growth factors. J Cell Sci 92(3):513
24. Ashton AW et al (1999) Inhibition of endothelial cell migration, intercellular communication, and vascular tube formation by thromboxane A(2). J Biol Chem 274(50):35562–35570
25. Kramer N et al (2013) In vitro cell migration and invasion assays. Mut Res 752(1):10–24
26. Cohen DM et al (2006) A conformational switch in vinculin drives formation and dynamics of a talin-vinculin complex at focal adhesions. J Biol Chem 281(23):16006–16015

Chapter 19

Isolation and Characterization of Mesenchymal Stem/Stromal Cells Derived from Human Third Trimester Placental Chorionic Villi and *Decidua Basalis*

Gina D. Kusuma, Mohamed H. Abumaree, Mark D. Pertile, and Bill Kalionis

Abstract

The *decidua basalis* and placental chorionic villi are critical components of maternal-fetal interface, which plays a critical role in normal placental development. Failure to form a proper maternal-fetal interface is associated with clinically important placental pathologies including preeclampsia and fetal growth restriction. Placental trophoblast cells are well known for their critical roles in establishing the maternal-fetal interface; however accumulating evidence also implicates mesenchymal stem/stromal cells that envelop the maternal and fetal blood vessels as playing an important role in the formation and efficient functioning of the interface. Moreover, recent studies associate abnormal mesenchymal stem/stromal cell function in the development of preeclampsia. Further research is needed to fully understand the role that these cells play in this clinically important placental pathology.

The intimate relationship between maternal and fetal tissues at the interface poses significant problems in the enrichment of *decidua basalis* and chorionic villous mesenchymal stem/stromal cells without significant cross-contamination. The protocols described below for the enrichment and characterization of mesenchymal stem/stromal cells from the maternal-fetal interface produce highly enriched cells that conform to international standards and show minimal cross-contamination.

Key words Mesenchymal stem/stromal cells, Placenta, Chorionic villi, *Decidua basalis*, Isolation, Characterization, Cell culture, Differentiation, Colony-forming unit, Fluorescence in situ hybridization

1 Introduction

1.1 The Maternal-Fetal Interface

The human placenta orchestrates a myriad of functions during the course of pregnancy to ensure the outcome of a healthy baby. Key functions are the provision of adequate nutrition to the developing fetus, removal of waste products, and maintenance of an immunological barrier between the mother and fetus [1]. Achieving these functions demands the establishment and maintenance of an interface with the mother's uterus. Specialized placental trophoblast

Padma Murthi and Cathy Vaillancourt (eds.), *Preeclampsia: Methods and Protocols*, Methods in Molecular Biology, vol. 1710, https://doi.org/10.1007/978-1-4939-7498-6_19,

cells migrate and invade into the uterus, specifically the *decidua basalis* and underlying myometrium, and modify maternal spiral arterioles to increase blood flow to the placenta. Disruption of placental development and shallow trophoblast invasion with subsequent inadequate maternal spiral arteriole modification underlie significant, clinically important placental pathologies such as preeclampsia and fetal growth restriction.

Research over many decades has justifiably focused on trophoblast stem cells because of the critical role they play in establishing and maintaining the fetal component of the maternal-fetal interface. However, more recent studies identified two mesenchymal cell populations with stem cell-like properties at the maternal-fetal interface of third trimester placentae, which could potentially play important roles in normal and pathological placental development. These two cell populations were isolated from the maternal *decidua basalis* [2–9] and the fetal chorionic villi [2, 10–16].

1.2 Mesenchymal Stem/Stromal Cell Populations at the Maternal-Fetal Interface

The stem cell-like features of these mesenchymal cells include multipotent differentiation potential, mesenchymal stem cell-like immunophenotype, and colony-forming ability. These cells have been variously referred to as mesenchymal stem/stromal or multipotent stem/stromal cells but are now generally referred to as MSCs. Initially, the isolation and characterization of MSCs from the maternal-fetal interface were complicated by different isolation protocols from numerous laboratories, the use of varying combinations of MSC genes and cell surface marker proteins, and inconsistencies in verifying multipotent differentiation potential [17]. This issue was addressed by the International Society for Cellular Therapy (ISCT) by establishing minimal criteria to define human MSCs [18]. The criteria stipulated that MSCs must adhere to untreated plastic surfaces; should express CD105, CD73, and CD90 but lack expression of CD34, CD14, CD19, CD11b, CD79α, or HLA-DR; and should form different functional cell types of the mesenchymal lineages (i.e., at least into osteocytes, chondrocytes, and adipocytes) to confirm their multipotency.

The close juxtaposition of tissues at maternal-fetal interface presented a unique challenge for the isolation of fetal chorionic villous MSCs (CMSCs) since contamination with fast growing maternal cells, which were most likely derived from the maternal *decidua basalis*, was a common problem. Parolini et al. [10, 19] proposed similar criteria to those of the ISCT, for defining MSCs of placental origin, and further specified that MSCs from the fetal components from the placenta (i.e., chorionic villi, amnion, and umbilical cord) should be of fetal origin, with <1% maternal cell contamination. Common methods for determining the origin of CMSCs and DMSCs are fluorescence in situ hybridization (FISH, see protocol below) [20] and reverse transcriptase polymerase chain reaction [16].

The protocol described below allows the preparation of CMSCs from the chorionic plate that conform to the ISCT and Parolini et al. criteria [10, 19]. The method for obtaining DMSCs from the maternal *decidua basalis* that remains attached to the maternal side of the placenta following delivery obviates the need for invasive decidual biopsies as a source of tissue for DMSC preparation. The preparation of highly enriched CMSC and DMSC preparations with minimal cross-contamination of cells was instrumental in demonstrating differences between the two MSC types with regard to gene expression/growth factor/cytokines expression differences, functional differences [20–22], and differences in their interactions with immune cells [23, 24].

The primary CMSCs and DMSCs produced by these protocols are capable of differentiation in vivo as shown by their ability to form ectopic bone in a murine animal model [25]. Two cell lines, DMSC23 and CMSC29, made by viral transduction of the hTERT (i.e., human telomerase reverse transcriptase) gene into DMSCs and CMSCs, respectively, showed extended lifespan and maintained many of the important differences between the two cell types [26].

1.3 The Role of DMSCs and CMSCs at the Maternal-Fetal Interface

Multiple lines of evidence suggest a role for DMSCs and CMSCs in preeclampsia. The specialized microenvironment, or niche, for DMSCs and CMSCs at the maternal-fetal interface is vascular, with both MSC types in close proximity to endothelial cells that comprise the vessel walls [6, 14, 27]. This close association suggests DMSCs and CMSCs may contribute to angiogenesis and vessel function. Tran et al. [28] showed CMSCs could promote angiogenesis by paracrine effects on endothelial cells and/or by direct differentiation into endothelial cells. Ohlsson et al. [29] showed defects in maternal and fetal placental vessel maturation and function when the platelet-derived growth factor receptor (PDGFR)-β gene was inactivated in a mouse model. PDGFR-β is specifically expressed in MSCs and pericytes in the vascular niche, and this knockout suggested DMSCs and CMSCs play important roles in normal placental development and potentially in placental pathologies that involve the vasculature such as preeclampsia and fetal growth restriction.

Furthermore, Kusuma et al. [6] showed a vascular niche for DMSCs in the spiral arterioles of the *decidua basalis* and underlying myometrium and determined their fate after establishment of the maternal-fetal interface. Following trophoblast cell invasion, migration, and remodeling of the spiral arterioles, the DMSC niche is destroyed or replaced. Kusuma et al. [6] postulated that DMSCs play a role not only in the establishment of the normal maternal-fetal interface but also in the placental pathologies associated with failure to adequately remodel the maternal spiral arterioles such as preeclampsia and fetal growth restriction.

1.4 The Role of DMSCs and CMSCs in Preeclampsia

Recent studies provide more direct evidence that DMSCs and CMSCs play a role at the maternal-fetal interface. Hwang et al. [30] showed differential expression of various cytokines (e.g., soluble intracellular adhesion molecule-1 and stromal-derived factor-1) in normotensive DMSCs and preeclampsia-affected DMSCs (PE-DMSCs). Liu et al. [31] determined the microRNA (miR) profiles and showed high level expression of miR-181a and miR-16 in PE-DMSCs compared to DMSCs. Wang et al. [31] showed that miR-16 was expressed at high levels in PE-DMSCs and demonstrated that miR-16 overexpression reduced DMSC proliferation and migration, blood vessel formation, and trophoblast cell migration. Subsequent studies provided evidence that miR-494 was highly expressed in PE-DMSCs and was responsible for their abnormal cell cycle progression in these cells [32, 33].

We subsequently provided evidence that PE-DMSCs have reduced colony-forming unit ability and reduced resistance to oxidative stress. The oxidative stress response was shown to be a consequence of reduced levels of aldehyde dehydrogenase (ALDH) 1A1 levels in PE-DMSCs [34]. Members of the ALDH family of enzymes are responsible for detoxifying aldehydes, which are at high levels in the blood of preeclamptic patients. Kusuma et al. [6] proposed that in the early stages of preeclampsia, shallow invasion of trophoblast cells and subsequent failure to adequately remodel the maternal spiral arterioles result in increased exposure of non-transformed spiral arteriole vessel walls and consequently increased numbers of abnormal PE-DMSCs in the vascular niche of these vessels, which could contribute to the pathogenesis of preeclampsia.

Abnormalities in CMSCs, which are derived from the fetal component of the interface, have also been reported, and these may also contribute to the pathogenesis of preeclampsia. Comparisons of growth parameters and cytokine expression patterns of CMSCs and PE-CMSCs prepared from chorionic villi of normotensive and preeclamptic third trimester placentae, respectively, showed significant differences in growth parameters and cytokine profiles [35]. When the conditioned medium from PE-CMSCs was added to chorionic villous explants, physiological changes observed in PE-affected chorionic villi were detected. Portmann-Lanz et al. [36] also reported differential expression of MSC surface markers (CD105, CD90, CD73, and CD44) between CMSCs isolated from PE and normotensive placentae. Clearly, further studies are needed to understand the role of DMSCs and CMSCs at the maternal-fetal interface in normotensive and preeclamptic pregnancies, and these studies require reproducible methods to routinely prepare highly enriched MSC populations with minimal cross-contamination between DMSCs and CMSCs.

1.5 DMSCs as Therapeutic Tools

Further investigations into the role of CMSCs and DMSCs will increase our understanding of their role in normal and pathological placental development. DMSCs in particular have potential as therapeutic tools to treat preeclampsia. For example, Liu et al. [37] infused human DMSCs into T helper 1 (Th1)-induced mice, which are used to model preeclampsia in humans. Following infusion of DMSCs, preeclamptic-like symptoms were reduced. More recently, Chatterjee et al. [38] induced hypertension and preeclampsia-like symptoms in pregnant mice using Toll-like receptor 3 (TLR3) agonist poly(I:C) or TLR7 agonist R837. Intramuscular injections of placenta-derived, mesenchymal-like, adherent stromal cells (called PLX-PAD, which have the same characteristics of CMSCs) could reduce hypertension, endothelial dysfunction, and other preeclampsia-like symptoms in this murine model. The mechanism of action of PLX-PAD in this murine model is not fully understood. Thus, MSCs from the maternal-fetal interface have the potential for incorporation into novel therapeutic strategies to treat preeclampsia. Such strategies will benefit from a greater understanding of the properties of highly enriched PE-DMSCs and PE-CMSCs using protocols such as those described below.

2 Materials

2.1 Chorionic Villous MSCs (CMSCs) Isolation and Expansion

1. Placentae are obtained from preeclamptic and/or normotensive patients who give informed, written consent prior to collection. Preeclamptic patients should be gestation matched to healthy, normotensive patients when possible. Preeclampsia is diagnosed when there was new onset hypertension (blood pressure >140/90 mmHg occurred after 20 weeks' gestation) and is accompanied by new onset proteinuria of >0.3 g/24 h [39]. MSC preparation is usually carried out as soon as possible after delivery (*see* **Note 1**).
2. Stereo dissecting microscope.
3. Tissue culture plasticwares (sterile 100 mm petri dishes and uncoated tissue culture flasks) and sterile, disposable supplies (centrifuge tubes, disposable syringes, and 21-gauge needles).
4. Sterilized instruments: scalpel blades, scissors, and forceps.
5. 1× Phosphate-buffered saline (PBS).
6. 2.5% 10× Trypsin.
7. Heat-inactivated fetal bovine serum (FBS).
8. Complete AmnioMax: 450 mL AmnioMax C-100 basal medium supplemented with 75 mL AmnioMax C-100 supplement.

2.2 Decidua Basalis MSCs (DMSCs) Isolation and Expansion

1. Placentae are collected from preeclamptic and/or normotensive patients with written informed patient consent as described above (*see* **Note 1**).
2. Tissue culture plasticwares and sterile, disposable supplies.
3. Sterilized instruments: 100 μm stainless steel sieves, 1 L glass beaker, scalpel blades, scissors, and forceps.
4. 1× PBS.
5. FBS.
6. Hank's Balanced Salt Solution (HBSS) (−): no calcium, no magnesium, and no phenol red.
7. HBSS (+): calcium, magnesium, and no phenol red.
8. 2.5% 10× Trypsin.
9. Penicillin/streptomycin (10,000 U/mL penicillin and 10,000 mg/mL streptomycin).
10. 200 mM 100× L-glutamine.
11. 10 mg/mL DNase 1 (stock solution).
12. 10 mg/mL Collagenase type 1 (stock solution).
13. Histopaque, density: 1.077 g/mL.
14. Red blood cells (RBC) lysis buffer: 0.25 M EDTA, 1 M $NaHCO_3$, and 1 M NH_4Cl. Autoclave or filter-sterilized.
15. Complete minimum essential medium with Alpha modification (α-MEM): α-MEM supplemented with 10% FBS, penicillin/streptomycin (P/S, 100 U/mL and 100 mg/mL respectively), and 2 mM L-glutamine.

2.3 Cell Expansion and Passaging

1. 1× TrypLE Express Enzyme, no phenol red.
2. Cell-counting materials: cell counting chamber slides and trypan blue.
3. HBSS (−) with P/S.
4. Complete AmnioMax medium.
5. Complete α-MEM medium.

2.4 MSC Characterization

2.4.1 Colony-Forming Unit Fibroblast (CFU-F) Assay

1. 10% Formalin.
2. Giemsa stain.
3. 1× PBS.

2.4.2 In Vitro Differentiation

1. Chamber slides (8-well).
2. 15 mL Polypropylene tubes.
3. Complete α-MEM medium.

4. Complete Dulbecco's MEM/F-12 medium (DMEM/F-12): DMEM/F-12 supplemented with 1% ITS supplement (insulin, transferrin, selenious acid, bovine serum albumin, and linoleic acid), penicillin/streptomycin (100 U/mL and 100 mg/mL, respectively), and 2 mM L-glutamine.

   The following are commercially available differentiation supplements (*see* **Note 2**):

5. Adipogenic induction medium: complete α-MEM medium supplemented with hydrocortisone, isobutylmethylxanthine, and indomethacin.
6. Osteogenic induction medium: complete α-MEM medium supplemented with dexamethasone, ascorbate-phosphate, and β-glycerophosphate.
7. Chondrogenic induction medium: complete DMEM/F-12 medium supplemented with dexamethasone, ascorbate-phosphate, proline, pyruvate, and TGF-β3.
8. Oil Red O staining solution: 30 mg Oil Red O powder dissolved into 10 mL isopropanol and 6.7 mL distilled water, filter-sterilized.
9. Alizarin Red staining solution: 2 g Alizarin Red powder dissolved into 100 mL distilled water, pH adjusted to 4.2, and filter-sterilized.
10. Safranin O staining solution: 0.1% (w/v) Safranin O in distilled water.
11. 10% formalin.
12. 70% ethanol.

2.4.3 Flow Cytometry

1. Directly conjugated antibodies for flow cytometry: panel of six positive MSC markers, i.e., CD90, CD146, CD166, CD44, CD73, CD105, and three negative MSC markers (hematopoietic, endothelial), i.e., CD45, HLA-DR, and CD19.
2. 5 mL round bottom polystyrene tubes with cell strainer cap.
3. Human serum.
4. DAPI.
5. Wash buffer: HBSS (−) with P/S and 2% FBS.

2.5 FISH Analysis of CMSCs and DMSCs

2.5.1 Slide Preparation

1. Polysine slides or pre-cleaned glass slides.
2. 1× PBS.
3. Carnoy's fixative, methanol/glacial acetic acid (3:1) (v/v).
4. 4.5 mL conical base centrifuge tubes.
5. Permanent marker or diamond tip pen.

2.5.2 Slide Pretreatment

1. 20× standard saline citrate (SSC) stock solution: 3.0 M NaCl, 0.3 M Na-citrate. Dissolve 175.3 g NaCl + 88.2 g in dH_2O. Adjust to pH 7.0 and autoclave.
2. 2× SSC: 100 mL 20× SSC + 900 mL sterile dH_2O.
3. Pepsin diluent 0.01 M HCl: 990 mL dH_2O + 10 mL 1 M HCl.
4. Pepsin stock solution 10% (w/v): 0.05 g pepsin (lyophilized stock at 2500 units/mg) + 0.5 mL dH_2O.
5. Pepsin working solution: add 30 μL 10% pepsin stock to 30 mL preheated pepsin diluent (0.01 M HCl) immediately prior to use. Active at 37 °C for up to 1 h.
6. Ethanol series: 70% pre-rinse, 70%, 85%, and 95% solutions. Working solutions can be kept in air tight Coplin jars and changed fortnightly. Change pre-rinse more frequently.
7. Formaldehyde diluent: 6 g $MgCl_2$ + 1 L PBS (without Ca^{2+} or Mg^{2+}).
8. Formaldehyde working solution 1% (v/v): 1 mL formaldehyde (37% formalin solution) + 30 mL formaldehyde diluent.
9. Coplin jars.

2.5.3 Specimen and Probe Co-denaturation

1. Vysis AneuVysion DNA probe kit: this kit includes directly labeled FISH probes for chromosomes 13, 21, and X,Y,18 (*see* **Note 3**). A kit is available with probes for X and Y only but note the X and Y probe colors are reversed.
2. Round coverslips (10 or 13 mm).
3. Rubber sealant—bicycle tire repair glue.
4. Hybridization chamber (*see* **Note 4**).

2.5.4 Post-hybridization (Stringency) Wash

1. 0.4× SSC/0.3% NP40: 200 mL 2× SSC + 800 mL dH_2O. Add 3 mL NP40 and mix well. Adjust pH to 7.
2. 2× SSC.
3. Forceps.

2.5.5 Slide Counterstaining and Mounting

1. DAPI counterstain in Vectashield antifade mounting medium: 15 μL 80 μg/mL DAPI + 1.5 mL Vectashield antifade mounting medium.
2. 24 mm × 60 mm coverslips.

3 Methods

3.1 CMSCs Isolation and Expansion

3.1.1 Day 1 Procedure

1. With the fetal side of the placenta facing up, near the umbilical cord insertion site, make an incision through the membranes (*see* **Note 5**).

2. With forceps and scissors, dissect out a small amount of chorionic tissue (approx. 1 g) from below the chorionic plate.
3. Place in a sterile 100 mm petri dish and add a small amount of 1× PBS dropwise.
4. Under a stereo dissecting microscope, use two syringes fitted with 21-gauge needles to tease apart chorionic tissue to obtain the typical villous "tree-like" morphology while removing non-villous tissue and red blood cells (Fig. 1).
5. Following careful dissection villous tissue should be uniform in color and free of attached material. Move the tissue to a sterile 100 mm petri dish with PBS and add 500 μL of 0.25% cold trypsin.
6. Mince the villi finely (1 mm^3 pieces) with scalpel blades and add about 1 mL more of the 0.25% trypsin.
7. Transfer the villi and trypsin suspension into a 15 mL centrifuge tube.
8. Cap the tube and incubate at 37 °C for 45 min (*see* **Note 6**).
9. Inactivate the trypsin with 500 μL FBS, mix thoroughly with a pipette, and centrifuge at 600 × *g* room temperature (RT) for 5 min.
10. Wash with 5 mL HBSS (−) + P/S + 1% FBS.
11. Centrifuge 600 × *g* at RT for 5 min to pellet the villi.
12. Carefully aspirate the supernatant with a pipette.
13. Resuspend the villi in 3 mL of pre-warmed complete AmnioMax medium and add to a T25cm^2 flask (*see* **Note 7**).
14. Place the flask in the humidified 37 °C incubator with 5% CO_2.

3.1.2 Day 2 Procedure

1. After overnight incubation, add another 2 mL of complete AmnioMax medium to each flask.
2. Monitor the culture for the presence of adherent cells arising from the perimeter of the attached tissue explants. Carefully change the medium to avoid dislocating the attached tissue explants and add just enough medium to cover the surface of the flask. This culture is designated passage 0 (P0) cells.
3. Remove the tissue explants after 1–2 weeks in culture (*see* **Note 8**).
4. If no migrating cells appear within 2–3 weeks, discard the culture.

3.2 DMSCs Isolation and Expansion

3.2.1 Day 1 Procedure

1. Collect 8 g of tissue from a central cotyledon on the maternal side of the placenta while avoiding any area of obvious calcification and manually remove blood clots (*see* **Note 5**; Fig. 1).
2. Finely mince the tissues with sterile scissors.

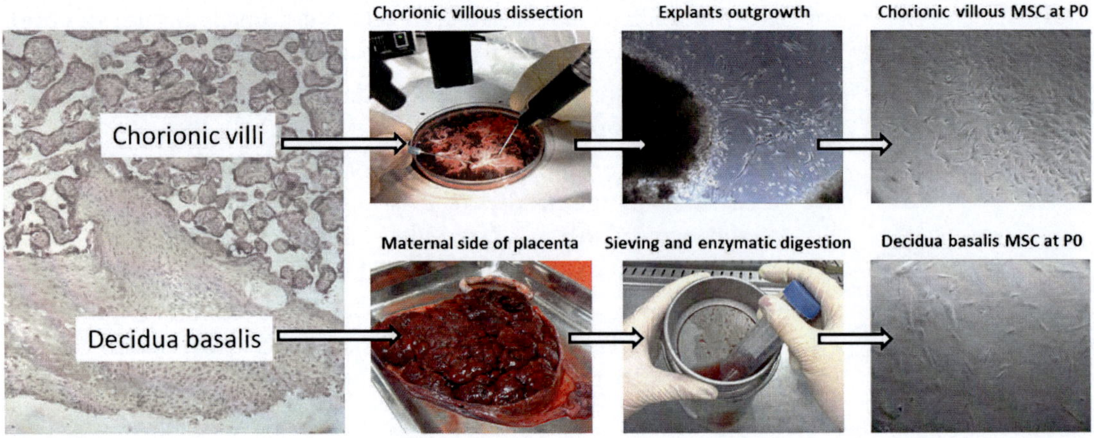

Fig. 1 MSCs isolation from human term placenta. Flow diagram showing the histological cross section of human term placenta and the preparation of chorionic villous MSCs (*top row*) and *decidua basalis* MSCs (*bottom row*)

3. Place in a 50 mL polypropylene tube and make up the volume to 50 mL with 1× PBS.
4. Centrifuge 200 × *g* for 5 min at RT.
5. Aspirate the supernatant without disturbing the pellet.
6. Repeat PBS wash step for three more times.
7. Aspirate the supernatant, and add 17.9 mL HBSS (−).
8. Add 2 mL of 10× trypsin and 100 μL DNase 1.
9. Digest the tissue overnight at 4 °C on a rocking platform.

3.2.2 Day 2 Procedure

1. Place 4.5 mL Histopaque into a 15 mL polypropylene tube. Allow to come to RT.
2. Retrieve tissue from the rocking platform, add 2 mL FBS, and make up volume to 50 mL with HBSS (+).
3. Centrifuge the tube at 400 × *g* for 5 min at RT. Aspirate the supernatant.
4. Add 10 mL of HBSS (+) and mix.
5. Centrifuge the tube at 400 × *g* for 5 min at RT. Aspirate the supernatant.
6. Add 10 mL of HBSS (+) with 1% P/S + 1% FBS.
7. Add 300 μL of 100 μg/μL collagenase type 1 and 50 μL of 10 mg/mL DNase 1, and mix and digest for 10 min in a 37 °C shaking water bath with gentle shaking.
8. Sieve the digest through 100 μM stainless steel sieve and retrieve the collected filtrate in a 10 mL syringe.
9. Layer the filtrate on top of the Histopaque solution in a 15 mL polypropylene tube.

10. Centrifuge the solution at 400 × *g* for 30 min at RT.
11. Using a 10 mL pipette, transfer the buffy coat interface (plasma and cells) and place into a new 15 mL polypropylene tube.
12. Centrifuge the tube at 200 × *g* for 5 min at RT.
13. Remove supernatant with pipette and add 10 mL of RBC lysis buffer.
14. Mix by pipette and centrifuge at 200 × *g* for 10 min at RT.
15. Remove supernatant with pipette and wash with 10 mL HBSS (−) with 1% P/S and 1% FBS. Pipette to mix.
16. Centrifuge the tube at 400 × *g* for 5 min at RT. Remove supernatant with a pipette.
17. Resuspend in 10 mL of complete α-MEM medium and plate into a T75cm^2 flask. Label flask with passage number, cell type, media, and date. This culture will be designated as passage 0 (P0).
18. Place the flask in the humidified 37 °C incubator with 5% CO_2.
19. Monitor the culture for the presence of adherent fibroblast-like cells (*see* **Note 9**). If no cells or colonies appear within 1–2 weeks, discard the culture.

3.3 Cell Expansion and Passaging

1. Passage cells when they reached ~70% confluency.
2. Remove the culture medium and rinse the cell monolayer twice with pre-warmed HBSS (−) with P/S.
3. Add TrypLE Express reagent to completely cover the monolayer and incubate at 37 °C for 5 min.
4. Centrifuge the cell suspension at 300 × *g* for 5 min. Aspirate the supernatant.
5. Replate the cells at subsequent passages at a cell seeding density of 1000 cells/cm^2 in their respective culture medium.
6. Perform a media change twice a week.
7. Cultures should be routinely monitored to check any morphological alterations or contaminants. Both CMSCs and DMSCs appear as fibroblast-shaped cells (Fig. 2a, b). When MSCs reach senescence, their morphology will become flatter and rounder.

3.4 CMSC and DMSC Characterization

3.4.1 CFU-F Assay

1. CFU-F assay can be performed with CMSCs and DMSCs at passage 1 or later to determine the cloning efficiency.
2. Plate 400 cells/well into 6-well plates in their respective medium and incubate for 14 days without a media change.
3. After 14 days, remove the medium and rinse the cells with PBS.
4. Fix the cell monolayer with 10% formalin for 10 min at RT.

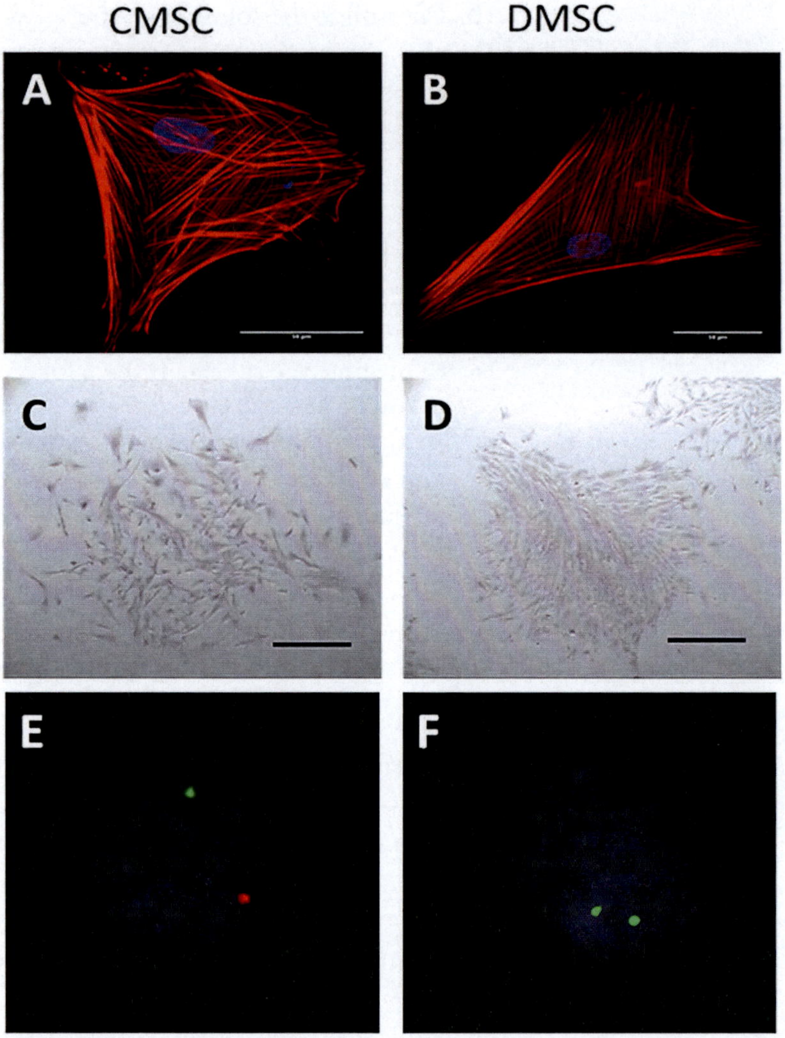

Fig. 2 CMSCs and DMSCs morphology. Fluorescence staining of actin cytoskeleton (phalloidin) of CMSCs (**a**) and DMSCs (**b**). White scale bar is 50 μm. A typical colony of CMSCs (**c**) and DMSCs (**d**) formed after CFU-F assay and stained with Giemsa. Black scale bar is 500 μm. Representative FISH analysis on nuclei from cells isolated from placenta of male newborn, (**e**) CMSCs showed one X chromosome (SpectrumGreen) and one Y chromosome (SpectrumOrange), and (**f**) DMSCs showed two X chromosomes (SpectrumGreen)

5. Stain with Giemsa to visualize the cells.
6. Count CFU-F colonies containing 50 or more cells, with a defined colony margin under the microscope.

3.4.2 In Vitro Differentiation

1. For adipogenic induction, seed cells at a density of 2×10^4 cells/cm^2 into chamber slides in their respective complete medium.
2. After reaching 100% confluency, replace the medium with adipogenic induction medium to induce adipogenesis. As a

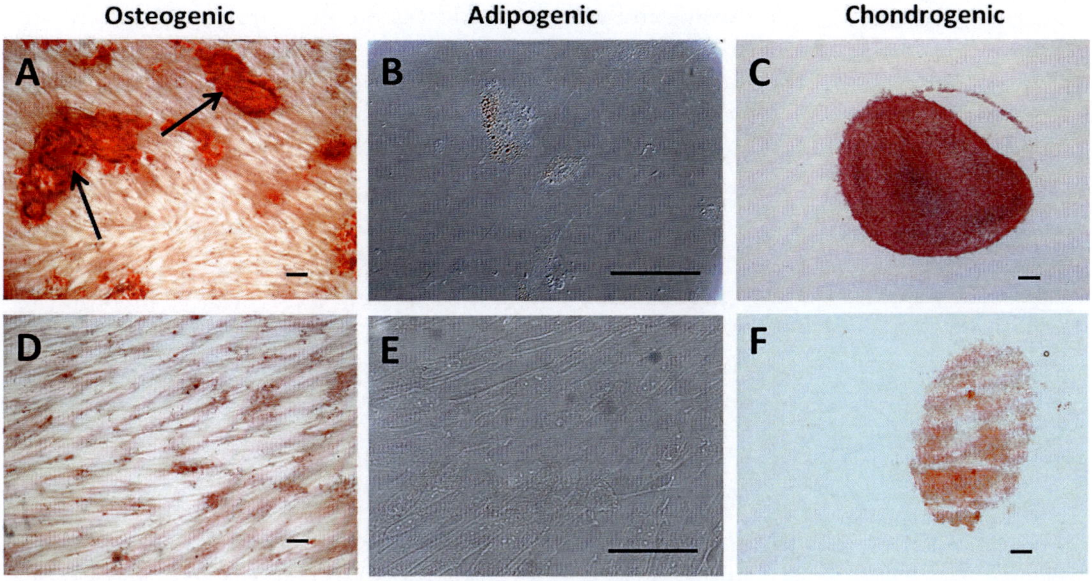

Fig. 3 Representative photomicrographs of DMSCs isolated from preeclamptic placentae differentiation into mesenchymal lineage. *Top row*: differentiated DMSCs (**a**–**c**). *Bottom row*: negative controls, undifferentiated DMSCs (**d**–**f**), and corresponding controls with no added differentiation medium supplements. (**a**) Alizarin Red staining of calcium deposits after osteogenic differentiation and (**d**) control. (**b**) Oil Red O staining of lipid droplets after adipogenic differentiation and (**e**) control. (**c**) Safranin O staining of proteoglycans after chondrogenic differentiation and (**f**) control. Scale bar is 100 μm

negative control, maintain some cultures in complete medium only.

3. Replace adipogenic induction medium every 3–4 days. After 14–21 days, fix the cells with 10% formalin and stain with Oil Red O staining solution for 15 min to detect lipid droplets. Rinse cells with distilled water (*see* **Note 10**; Fig. 3b, e).
4. For osteogenic induction, seed cells at a density of 4×10^3 cells/cm^2 into chamber slides in their respective complete medium.
5. At 50% confluency, replace the medium with osteogenic induction medium to induce osteogenesis. As a negative control, maintain some cultures in complete medium only.
6. Replace osteogenic induction medium every 3–4 days. After 14–21 days (or when cells start to detach), fix the cells with 70% ethanol and stain with Alizarin Red staining solution for 30 min to detect calcium deposits (Fig. 3a, d).
7. For chondrogenesis induction, cells are prepared in a 3D pellet culture at a density of 2.5×10^5 cells per 15 mL polypropylene conical tube (*see* **Note 11**).
8. Centrifuge the cells at $200 \times g$ for 5 min. Aspirate the supernatant.

9. Resuspend cells in chondrogenic induction medium and centrifuge at 200 × *g* for 5 min to form a free-floating pellet. Loosen the tube cap to allow gas exchange, and within 24 h of culture, the cells should form a spherical aggregate, which does not adhere to the walls of the tube.
10. Replace chondrogenic induction medium three times a week without disturbing the cell pellet. Culture cells in DMEM/F12 medium as a negative control.
11. After 21 days, embed the pellet in a cryofixative medium, section in a cryostat (5 μm thickness) and fix the sections in 4% paraformaldehyde, and stain with Safranin O staining solution for 5 min (Fig. 3c, f).

3.4.3 Flow Cytometry

1. For each antibody, stain 1 × 10^5 cells per tube with the fluorescently labeled antibody and the matched isotype control.
2. Incubate the cells with blocking reagent such as human serum and appropriate antibody for 30 min at 4 °C in the dark.
3. Rinse the cells in HBSS (−) with 2% FBS.
4. Centrifuge the cells at 200 × *g* for 5 min. Aspirate the supernatant.
5. Resuspend the cells in HBSS (−) with 2% FBS and 1 μg/mL DAPI.
6. To obtain a single cell suspension, filter the solution through a 35 μm nylon mesh cell strainer cap into the 5 mL FACS tube.
7. Analyze using a flow cytometer. If cells cannot be analyzed on the same day, fix the cells with 4% paraformaldehyde.

3.5 FISH Analysis of DMSCs and CMSCs

FISH analysis was used to differentiate the maternal or fetal origin of DMSCs and CMSC, respectively, and therefore is only performed on placenta obtained from pregnancies with male newborns.

3.5.1 Slide Preparation

1. Mark two well-separated areas on the reverse side of a Polysine slide using a permanent marker or diamond pen to indicate the placement of the pooled cell suspension. The "P" marked on the Polysine slide should face upward, with the marked area on the reverse side. A pre-cleaned glass slide can be used if a Polysine slide is not available (*see* **Note 12**).
2. Centrifuge the cell suspension at 480 × *g* for 5 min.
3. Remove supernatant. Resuspend cells in 2 mL PBS and centrifuge at 480 × *g* for 5 min.
4. Remove supernatant. Add 60 μL PBS and resuspend the pellet. The pellet should look slightly turbid. Adjust the concentration of the pellet with additional PBS if needed.

5. Place ~20 μL of the cell suspension onto each of the marked areas on the slide. Leave the cells to settle for approximately 2 min.
6. Gently add 1–2 μL of Carnoy's fixative to the center of the cell bubbles. Leave for 2 min.
7. Drain excess fluid from the slide by tilting on its long edge and tapping gently against tissue paper.
8. Tilt slide and add approximately 60 μL of fixative so that it washes over the areas of cell adhesion. Drain excess fixative. Repeat this step and allow slides to dry upright for a minimum 5 min. In high humidity, slides may take longer to dry completely.
9. Check cell density under a phase contrast microscope. Approximately 50–100 cells per field of view using a 10× objective are ideal.
10. On the reverse of the slide, use a permanent marker or diamond pen to draw a 10 mm circle around the area where the density of cells is most suitable for the probe to be placed.
11. Proceed directly to pretreatment.

3.5.2 Slide Pretreatment (Undertake in Fume Hood Due to Use of Formaldehyde)

1. Place slides into a Coplin jar of preheated 2× SSC for 2 min at 73 °C ± 2 °C.

   Transfer slides to a Coplin jar containing 30 mL of preheated pepsin working solution for 5 min at 37 °C. The pepsin (30 μL) should be added to the diluent just prior to the addition of slides and will retain activity for up to 1 h.
2. Transfer slides to a Coplin jar of PBS at RT and agitate briefly.
3. Transfer slides to a Coplin jar containing 30 mL of 1% formaldehyde solution for 5 min at RT.
4. Agitate slides briefly in PBS at RT.
5. Run slides briefly through the ethanol series at RT; rinse in 70% ethanol for 1 min; repeat with 85% ethanol for 1 min, followed by 95% ethanol; drain excess ethanol; and air-dry.

3.5.3 Specimen and Probe Co-denaturation

1. Vortex and pulse microfuge the XY probe mix (*see* **Note 13**).
2. Add 1 μL of probe to the target area on the slide. Place a 10 mm round coverslip over the probe. Alternatively, add 1.5–2 μL of probe to each target area if using a 13 mm round coverslip (*see* **Note 14**).
3. Ensure there are no air bubbles under the coverslip, and seal generously with rubber cement. Use a glass pipette to expel the rubber cement so it creates a complete seal between the edge of the coverslip and the glass slide.

4. Co-denature the probe and target by placing the slide on a hotplate at 75 °C ± 1 °C for 5 min.
5. Place slide into a moistened hybridization chamber and hybridize overnight at 37 °C.

3.5.4 Post-hybridization (Stringency) Wash

1. Next morning, preheat a Coplin jar of 0.4× SSC/0.3% NP40 to 73 °C.
2. Take slides from hybridization chamber and use forceps to remove the rubber cement and coverslip from the FISH slides.
3. Wash slide for 2 min in 0.4× SSC/0.3% NP40 at 73 °C without agitation.
4. Remove slides and wash in 2× SSC for 1 min at RT.
5. Drain slide by standing upright and proceed to mounting.

3.5.5 Slide Counterstaining and Mounting

1. While the slide is still damp, mount slide in 8 μL DAPI working solution in fluorescence mounting medium.
2. Cover with a 24 mm × 60 mm coverslip, ensuring there are no air bubbles. Blot off excess fluorescence mounting medium/DAPI before use.
3. Place slides in a covered tray out of the direct light ready for analysis.

3.5.6 Analysis

1. Interphase FISH analysis can be undertaken using a fluorescence microscope fitted with appropriate filters for visualizing DAPI, SpectrumGreen, and SpectrumOrange.
2. Localize the cells under low power (10× objective) using the DAPI filter. Once localized score cell nuclei at a higher magnification (e.g., 63× objective).
3. Female cells such as DMSCs will exhibit two green (X) signals (Fig. 2f). Male cells such as CMSCs will exhibit one green (X) and one orange (Y) signal (Fig. 2e). Score a minimum of 200 cell nuclei.

4 Notes

1. Placenta tissue may contain blood-borne pathogenic microorganisms, and therefore utmost care must be taken to avoid exposure, splashing, or spills. The risk can be decreased by PC2 biohazard training. Personal protective equipment should be used and gloves worn to protect the exposed skin. Wearing a double layer of latex gloves provides added protection and enables easy removal of gloves.
2. A range of commercial MSCs differentiation kits are available. We tested several and achieved reproducible results with the

human MSCs functional identification kit (R&D Systems). Detailed protocols for using the differentiation supplements can be found at the manufacturer's website.

3. The Vysis AneuVysion DNA probe kit also includes DAPI II counterstain, NP40, and 20× SSC, which can be substituted for the equivalent reagents above.
4. An airtight plastic container provides an inexpensive and effective hybridization chamber. Place a moistened paper towel into the bottom of the plastic container, and place two icy pole sticks or tongue depressors on top of the paper towel. Rest the FISH slides across the icy pole sticks and seal the plastic container lid firmly. Place in a 37 °C incubator to hybridize.
5. MSCs isolation from preeclamptic placentae can be hindered by a low recovery efficiency of fibroblast-like cells. Therefore, we suggest using placenta tissue as fresh as possible. At least 50% isolation success has been achieved by processing placenta tissues stored at 4 °C <16 h after placenta delivery. If necessary, fibronectin precoating could also assist in improving MSCs isolation efficiency by promoting cell adherence. Incubate the tissue culture flasks using 10 μg/mL of fibronectin for 1 h at 37 °C.
6. With the explant method for CMSCs isolation, the digestion step could also be performed with 2.5% trypsin and 271 units/mL DNase with gentle agitation at 4 °C for overnight.
7. With the explant method for CMSCs isolation, scratching the surface of the well plates or tissue culture flasks is recommended to aid explant attachment and avoid floating tissue during the first few weeks of culture.
8. With the explant method for CMSCs isolation, digested tissue explants should be removed from tissue culture flasks after 1–2 weeks; however if fungal contamination is a recurring problem during the first 2 weeks of culture, add 0.5% fungizone and/or 1% tylosin to the culture medium.
9. During the final steps of DMSCs isolation, the cell pellet can contain a heterogeneous population of cells at passage 0 that may include endothelial cells and epithelial cells. During routine medium change and cell passaging, the presence of these contaminating cells will decrease over time, and more homogenous populations of fibroblast-like cells will be obtained.
10. It should be noted that adipogenic differentiation of placenta-derived MSCs such as CMSCs and DMSCs is not as efficient as MSCs from other tissue sources such as human bone marrow and adipose tissue.
11. For chondrogenic differentiation, the use of polypropylene tube is crucial for the cells to form a spherical pellet. The use

of polystyrene tubes, for example, will result in cells being attached to the tube surface, and they would not form a spherical pellet.

12. The pooled cell suspensions can be from the same sample or different samples. Ensure position on the slide is recorded accurately if using different samples.
13. Exposure of fluorescence probes to harsh light results in photo bleaching and should be avoided. However, experience has shown that all incubations, washes, and slide drying can be undertaken in normal indoor lighting conditions without adversely affecting the quality of results. Shield slides from light once prepared.
14. The use of a small target region reduces probe cost substantially (1–2 μL FISH probe applied per test instead of 10 μL).

Acknowledgments

We greatly acknowledge the work of Dr Rishika Anne Pace, Dr Sharon Qin, Melissa Duggan, and Anthony Borg who contributed to the optimization of these protocols.

References

1. Gude NM, Roberts CT, Kalionis B, King RG (2004) Growth and function of the normal human placenta. Thromb Res 114:397–407. https://doi.org/10.1016/j.thromres.2004.06.038
2. in't Anker PS, Scherjon SA, Kleijburg-van der Keur C et al (2004) Isolation of mesenchymal stem cells of fetal or maternal origin from human placenta. Stem Cells 22:1338–1345. https://doi.org/10.1634/stemcells.2004-0058
3. Wulf GG, Viereck V, Hemmerlein B et al (2004) Mesengenic progenitor cells derived from human placenta. Tissue Eng 10:1136–1147. https://doi.org/10.1089/ten.2004.10.1136
4. Macias MI, Grande J, Moreno A et al (2010) Isolation and characterization of true mesenchymal stem cells derived from human term decidua capable of multilineage differentiation into all 3 embryonic layers. Am J Obstet Gynecol 203:495.e9–495.e23
5. Kanematsu D, Shofuda T, Yamamoto A et al (2011) Isolation and cellular properties of mesenchymal cells derived from the decidua of human term placenta. Differentiation 82:77–88. https://doi.org/10.1016/j.diff.2011.05.010
6. Kusuma GD, Manuelpillai U, Abumaree MH et al (2015) Mesenchymal stem cells reside in a vascular niche in the decidua basalis and are absent in remodelled spiral arterioles. Placenta 36:312–321. https://doi.org/10.1016/j.placenta.2014.12.014
7. Oliver C (1999) Human decidual stromal cells express alpha-smooth muscle actin and show ultrastructural similarities with myofibroblasts. Hum Reprod 14:1599–1605. https://doi.org/10.1093/humrep/14.6.1599
8. Indumathi S, Harikrishnan R, Mishra R et al (2013) Comparison of feto-maternal organ derived stem cells in facets of immunophenotype, proliferation and differentiation. Tissue Cell 45:434–442. https://doi.org/10.1016/j.tice.2013.07.007
9. Castrechini NM, Murthi P, Qin S et al (2012) Decidua parietalis-derived mesenchymal stromal cells reside in a vascular niche within the choriodecidua. Reprod Sci 19:1302. https://doi.org/10.1177/1933719112450334
10. Parolini O, Alviano F, Bagnara GP et al (2008) Concise review: isolation and characterization of cells from human term placenta: outcome of the first international Workshop on Placenta Derived Stem Cells. Stem Cells 26:300–311.

https://doi.org/10.1634/stemcells.2007-0594
11. Fukuchi Y, Nakajima H, Sugiyama D et al (2004) Human placenta-derived cells have mesenchymal stem/progenitor cell potential. Stem Cells 22:649–658. https://doi.org/10.1634/stemcells.22-5-649
12. Igura K, Zhang X, Takahashi K et al (2004) Isolation and characterization of mesenchymal progenitor cells from chorionic villi of human placenta. Cytotherapy 6:543–553. https://doi.org/10.1080/14653240410005366
13. Zhang X, Mitsuru A, Igura K et al (2006) Mesenchymal progenitor cells derived from chorionic villi of human placenta for cartilage tissue engineering. Biochem Biophys Res Commun 340:944–952. https://doi.org/10.1016/j.bbrc.2005.12.091
14. Castrechini NM, Murthi P, Gude NM et al (2010) Mesenchymal stem cells in human placental chorionic villi reside in a vascular Niche. Placenta 31:203–212. https://doi.org/10.1016/j.placenta.2009.12.006
15. Nazarov I, Lee JW, Soupene E et al (2012) Multipotent stromal stem cells from human placenta demonstrate high therapeutic potential. Stem Cells Transl Med 1:359–372. https://doi.org/10.5966/sctm.2011-0021
16. Abumaree MH, Al Jumah MA, Kalionis B et al (2013) Phenotypic and functional characterization of mesenchymal stem cells from chorionic villi of human term placenta. Stem Cell Rev Rep 9:16–31. https://doi.org/10.1007/s12015-012-9385-4
17. Heazlewood CF, Sherrell H, Ryan J et al (2014) High incidence of contaminating maternal cell overgrowth in human placental mesenchymal stem/stromal cell cultures: a systematic review. Stem Cells Transl Med 3:1305–1311
18. Dominici M, Le Blanc K, Mueller I et al (2006) Minimal criteria for defining multipotent mesenchymal stromal cells. The International Society for Cellular Therapy position statement. Cytotherapy 8:315–317. https://doi.org/10.1080/14653240600855905
19. Parolini O, Alviano F, Bergwerf I et al (2010) Toward cell therapy using placenta-derived cells: disease mechanisms, cell biology, preclinical studies, and regulatory aspects at the round table. Stem Cells Dev 19:143–154. https://doi.org/10.1089/scd.2009.0404
20. Kusuma GD, Abumaree MH, Pertile MD et al (2016) Mesenchymal stem/stromal cells derived from a reproductive tissue niche under oxidative stress have high aldehyde dehydrogenase activity. Stem Cell Rev Rep 12:285–297. https://doi.org/10.1007/s12015-016-9649-5
21. Abumaree MH, Abomaray FM, Alshehri NA et al (2016) Phenotypic and functional characterization of mesenchymal stem/multipotent stromal cells from decidua parietalis of human term placenta. Reprod Sci 23:1193. https://doi.org/10.1177/1933719116632924
22. Gonzalez PL, Carvajal C, Cuenca J et al (2015) Chorion mesenchymal stem cells show superior differentiation, immunosuppressive, and angiogenic potentials in comparison with haploidentical maternal placental cells. Stem Cells Transl Med 4:1109–1121
23. Abumaree MH, Al JM a, Kalionis B et al (2013) Human placental mesenchymal stem cells (pMSCs) play a role as immune suppressive cells by shifting macrophage differentiation from inflammatory M1 to anti-inflammatory M2 macrophages. Stem Cell Rev Rep 9:620–641. https://doi.org/10.1007/s12015-013-9455-2
24. Abomaray FM, Al Jumah MA, Kalionis B et al (2015) Human chorionic villous mesenchymal stem cells modify the functions of human dendritic cells, and induce an anti-inflammatory phenotype in CD1+ dendritic cells. Stem Cell Rev 11:423. https://doi.org/10.1007/s12015-014-9562-8
25. Kusuma GD, Menicanin D, Gronthos S et al (2015) Ectopic bone formation by mesenchymal stem cells derived from human term placenta and the decidua. PLoS One 10:e0141246. https://doi.org/10.1371/journal.pone.0141246
26. Qin SQ, Kusuma GD, Al-Sowayan B et al (2016) Establishment and characterization of fetal and maternal mesenchymal stem/stromal cell lines from the human term placenta. Placenta 39:134–146. https://doi.org/10.1016/j.placenta.2016.01.018
27. Liu H, Murthi P, Qin S et al (2014) A novel combination of homeobox genes is expressed in mesenchymal chorionic stem/stromal cells in first trimester and term pregnancies. Reprod Sci 21:1382–1394
28. Tran TC, Kimura K, Nagano M et al (2011) Identification of human placenta-derived mesenchymal stem cells involved in re-endothelialization. J Cell Physiol 226:224–235. https://doi.org/10.1002/jcp.22329
29. Ohlsson R, Falck P, Hellstrom M et al (1999) PDGFB regulates the development of the labyrinthine layer of the mouse fetal placenta. Dev Biol 212:124–136. https://doi.org/10.1006/dbio.1999.9306
30. Hwang JH, Lee MJ, Seok OS et al (2010) Cytokine expression in placenta-derived mes-

enchymal stem cells in patients with preeclampsia and normal pregnancies. Cytokine 49:95–101. https://doi.org/10.1016/j.cyto.2009.08.013

31. Wang Y, Fan H, Zhao G et al (2012) miR-16 inhibits the proliferation and angiogenesis-regulating potential of mesenchymal stem cells in severe pre-eclampsia. FEBS J 279:4510–4524. https://doi.org/10.1111/febs.12037
32. Zhao G, Zhou X, Chen S et al (2014) Differential expression of microRNAs in decidua-derived mesenchymal stem cells from patients with preeclampsia. J Biomed Sci 21:81. https://doi.org/10.1186/s12929-014-0081-3
33. Chen S, Zhao G, Miao H et al (2015) MicroRNA-494 inhibits the growth and angiogenesis-regulating potential of mesenchymal stem cells. FEBS Lett 589:710–717. https://doi.org/10.1016/j.febslet.2015.01.038
34. Kusuma GD, Abumaree MH, Perkins AV et al (2017) Reduced aldehyde dehydrogenase expression in preeclamptic decidual mesenchymal stem/stromal cells is restored by aldehyde dehydrogenase agonists. Sci Rep 7:42397. https://doi.org/10.1038/srep42397
35. Rolfo A, Giuffrida D, Nuzzo AM et al (2013) Pro-inflammatory profile of preeclamptic placental mesenchymal stromal cells: new insights into the etiopathogenesis of preeclampsia. PLoS One 8:e59403
36. Portmann-Lanz CB, Baumann MU, Mueller M et al (2010) Neurogenic characteristics of placental stem cells in preeclampsia. Am J Obstet Gynecol 203(399):e1–e7. https://doi.org/10.1016/j.ajog.2010.06.054
37. Liu L, Zhao G, Fan H et al (2014) Mesenchymal stem cells ameliorate Th1-induced preeclampsia-like symptoms in mice via the suppression of TNF-alpha expression. PLoS One 9:e88036. https://doi.org/10.1371/journal.pone.0088036
38. Chatterjee P, Chiasson VL, Pinzur L, Raveh S, Abraham EEA (2016) Human placenta-derived stromal cells decrease inflammation, placental injury, and blood pressure in hypertensive pregnant mice. Clin Sci (Lond) 130:513–523. https://doi.org/10.1042/CS20150555
39. National High Blood Pressure Education Program Working Group on High Blood Pressure in P (2000) Report of the National High Blood Pressure Education Program Working Group on high blood pressure in pregnancy. Am J Obstet Gynecol 183:s1–s22. https://doi.org/10.1067/mob.2000.107928

Chapter 20

An Electrical Impedance-Based Assay to Examine Functions of Various Placental Cell Types In Vitro

Tejasvy Chollangi, Hélène Clabault, Andrée-Anne Hudon Thibeault, Hannah E.J. Yong, Shagun Narula, Ellen Menkhorst, J. Thomas Sanderson, Cathy Vaillancourt, and Padma Murthi

Abstract

In vitro functional analyses of cells are widely used to investigate the molecular mechanisms involved in preeclampsia. Common cellular functions studied include adhesion, apoptosis, proliferation, migration, and invasion. At present, most researchers will use endpoint experimental assays that only allow the determination of cell function at a single time point, with the need to repeat the experiment for an alternate time point. Here, we describe an electrical impedance-based tool that allows real-time monitoring of cells, which enables the efficient assessment of multiple time points over the duration of a single experiment.

Key words Functional assays, Adhesion, Proliferation, Apoptosis, Migration, Invasion, xCELLigence® RTCA systems

1 Introduction

A large variety of cell types are involved in placentation. Understanding how these cells function is imperative to further the current knowledge of placental disorders such as preeclampsia. For example, much research performed has focused on the migration and invasion of extravillous trophoblast cells into the decidua. Another example would be determining apoptosis of endothelial cells in the context of endothelial dysfunction. Current assays that are commonly used, such as migration scratch assays and cell viability assays, are tedious and require multiple experiments to measure different time points. In this chapter, we describe the use of the xCELLigence® real-time cell analysis (RTCA) systems (ACEA

Cathy Vaillancourt and Padma Murthi share joint senior authorship.
Tejasvy Chollangi, Hélène Clabault, Andrée-Anne Hudon Thibeault, and Hannah E.J. Yong, contributed equally to this study.

Padma Murthi and Cathy Vaillancourt (eds.), *Preeclampsia: Methods and Protocols*, Methods in Molecular Biology, vol. 1710, https://doi.org/10.1007/978-1-4939-7498-6_20, © Springer Science+Business Media LLC 2018

Biosciences Inc., San Diego, CA), which offer the opportunity to continuously monitor cellular behavior and explore multiple cell functions in real time [1]. The xCELLigence® RTCA systems can be used to study basic cell behaviors, such as adhesion, apoptosis, migration, proliferation, and invasion, as well as be customized to determine specialized cell functions. These systems enable cell activity and kinesis to be measured and quantified as changes in the impedance of an electric current (Fig. 1). Gold microelectrodes embedded in the base of the wells of a cell culture plate transmit the current at specific intervals. The presence of adherent cells impedes the flow of electrons when current is applied. This impedance in the conduction of electricity is measured as a quantifiable signal referred to as the cell index (Fig. 1a). The cell index is an arbitrary unit of measurement defined as $\frac{R(t)-R(t_0)}{15}$. $R(t_0)$ represents the background impedance in the well with only medium, while $R(t)$ reflects the impedance at any given time point when the cells are present [2, 3]. The cell index accounts for background impedance through the use of an initial "blanking" step, which enables the system to correct for the impedance caused by medium alone. The cell index rises as cells spread across the electrodes (Fig. 1b). Eventually, when the cells reach confluence in the well, the cell index will plateau for a period of time. Any subsequent decline will reflect the cell death or detachment. Therefore, the real-time monitoring of cell activity allows users to select the optimal time points for other endpoint experiments.

There are seven different xCELLigence® RTCA models, with different plate compatibilities. For placental studies, the most popular models are the xCELLigence® dual plate (DP), single plate (SP), and multiple plate (MP) (Table 1). Customized plates allow various functions to be tested. The E-plate can contain anywhere from 8 to 384 wells depending on the xCELLigence® RTCA model with the most popular plates having 16 or 96 wells. E-plates can be used to measure events such as cell adhesion, proliferation, and apoptosis (Table 1). E-Plates are similar to regular cell culture plates except that the base of each well contains electrodes. The alternative cell invasion/migration (CIM)-plate, which is only available in 16-well format, is used to determine cell migration or invasion in wells that are pre-coated with a gel matrix. The CIM-plate utilizes a modified Boyden chamber, and each well consists of an upper and lower chamber separated by a microporous membrane (8 μm pore). The microelectrodes are present at the underside of the upper chamber to detect electrical impedance change caused by migratory and invasive cells that have passed through the membrane. E-Plate inserts, which are to be used for co-culture assays, are also available can be added on top of a 16- or 96-well E-plate. There is no impedance monitoring in the insert. E-plate

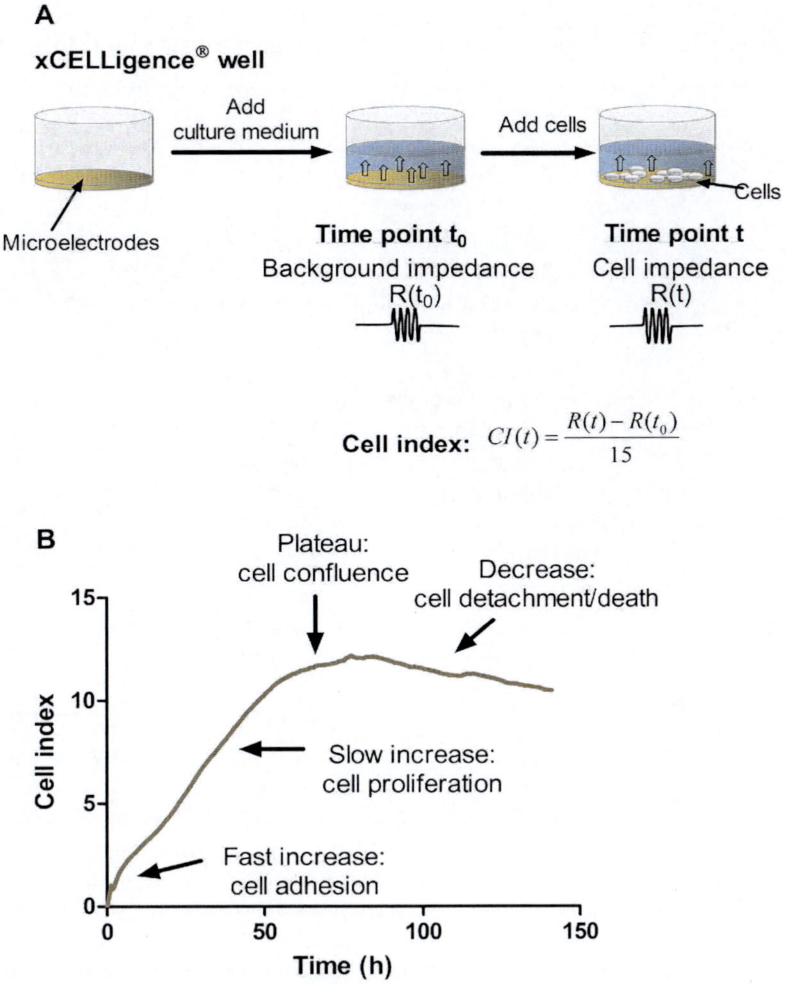

Fig. 1 Basic principles of the xCELLigence® RTCA systems. (**a**) Impedance and cell index measurements. The xCELLigence® RTCA systems utilize differences in electrical impedance caused by cell attachment to provide a measurement of cell function expressed as a cell index. The background impedance ($R(t_0)$) is determined at the start of the experiment, with its cell index always rendered to a value of 0. Any subsequent measurements of impedance caused by cell attachment are then reflected in positive cell index values ($R(t)$). (**b**) A typical real-time impedance curve

inserts are rather used to evaluate the influence of another cell type on the cells in the E-plate wells.

The use of xCELLigence® RTCA instruments can be challenging when setting up experiments with non-adherent or non-proliferative cells. Cell impedance monitoring is also sensitive to any change in the atmospheric conditions, and experiments can be affected by humidity and temperature changes in the incubator due to door opening, for instance. Consumables can also be expensive (*see* **Note 1**). Nevertheless, xCELLigence® RTCA systems have

Table 1
Description of the most commonly used xCELLigence instruments to study placental cell lines

Instrument	Assays: – Cell characterization – Proliferation and cytotoxicity – Adhesion – Receptor signaling – Cell interaction: co-culture – Hypoxia studies – Phenotypic screening (mode of action of drugs)	Assays: – Invasion – Migration	Format	Compatible plate
RTCA DP	Yes	Yes	3 × 16 wells	– CIM-plate 16 – E-plate 16 (±View and ±PET) – E-plate insert
RTCA SP	Yes	No	1 × 96 wells	– E-plate 96 (±View and ±PET) – E-plate insert
RTCA MP	Yes	No	3 × 96 wells	

RTCA real-time cell analyzers, *DP* dual plate, *SP* single plate, *MP* multiple plates, *CIM* cell invasion/migration, *View* wells have a clear inspection window to visualize cells (no electrode in this window), *PET* bottomed plates, polyethylene terephthalate is an alternative to more expensive glass-bottomed plates. Offered only for E-plate 16 and 96 VIEW

numerous advantages over conventional end-point-based cell assays. The benefits of xCELLigence® RTCA systems include considerable time savings and the ability to continuously measure cellular events without the use of invasive cell labels. Furthermore, xCELLigence® RTCA systems have the capacity to adapt a running protocol in real-time response to the collected data. It is also possible to harvest the conditioned medium and the cells after xCELLigence monitoring to perform other analyses such as the staining of cell markers or measurement of cell secretions, such as human chorionic gonadotropin (hCG), human placental lactogen (hPL), or steroid hormones.

2 Material

In the present chapter, we will focus on three xCELLigence® models: DP, SP, and MP.

2.1 Cell Passage and Counting

1. Cells of interest.
2. Phosphate-buffered saline (PBS); pH 7.4.

3. Trypsin or other cell dissociation buffers.
4. Cell culture medium.
5. Treatment (optional).
6. Manual or automated cytometer.
7. Trypan blue (optional).

2.2 The xCELLigence Assays

1. The xCELLigence® RTCA instrument: dual plate (DP, 16 wells × 3 cradles), single plate (SP, 96 wells × 1 cradle), or multiple plate (MP, 96 wells × 6 cradles) (ACEA Biosciences).
2. E-Plates 16 or 96 for adhesion, proliferation, and apoptosis assays (ACEA Biosciences).
3. CIM-plates 16 for migration and invasion assays (ACEA Biosciences).
4. Extracellular matrix (e.g., Matrigel™) for invasion assays.

3 Methods

Handle all materials in a sterile hood. The xCELLigence instrument® RTCA should be placed in an incubator and maintained at standard humidified conditions (37 °C/5% CO_2). Ensure that the instrument is properly connected to the computer and functional before starting the experiment (*see* **Note 2**). Optimal time points and cell densities must be determined for each cell type to be used. The following steps are a guide only; the xCELLigence user manual should be consulted before use.

3.1 Adhesion/Proliferation Assay

1. Add 100 μL of medium to each well (*see* **Notes 3–5**). Leave E-plate to equilibrate for 30 min at room temperature.
2. During plate equilibration, trypsinize cells and resuspend in culture medium to obtain the appropriate dilution of cell suspension (100 μL per well will be necessary). The ideal cell density has to be optimized for each cell type studied (Fig. 2 and Table 2).
3. Once the plate is equilibrated, do a background measurement in the xCELLigence instrument (*see* Subheading 3.3).
4. Add 100 μL of cell suspension and allow cells to settle on the base of the well for 30 min at room temperature (*see* **Note 6**).
5. Place plate into the instrument cradle and begin the experiment (*see* **Notes 7–9**). If performing a co-culture experiment, *see* Subheading 3.2 in Chapter 23 for a detailed protocol.

3.2 Migration/Invasion Assay

1. When performing an invasion assay, pre-coat the upper chamber with Matrigel™ or another desired gel matrix (*see* **Note 10**).

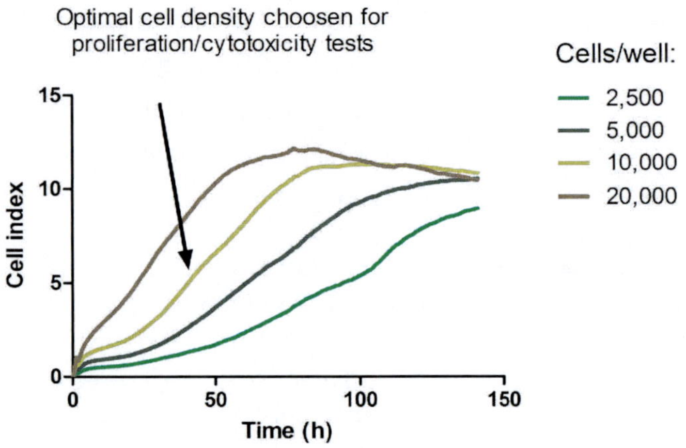

Fig. 2 The xCELLigence® RTCA system can be used to produce typical cell titration curves to determine optimal cell densities and time points for other experiments (an example is given for the proliferation of BeWo cells, 200 μL of medium by well)

Table 2
Optimal cell densities for placental cell lines using an xCELLigence® RTCA system

Cell line	Plate type	Cell concentration (cells/well)	References
Proliferation tests			
BeWo	E-plate 16	1×10^4	[5]
JEG-3	E-plate 96	2.5×10^3 and 5×10^3	[6] (Clabault data not published)
HIPEC	E-plate 96	2.5×10^3	(Clabault data not published)
HTR8/SVneo	E-plate 16	4×10^3–4×10^4	[3, 7]
SGHPL-4	E-plate 16	1.25×10^3–4×10^4	[3]
BeWo/H295R co-culture	E-plate 16 and E-plate insert	H295R (well): 2×10^4 BeWo (insert): 1×10^4	[5]
Migration/invasion tests			
HTR8/SVneo migration	CIM-plate 16	4×10^4–2×10^5	[3, 7–9]
HTR8/SVneo invasion	CIM-plate 16	4×10^4	[8]

2. Add 165 μL of culture medium to the bottom chamber of each well. Attach the upper chamber and add a further 50 μL of culture medium to the upper chamber of each well (*see* **Note 11**). Leave CIM-plate to equilibrate for 1 h in the xCELLigence instrument.
3. During plate equilibration, trypsinize cells and resuspend in culture medium to obtain the appropriate cell density. The ideal number of cells has to be optimized for each cell type studied (Table 2).

4. Once the plate is equilibrated, do a background measurement of medium alone in the xCELLigence instrument (*see* Subheading 3.3).
5. After the background check, add 100 μL of cell suspension and allow cells to settle on the base of the upper chamber of each well for 30 min at room temperature. This is a critical step as convection currents from the warm medium (37 °C) may affect cell attachment and introduce variations into the experimental results.
6. Place plate into the instrument cradle and begin the experiment.

3.3 Using the xCELLigence Software

1. Create a new experiment.
2. Enter the relevant information such as treatment conditions, cell types, cell density, and number of replicates in the "Layout" tab.
3. In the "Schedule" tab, add at least two steps. The first step is the background measurement step and the default settings should not be modified. The second step is the start of the experiment and can be split into sub-steps if desired to, for example, require readings to be taken every 5 min in the first hour (12 sweeps during 1 h) and once an hour for the next 48 h (48 sweeps during 48 h). Experimental protocols can be set up and saved in the computer software beforehand.
4. After placing the plate into the instrument cradle, check the "Message" tab to ensure that all connections are good. The message should say "Plate scanned. Connections ok." Usually at this step, pressing the "Play" button will prompt the software to ask if you wish to save the experiment. Click "Yes" and the background measurement will be recorded and accounted for. When completed, remove the plate and proceed to add the cells.
5. After cells have been added to the wells and allowed to settle, place the plate back into the cradle to begin the experiment. Before pressing the "Play" button, ensure that there are no connection errors in the "Message" tab as above. When the plate has to be removed from the instrument cradle (e.g., for treatments), press the "Pause" button.
6. When the experiment is finished (either at the end of the last step or after abortion of the experiment), problematic curves may be repaired using the curve adjustment tool (shift or line fit) under the "Plot" tab in the xCELLigence software.
7. Data can be normalized relative to a given time point, usually at the beginning of the experiment after the cells have settled down. Normalization corrects for well-to-well variation in initial cell densities that are not due to experimental conditions/treatments. It is also possible to express cell index as the

difference between an experimental condition and a baseline at each given time point, which is called delta cell index.

8. Analyze data using the data analysis tool.

4 Notes

1. Plates may potentially be reused to minimize costs [4]. It is up to the end user to decide if they wish to do so. However, we personally would not recommend it as there is a substantial risk of contamination once the plate is placed in the incubator and exposed to a non-sterile environment. Additionally, the process of removing the cells and spent medium may damage the sensitive electrodes within the wells, which would affect subsequent experimental results.
2. The instrument must be regularly maintained as per manufacturer's instructions. Routinely check for any corrosion of cradle pins as this will likely affect experimental results. Ensure that control plates (supplied with the instrument) are run to identify any problems if the instrument has not been used for a significant period of time.
3. It is possible to add PBS in the gaps between the wells to minimize evaporation from the wells.
4. The incubator housing the xCELLigence instrument should have sufficient water in the water tray to ensure high humidity, as the electrodes are highly sensitive to fluctuations in surrounding humidity. Care should be taken to recognize a potential "edge effect" in the plate, as wells on the periphery of the plate are not exposed to the same humidity level as the wells within, which may affect cell behavior depending on the cell type studied.
5. If not all the wells are used in an experiment, the unused wells can be kept sterile with a sealing adhesive film (e.g., PCR sealing film).
6. Ensure that no air bubbles are present after pipetting the culture medium into the wells. The air bubbles can affect the electrical impedance detected in the well and give an inaccurate background measurement. Be extra careful when pipetting medium containing fetal calf serum, which can produce a lot of bubbles. One method to avoid air bubbles is to perform reverse pipetting, which will allow the target volume to be released without introducing any air.
7. If you need to treat the cells, pause the cell impedance monitoring step, remove the plate from the station and add the test compounds to the culture medium or replace the culture

medium in the wells with pretreated culture medium. Another possibility is to plate cells directly in pretreated culture medium at the beginning of the experiment, but be aware that treatments may affect cell adhesion.

8. If at any time point of the experiment, the culture medium needs to be removed to either renew the medium or to add pretreated culture medium to the wells, avoid touching the bottom of the wells with the pipet tip as it could detach cells and introduce additional variability to the experiment. This can be done by leaving a small amount of culture medium (10 μL) in each well. Fresh culture medium should be added carefully, ideally by pipetting down slowly against the inside wall of the well.
9. Using E-Plate View, it is possible to visually inspect the cells (e.g., morphology, proliferative state), while pausing the experiment.
10. When coating the wells with Matrigel™ for the invasion assays, ensure that ice-cold medium is used to dilute the Matrigel™. It is also imperative that there are no air bubbles in the Matrigel™ coating, as these will interfere with cell movement through the matrix. From our experience, the best technique to ensure this is by reverse pipetting. The coated plate can then be incubated for 30 min at 37 °C or left in the cell culture cabinet overnight at room temperature to set. If using the incubator, do not leave the gel to set for more than 2 h as the coating may dry out.
11. There should be a clear meniscus on top of the wells in the lower chamber. This comes into direct contact with the electrodes. A "click" sound should be heard when attaching the upper and lower chambers together.

Acknowledgment

The authors would like to thank the Department of Maternal-Fetal Medicine, Pregnancy Research Centre at the Royal Women's Hospital for its financial support for the purchase of an xCELLigence (DP) system. This work was further supported by March of Dimes Social and Behavioral Sciences Research (grant no. 12-FY12-179) both awarded to J.T.S. and C.V.; Natural Sciences and Engineering Research Council (NSERC) of Canada Discovery grants to C.V. (03948-2014) and J.T.S. (313313-2012), as well as studentships to H.C. from the *Réseau Québécois en Reproduction-NSERC-CREATE* and the *Fondation Universitaire Armand-Frappier INRS*, and to A.A.H.T. from the Canadian Institutes of Health Research (CIHR).

References

1. ACEA Biosciences Inc (2016) xCELLigence RTCA systems. ACEA Biosciences Inc, San Diego, CA
2. Ke N, Wang X, Xu X, Abassi YA (2011) The xCELLigence system for real-time and label-free monitoring of cell viability. Methods Mol Biol 740:33–43
3. Keogh RJ (2010) New technology for investigating trophoblast function. Placenta 31: 347–350
4. Stefanowicz-Hajduk J, Adamska A, Bartoszewski R, Ochocka JR (2016) Reuse of E-plate cell sensor arrays in the xCELLigence real-time cell analyzer. BioTechniques 61:117–122
5. Thibeault AA, Deroy K, Vaillancourt C, Sanderson JT (2014) A unique co-culture model for fundamental and applied studies of human fetoplacental steroidogenesis and interference by environmental chemicals. Environ Health Perspect 122:371–377
6. Kaitu'u-Lino TJ, Pattison S, Ye L, Tuohey L, Sluka P, MacDiarmid J, Brahmbhatt H, Johns T, Horne AW, Brown J, Tong S (2013) Targeted nanoparticle delivery of doxorubicin into placental tissues to treat ectopic pregnancies. Endocrinology 154:911–919
7. Peng W, Chen Y, Luo X, Shan N, Lan X, Olson D, Zhang H, Ding YB, Qi HB (2016) DNA methylation-associated repression of MEST/PEG1 expression contributes to the invasion of extravillous trophoblast cells. Placenta 46:92–101
8. Chau SE, Murthi P, Wong MH, Whitley GS, Brennecke SP, Keogh RJ (2013) Control of extravillous trophoblast function by the eotaxins CCL11, CCL24 and CCL26. Hum Reprod 28:1497–1507
9. Nystad M, Sitras V, Larsen M, Acharya G (2014) Placental expression of aminopeptidase-Q (laeverin) and its role in the pathophysiology of preeclampsia. Am J Obstet Gynecol 211(686): e681–e631

Chapter 21

In Vitro Induction of Hypoxia/Reoxygenation on Placental Cells: A Suitable Model for Understanding Placental Diseases

Lucas Sagrillo-Fagundes, Laetitia Laurent, Josianne Bienvenue-Pariseault, and Cathy Vaillancourt

Abstract

Lack of blood flow and aberrant levels of oxygenation in placentas are recurrent in pregnancy diseases, such as preeclampsia. These alterations generate situations of hypoxia and hypoxia/reoxygenation (H/R) and consequent oxidative stress, increased cell death, and inflammation in trophoblasts. The models used to understand the effects of hypoxia and H/R on trophoblasts require a rather big structure. This chapter describes the details of a suitable and reasonable approach with hypoxia chambers to expose human placental trophoblasts to variable conditions of oxygenation.

Key words Normoxia, Hypoxia, Hypoxia/reoxygenation, Villous trophoblast, Extravillous trophoblast, Syncytiotrophoblast

1 Introduction

Across the first trimester of pregnancy, hypoxia has a key role in the uterine invasion. This stimulus is essential for the invasion of extravillous trophoblasts (evTB) and the achievement of endovascular trophoblasts toward the enlargement of uteroplacental arteries and consequent increased placental blood flow. Low concentrations of oxygen (15–20 mmHg or <2% O_2) during the placentation are gradually increased, and the end of the pregnancy is coincident with relatively high levels of oxygen (55–60 mm Hg or <8% O_2) [1, 2]. This increase is tightly regulated and is correlated with successful pregnancy outcomes. The lack of regulation in this process leads to alterations such as preeclampsia and intrauterine growth restriction (IUGR) [3]. The etiology of preeclampsia is still a source of debates and some epidemiological studies suggest that it has a genetic and immunological origin. Regardless of its origin, the effects of preeclampsia are well characterized with several

Padma Murthi and Cathy Vaillancourt (eds.), *Preeclampsia: Methods and Protocols*, Methods in Molecular Biology, vol. 1710, https://doi.org/10.1007/978-1-4939-7498-6_21,

effects for maternal and fetal health according to its intensity and mainly with its onset point [4, 5]. Just as preeclampsia, IUGR is a major morbidity during the pregnancy. Both of these diseases are associated with an abnormal first-trimester trophoblast differentiation. This happening is related with a shallow placental invasion and decreased remodeling of maternal spiral arteries and a consequent failure at the uteroplacental perfusion. Reduced perfusion leads to episodes of hypoxia or hypoxia/reoxygenation (H/R), correlated with inflammatory processes, aberrant cell death, and oxidative stress in trophoblasts [2, 5]. The comprehension of the effect of aberrant oxygenation during the pregnancy has been a source of experimental and epidemiological studies.

Human placenta is classified as type haemomonochorial, only present in superior apes. In this kind of placenta, syncytiotrophoblast has a direct contact with the maternal blood and is able to produce the hormone human chorionic gonadotropin (hCG). The unique architecture of human placenta is a challenge for animal models as it varies drastically even in the order of primates. Usual animal models (e.g., rats and mice) can only reproduce some characteristics of preeclampsia under pharmacological induction. Only members of the family Homininae (humans, chimpanzees, and gorillas) have a similar pattern of deep evTB invasion and spiral artery remodeling [6, 7]. In this context, placental cell lines, primary isolated cytotrophoblast cells, and even placental explants have been shown as suitable models for the comprehension of H/R to the placental homeostasis. Moreover, these models have been used to understand the molecular events involving preeclampsia and IUGR [8–10]. A great variety of approaches have been developed to reproduce properly the placental environment under hypoxic conditions along the last decades with results with increasing levels of comprehension and complexity.

The procedure detailed in this chapter has been used in several approaches during the last years with consistent results and reproducibility and has a relatively affordable cost.

2 Materials

1. Modular incubator chamber (a set of two chambers is necessary for simultaneous induction of normoxia, hypoxia, and H/R).
2. Single flow meter.
3. 50 mm In-Line Filter (PTFE, pore: 1.0 μm).
4. Pro Star Gas Regulator.
5. Gas hose class VI clear 5/16 (three pieces with ~0.5 m).
6. 17 mm adjustable gas hose clamp.

7. Gas cylinder size K:
   (a) Normoxia (third trimester's composition: 5% CO_2, 8% O_2, Bal. N_2).
   (b) Normoxia (first trimester's composition: 5% CO_2, 2% O_2, Bal. N_2).
   (c) Hypoxia (5% CO_2, 0.5% O_2, Bal. N_2).
8. Oxygen microelectrode.
9. Oxygen adapter.
10. pH-mV meter.

3 Methods

3.1 Hypoxia Chamber Assembling with the Flow Meter and a Cylinder of Gas (Fig. 1)

1. Attach a hose (*5*) with a clamp (*6*) to the gas cylinder (*7*) (*see* **Note 1**).
2. Insert the 1 μm pore size filter (*3*) between the hose attached to the cylinder (*5a*) and the inlet hose (*5b*) of the flow meter (*2*).
3. Connect the outlet hose (*5c*) of the flow meter to the inlet port of the hypoxia chamber (*1*).
4. Open the outlet port of the hypoxia chamber.

3.2 Hypoxia Chamber Operation (Fig. 1)

1. Inside a laminar flow hood, open the chamber and place a petri dish with sterile water to avoid dehumidification.
2. Place the plates or cell culture flasks previously prepared on the superior levels of the chamber.

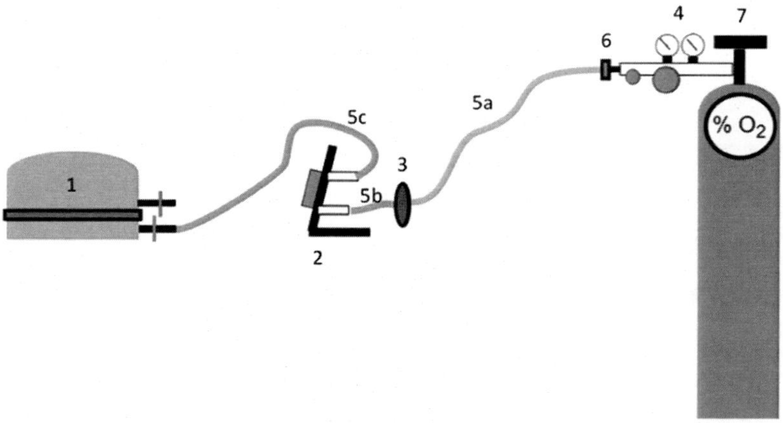

Fig. 1 Schematic representation of the components of a hypoxia/reoxygenation chamber. Hypoxia chamber and gas cylinder assembling: (*1*) modular incubator chamber; (*2*) flow meter; (*3*) inlet filter; (*4*) gas regulator; (*5a*) cylinder gas hose; (*5b*) inlet hose; (*5c*) outlet hose; (*6*) gas hose clamp; (*7*) gas cylinder (Modified from Sagrillo-Fagundes et al. 2016 [12])

3. Close the chamber inside the hood.
4. Outside the hood, attach the chamber (inlet port) by the gas hose (*5c*) to the set of source of gas (*7*) as described in Subheading 3.1. Open both inlet and outlet ports of the chamber. At this moment the gas regulator (*4*) should remain closed.
5. Carefully open the valve of the gas regulator (*4*) (*see* **Note 2**). The flow meter (*2*) will indicate the amount of air (L/min) that is accessing the chamber. A flush of 4 min with an amount of 25 L/min is necessary to completely change the gas inside the chamber.
6. After the intended time of air flow, close the gas regulator (*4*) and then close the inlet and outlet ports of the chamber.
7. Unplug the flow meter outlet hose (*5c*) from the inlet port of the chamber.
8. Set the chamber in a cell incubator at 37 °C.
9. The chamber must be filled with gas again 1 h afterward. The purpose of this last purge is to remove the air presumably present in the plates, flasks, and dissolved in the culture medium.
10. Repeat **steps 1–9** for chambers comprising other gas configurations.

3.3 Confirmatory Oxygen Measurement (Fig. 2)

1. To confirm the concentration of oxygen in the cell medium kept inside the chamber, it is necessary to use an oxygen electrode hooked up to an Oxygen Adapter. The oxygen electrode must be connected to a voltmeter or an mvMeter.
2. To create a calibration curve, expose cell media to a range of gas mixtures containing known concentrations of oxygen (e.g., expose to gas mixtures with 0% of oxygen and to 21% of oxygen). After acquiring a stable value at each point of the curve, the electrode is ready to be introduced in the medium exposed in the chamber. As the concentration of oxygen is dependent upon the depth within the medium, all the measurements must be held at the same depth [11, 12].

3.4 Induction of Normoxia, Hypoxia, or H/R: Placental Studies

1. After seeding placental cell lines, primary culture of trophoblasts or explants in appropriate flasks, plates, or petri dish, inductions can be performed as necessary (*see* **Note 3**), and every 24 h cells are reexposed to the desired gas mixture to reproduce a specific condition (Fig. 3a).
2. The physiological condition that evTB are exposed during the first trimester is also reproducible with modular incubator chambers [13, 14] (Fig. 3b).

A.

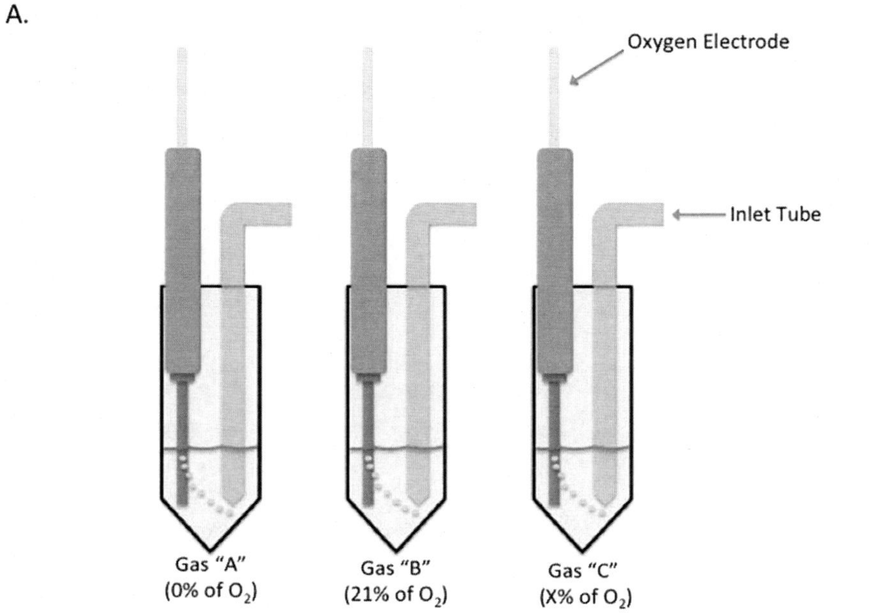

B.

	% of O_2	mV value	Confirmed % of O_2
◆	0%	0.573642	0%
O	?%	**0.432592**	**7.879888%**
■	21%	0.198243	21%

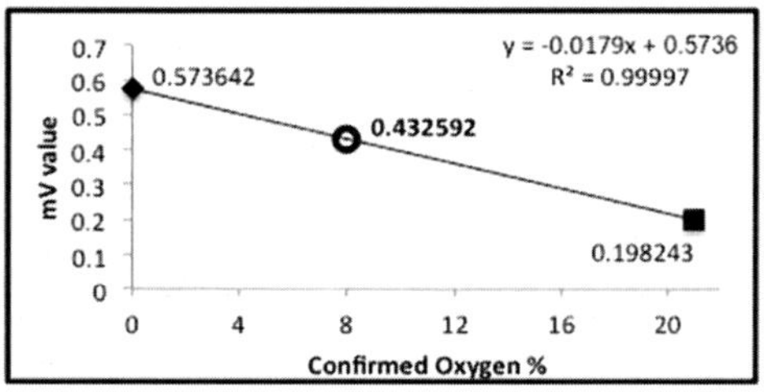

C.

Y= ax + b	?%= (0.432592 – 0.573642)/-0.0179
a= slope	?%= (-0.14105)/-0.0179
b= 0% mV value	?%= 7.879888% of O_2

Fig. 2 Representation of dissolved oxygen concentration. (**a**) Confirmation of oxygen concentration in a cell medium using other solutions with known concentration of oxygen. (**b**) The relative values obtained in the solutions "A" and "B" are plotted in a graphic of linear function to confirm the oxygen concentration in the solution "C." (**c**) Data obtained in the graphic are applied to a linear function determination to confirm the oxygen concentration in solution "C" (Modified from Sagrillo-Fagundes et al. 2016 [12])

4 Notes

1. During the assembling of the components, all valves must be closed.
2. Caution is advised for injecting gas inside the chambers due to their relative small size.

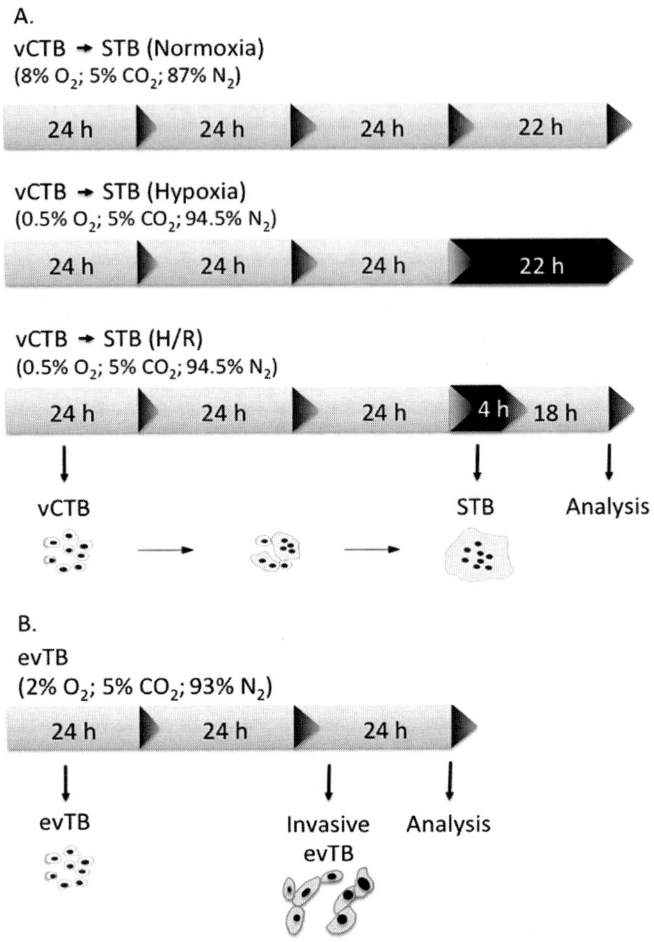

Fig. 3 Generic model of cell culture in modular incubator chamber. (**a**) Normoxia, hypoxia, and hypoxia/reoxygenation (H/R) are adequate methods to study pathological conditions in STB (*see* **Note 4**). Every 24 h (*black triangle*), gas should be renewed. Under hypoxic conditions, STB (from 72 h onward) are exposed continuously to 0.5% of O_2. Under H/R, STB are exposed during 4 h to hypoxia and then are reexposed to normoxia (8% O_2). (**b**) The rate of oxygenation that evTB are exposed during the first trimester of pregnancy is obtained using the adequate gas mixture with the modular incubator chamber. *vCTB* villous cytotrophoblast, *STB* syncytiotrophoblast, *evTB* extravillous trophoblasts

3. Incubation chambers allow performing any protocol of treatment/induction. However, every time that a chamber is opened to treat or change the medium of cells, the gas mixture must be reflushed as described in Subheading 3.2.
4. Figure 3a reproduces a generic protocol of hypoxia induction for STB. To induce the same conditions for vCTB, the time of incubation should be reduced to a maximum of 48 h [12].

Acknowledgments

This work was supported financially by the discovery grant of the Natural Sciences and Engineering Research Council of Canada (NSERC) (no. 262011-2009) and by the March of Dimes Foundation. L.S.F. received a studentship from Fonds Québécois de la Recherche sur la Nature et les Technologies (FQRNT).

References

1. Jauniaux E, Biernaux V, Gerlo E, Gulbis B (2001) Chronic maternal smoking and cord blood amino acid and enzyme levels at term. Obstet Gynecol 97:57–61
2. Soleymanlou N, Jurisica I, Nevo O, Ietta F, Zhang X, Zamudio S, Post M, Caniggia I (2005) Molecular evidence of placental hypoxia in preeclampsia. J Clin Endocrinol Metab 90:4299–4308
3. Ji L, Brkic J, Liu M, Fu G, Peng C, Wang YL (2013) Placental trophoblast cell differentiation: physiological regulation and pathological relevance to preeclampsia. Mol Asp Med 34:981–1023
4. Dekker G (2002) The partner's role in the etiology of preeclampsia. J Reprod Immunol 57:203–215
5. Roberts JM, Hubel CA (2009) The two stage model of preeclampsia: variations on the theme. Placenta 30(Suppl A):S32–S37
6. Crosley EJ, Elliot MG, Christians JK, Crespi BJ (2013) Placental invasion, preeclampsia risk and adaptive molecular evolution at the origin of the great apes: evidence from genome-wide analyses. Placenta 34:127–132
7. Robillard PY, Dekker GA, Hulsey TC (2002) Evolutionary adaptations to pre-eclampsia/eclampsia in humans: low fecundability rate, loss of oestrus, prohibitions of incest and systematic polyandry. Am J Reprod Immunol 47:104–111
8. MacLennan AH, Carty MJ, Sheppard BL, Sharp F (1975) An ultrastructural study of the reversibility of the effects of hypoxia on human trophoblast maintained in organ culture. J Reprod Fertil 43:501–504
9. Lanoix D, Lacasse AA, Reiter RJ, Vaillancourt C (2013) Melatonin: the watchdog of villous trophoblast homeostasis against hypoxia/reoxygenation-induced oxidative stress and apoptosis. Mol Cell Endocrinol 381:35–45
10. Tannetta DS, Sargent IL, Linton EA, Redman CW (2008) Vitamins C and E inhibit apoptosis of cultured human term placenta trophoblast. Placenta 29:680–690
11. Chen B, Longtine MS, Nelson DM (2013) Pericellular oxygen concentration of cultured primary human trophoblasts. Placenta 34:106–109
12. Sagrillo-Fagundes L, Clabault H, Laurent L, Hudon-Thibeault AA, Salustiano EM, Fortier M, Bienvenue-Pariseault J, Wong Yen P, Sanderson JT, Vaillancourt C (2016) Human primary trophoblast cell culture model to study the protective effects of melatonin against hypoxia/reoxygenation-induced disruption. J Vis Exp 113:27500522
13. Handschuh K, Guibourdenche J, Cocquebert M, Tsatsaris V, Vidaud M, Evain-Brion D, Fournier T (2009) Expression and regulation by PPARgamma of hCG alpha- and beta-subunits: comparison between villous and invasive extravillous trophoblastic cells. Placenta 30:1016–1022
14. Tarrade A, Lai Kuen R, Malassine A, Tricottet V, Blain P, Vidaud M, Evain-Brion D (2001) Characterization of human villous and extravillous trophoblasts isolated from first trimester placenta. Lab Investig 81:1199–1211

Chapter 22

Measurement of Oxidative Stress: Mitochondrial Function Using the Seahorse System

Dilys T.H. Leung and Simon Chu

Abstract

The Seahorse XFp Analyzer is a powerful tool for the assessment of various parameters of cellular respiration. Here we describe the process of the Seahorse Cell Phenotype Test using the Seahorse XFp Analyzer to characterize the metabolic phenotype of live cells. The Seahorse XFp Analyzer can also be coupled with other assays to measure cellular energetics. Given that mitochondrial dysfunction is implicated in preeclampsia, the Seahorse XFp Analyzer will serve as a useful tool for the understanding of pathological metabolism in this disorder.

Key words Respiration, Glycolysis, Metabolism, Mitochondrial function, Seahorse mito-stress

1 Introduction

The Seahorse XFp Analyzer measures respiration (oxygen consumption rate; OCR) and extracellular pH (extracellular acidification rate; ECAR) to provide information on mitochondrial function, oxidative stress, and metabolic dysfunction of viable cells [1]. Unlike the traditional oxygraph, which requires a large number of cells for analysis, the Seahorse XFp Analyzer offers a fast real-time analysis of metabolism with limited numbers of viable cells. These features make a powerful experimental tool to assess cellular respiration in various disorders of energy metabolism and mitochondrial function. One disorder in which disruption of mitochondrial metabolism has been implicated is preeclampsia. Mitochondria, as the major oxygen consuming organelle, produces reactive oxygen species (ROS) [2]. The inability of the cells to detoxify ROS intermediates results in a state of oxidative stress, which occurs in normal pregnancy [2]. However, oxidative stress is heightened in preeclampsia [2]. The literature has suggested that excess production of ROS by the malfunctioned mitochondrion may contribute to the pathogenesis of preeclampsia [2, 3]. Proteomic analysis of isolated placental mitochondria identified altered expression of

Padma Murthi and Cathy Vaillancourt (eds.), *Preeclampsia: Methods and Protocols*, Methods in Molecular Biology, vol. 1710, https://doi.org/10.1007/978-1-4939-7498-6_22, © Springer Science+Business Media LLC 2018

proteins involved in the regulation of oxidative stress and the respiratory chain [3]. The Seahorse XFp Analyzer should thus enable functional analysis to provide insight into the contribution of mitochondria dysfunction in the development of preeclampsia.

2 Materials

Agilent Technologies offer Seahorse XF Analyzers in three plate formats: Seahorse XFp Analyzer (8-well miniplate), Seahorse XFe24 Analyzer (24-well plate), and Seahorse XFe96 Analyzer (96-well plate). Each of these analyzers can be paired with various kits (*see* **Notes 1–4**) that the manufacturer (Agilent Technologies) supplies to study specific aspects of cellular energetics.

While these kits provide a standard method for the measurement of mitochondrial respiration in live cells, it is possible to design user-defined experiments that utilize alternative stressors, and these as well as the order of injections must be optimized as required by the experiment. The following protocol is based on the Cell Energy Phenotype Test using the Seahorse XFp Analyzer. However, the basic steps including preparation and cell seeding are applicable to other tests. Refer to the specific protocol regarding constitution of the compounds for respective kits.

2.1 Reagents and Consumables

1. Seahorse XF Calibrant.
2. Seahorse assay medium supplemented with 1 mM pyruvate, 2 mM glutamine, and 10 mM glucose in XFp Base Medium, pH 7.4.
3. Seahorse XFp Cell Culture Miniplates.
4. XFp Carrier Tray.
5. Sterile phosphate-buffered saline (PBS).
6. Hydrochloric acid (HCl).
7. Syringe and 0.22 μm filter.

2.2 Wave Desktop

The Wave Desktop is a data analysis software for both Seahorse XFp and XFe Analyzers. It can also be used to create and modify protocol as required for the experiment. The software can be downloaded at: http://www.agilent.com/en-us/products/cell-analysis-(seahorse)/software-download-for-wave-desktop.

3 Methods

3.1 Day Prior to Assay

Turn on Seahorse XFp Analyzer.

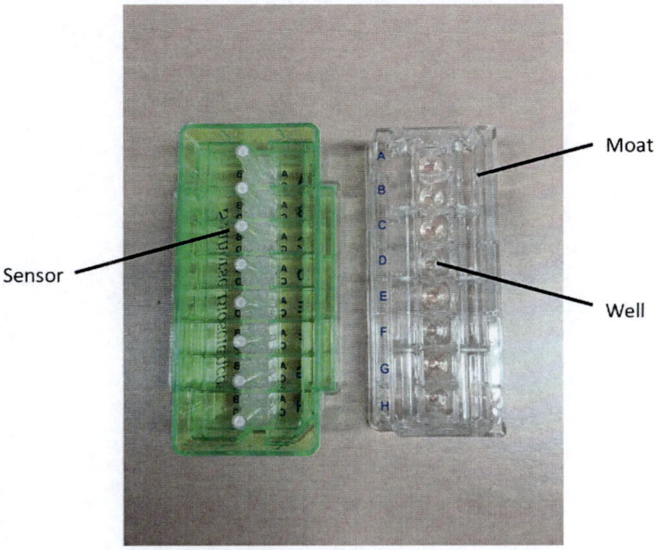

Fig. 1 Sensory cartridge (*left*) and utility plate (*right*)

3.1.1 Hydrate Sensor Cartridge for Assay

1. Lift sensory cartridge from the utility plate and place it upside down on the bench—avoid contact of the sensors (Fig. 1).
2. Add 200 μL of Seahorse XF Calibrant to each well of the utility plate.
3. Add 400 μL of Seahorse XF Calibrant to each moat around the wells.
4. Place the sensor cartridge (lid) back onto the utility plate so that the sensors are now submerged in the calibrant.
5. Place the cartridge assembly in a non-CO_2, humidified, 37 °C incubator overnight.

3.1.2 Cell Seeding

1. In a Seahorse XFp Cell Culture Miniplate (Fig. 2), add 80 μL of cell growth medium to wells A and H. These are background correction wells so they contain no cells.
2. Seed adherent cells at the desired density in 80 μL of cell growth medium into each of wells B to G the day prior to assay (*see* **Note 5**).
3. Determine the optimal cell seeding densities from the literature or consult the Seahorse Bioscience Cell Reference Database (http://www.seahorsebio.com/cell-reference-database/). Alternatively, optimize by testing. Typical cell density is between 5×10^3 and 4×10^4 cells per well. The seeding surface of each well is 0.106 cm^2, which is approximately 40% of that in a standard 96-well plate.
4. Fill the moat around the wells of the Seahorse XFp Miniplate with 400 μL of sterile Milli-Q or PBS.
5. Leave in a humidified, 37 °C incubator supplemented with 5% CO_2 overnight.

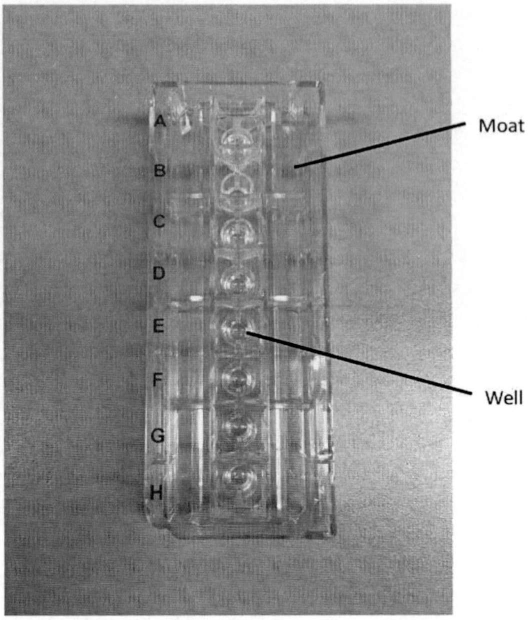

Fig. 2 Seahorse XFp cell culture miniplate

3.2 Day of the Assay

3.2.1 Prepare Assay Medium

1. Prepare 20 mL assay medium (*see* **step 2** in Subheading 2.1) for each assay.
2. Adjust to pH 7.4 with HCl.
3. Filter-sterilize XFp Base Medium containing the supplements (referred to as assay medium) and warm the assay medium to 37 °C prior to use.

3.2.2 Prepare XFp Cell Culture for Assay for Adherent Cells

1. Aspirate 60 μL of cell growth medium (with 20 μL remaining) and replace with 60 μL of assay medium. Repeat once.
2. Remove 60 μL of medium and fill well with assay medium to a final volume of 180 μL per well.
3. To de-gas, place the XFp Cell Culture Miniplate in a non-CO_2, humidified, 37 °C incubator for 45–60 min prior to the assay. This is an important step to prevent cellular CO_2 to contribute to background ECAR reading.

3.2.3 Prepare XFp Cell Culture for Assay for Suspension Cells

1. Add 50 μL assay medium to wells A and H without cells.
2. Harvest, count, and seed cells at the desired cell density in 50 μL of assay medium in wells B to G.
3. Centrifuge the miniplate in XFp Carrier Tray at 300 × *g* for 1 min.
4. Add 130 μL assay medium to a final volume of 180 μL per well.
5. To de-gas, place the XFp Cell Culture Miniplate in a non-CO_2, humidified, 37 °C incubator for 45–60 min prior to the assay.

Table 1
Stock solution of oligomycin and FCCP (Carbonyl cyanide 4-(trifluoromethoxy) phenylhydrazone)

	Volume of assay medium (μL)	Final concentration (μM)
Oligomycin	252	50
FCCP	288	50

Table 2
Optimization of stressor mix with oligomycin and FCCP (Carbonyl cyanide 4-(trifluoromethoxy) phenylhydrazone)

Desired FCCP concentration in well (μM)	Medium volume (μL)	Oligomycin stock volume (μL)	FCCP stock volume (μL)	Port concentration of oligomycin (μM)	Port concentration of FCCP (μM)
0.125	232.5	60	7.5	10	1.25
0.25	225	60	15	10	2.5
0.5	210	60	30	10	5.0
1	180	60	60	10	10
2	120	60	120	10	20

3.2.4 Prepare Stock Stressor Compounds

1. Thaw stressors (oligomycin and FCCP) in the pouch at room temperature for approximately 15 min prior to reconstitution.
2. Suspend the stressors with assay medium according to Table 1.
3. Refer to the Cell Characterization Data Table and Cell Reference Database to select a FCCP concentration appropriate for the experimental cell types. Alternatively, a FCCP titration can be performed as stated in Table 2. Optimization is required should the concentration of the compounds and order of injections be adjusted.

3.2.5 Load Sensor Cartridge

1. Stressors should be prepared and loaded 20 min prior to assay.
2. Load 20 μL stressor mix into every port of the hydrated sensor cartridge (Fig. 3). Ensure all corresponding ports for each stressor are loaded.
3. If using kits other than the Cell Energy Phenotype Test, load stressor mix in order according to the number of injection included in the protocol. For example, first stressor in port A,

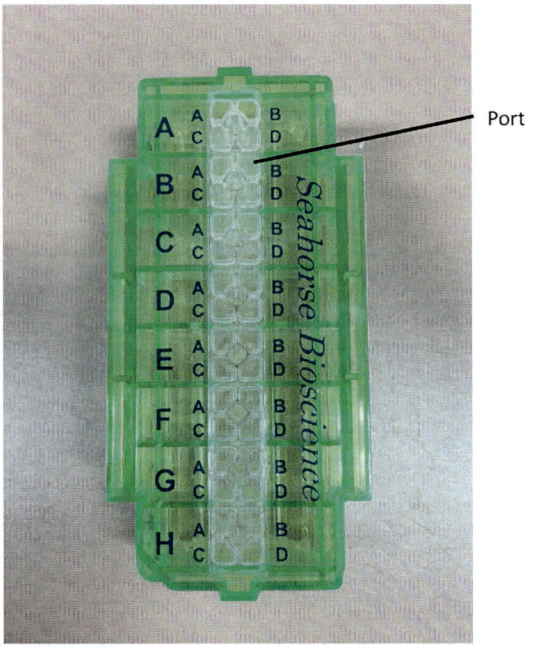

Fig. 3 Sensor cartridge

second stressor in port B, and so on. Maximum number of injections is four.

4. The utility plate-sensor cartridge assembly is now ready for calibration.

3.2.6 Running the Assay

1. To initiate calibration, select Cell Energy Phenotype Test on the Templates window and make the following adjustments to the protocol. Alternatively, insert a USB with the modified protocol.
2. At the protocol page, deselect the FCCP and rotenone/antimycin A injection steps.

   Increase the number of cycles of "oligomycin + FCCP" injection to "5."
3. Label control or experimental group accordingly. Note that additional experimental groups can only be added on the Wave software (prior with a modified protocol uploaded using a USB or after assay completion) but not at the Seahorse XFp Analyzer.
4. Select "Start Assay." This will initiate calibration of the utility plate-sensor cartridge assembly.
5. Remove the lid of the utility plate and place the assembly on the instrument tray with the correct orientation as instructed on the screen.

6. Select "Continue" to commence the 20 min calibration. The end of calibration should be the end of the 1 h de-gas period of the cells.
7. Remove the utility plate upon the completion of the calibration. Place the XFp Cell Culture Miniplate on the tray with the correct orientation as instructed on the screen.
8. The Cell Phenotype Test takes three OCR and ECAR readings at the basal level and five following injection of stressors (*see* **Note 6**). These parameters can be monitored during the run in the Overview window. Please refer to **Notes 7** and **8** for desired starting OCR.

3.2.7 Data Analysis

1. Remove the plate as instructed upon completion of the run.
2. Results of the run will be automatically saved in the Seahorse XFp Analyzer under Settings, then Assay Results. Alternatively, insert a USB drive and export in any of the three formats: Wave Assay Results, Microsoft Excel workbook, or GraphPad Prism.
3. Load the results in the Microsoft Excel workbook format on the XF Cell Energy Phenotype Test Report Generator (http://www.agilent.com/en-us/products/cell-analysis-(seahorse)/xf-cell-energy-phenotype-report-generator). The XF Cell Energy Phenotype Profile (Fig. 4) and metabolic potential graph will be generated.

3.2.8 Data Interpretation

1. Upon inhibition of ATP synthesis by oligomycin, there is an increase rate of glycolysis as a compensatory mechanism to meet energy demands. CO_2 production from glycolytic cells

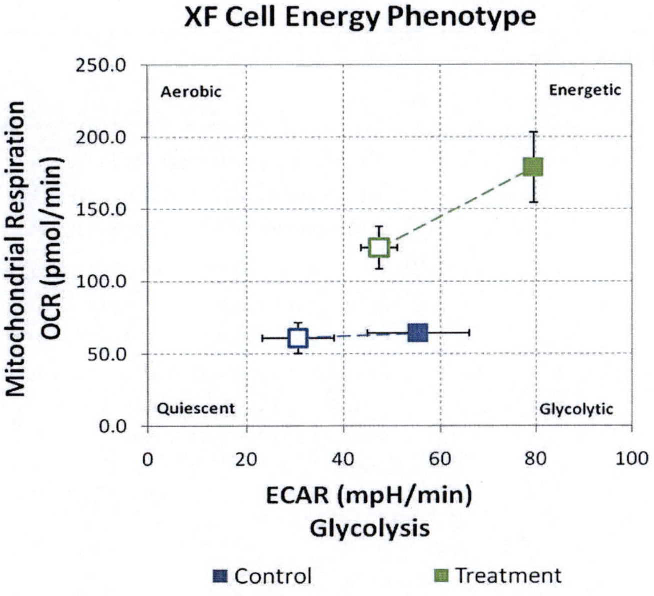

Fig. 4 The XF cell energy phenotype profile

contributes to ECAR; hence it is an indicator of the rate of glycolysis.

2. As FCCP depolarizes the mitochondrial membrane, the rate of mitochondrial respiration increases to restore the proton gradient. This is measured by OCR.
3. Baseline and stressed OCR and ECAR are presented in bar graphs in the XF Cell Energy Phenotype Test Report. Inability of cells to respond to stress may imply underlying mitochondrial dysfunction.
4. Baseline phenotype refers to the preferred pathway of metabolism of the cells in the non-stressed situation or in the presence of non-limiting quantity of substrates.
5. Stressed phenotype refers to the pathways of metabolisms when the cells undergo an increased energy demand—in the presence of stressor compounds such as oligomycin and FCCP.
6. The metabolic potential of the cells refers to the cells' ability to utilize respiration and/or glycolysis to meet an increased energy demand. The XF Cell Energy Phenotype Test Report Generator calculates the metabolic potential using the % stressed to baseline OCR or ECAR ratio, which is presented in a bar graph.
7. Cells can be characterized into four energy phenotypes depending on the pathway(s) they utilize to meet energy demand (Fig. 4): (a) quiescent, cells not being metabolically active; (b) energetic, cells utilize both aerobic respiration and glycolysis; (c) aerobic, cells utilize aerobic respiration; or (d) glycolytic, cells utilize glycolysis to meet energy demand.

4 Notes

1. The Cell Energy Phenotype Test provides an overview of the metabolic potential and energy phenotype of the tested cells. The kit contains oligomycin, an ATP synthesis inhibitor, and FCCP, a compound which depolarizes mitochondrial membrane.
2. The Mito Stress test measures key parameters of mitochondrial function including basal respiration, ATP-linked respiration, H^+ (Proton) Leak, maximal respiration, spare respiratory capacity, and non-mitochondrial respiration. The kit contains oligomycin, FCCP, and rotenone/antimycin A, an inhibitor of the electron transport chain.

3. The Glycolysis Stress test assesses glycolytic flux by measuring parameters such as the glycolytic capacity, glycolytic reserve, and non-glycolytic acidification. The kit contains oligomycin, glucose, and 2-deoxy-glucose.
4. The Mito Fuel Flex Test allows the study of substrate metabolism, in particular, the capability, dependency, and flexibility of cells in utilizing fuel pathways to meet metabolic demand. The kit contains inhibitors of three pathways: UK5099, BPTES, and Etomoxir to inhibit pathways that oxidizes glucose, glutamine, and fatty acids, respectively.
5. Suspension cells can be seeded on the day of assay.
6. The assay will run for approximately 1 h.
7. OCR should increase following injection. If not, perform a FCCP titration to determine the appropriate concentration. According to the manufacturer, a 10 μM working concentration of oligomycin is optimal for most experiments.
8. Starting OCR should be between 50 and 160 pmol/O_2/min. Readings below this range are regarded as background. Increase the cell number or perform a cell density optimization in order to obtain a higher OCR value as per the manufacturer's instructions.

Acknowledgment

D.L. is supported by the Endocrine Society of Australia through a Research Higher Degree Scholarship. S.C. is supported by the Ovarian Cancer Research Foundation and the Granulosa Cell Tumor of the Ovary Foundation. The Hudson Institute is supported by the Victorian Government's Operational Infrastructure Scheme.

References

1. Divakaruni AS, Paradyse A, Ferrick DA, Murphy AN, Jastroch M (2014) Analysis and interpretation of microplate-based oxygen consumption and pH data. Methods Enzymol 547:309–354. https://doi.org/10.1016/B978-0-12-801415-8.00016-3
2. Muralimanoharan S, Maloyan A, Mele J, Guo C, Myatt LG, Myatt L (2012) MIR-210 modulates mitochondrial respiration in placenta with preeclampsia. Placenta 33(10):816–823. https://doi.org/10.1016/j.placenta.2012.07.002
3. Shi Z, Long W, Zhao C, Guo X, Shen R, Ding H (2013) Comparative proteomics analysis suggests that placental mitochondria are involved in the development of pre-eclampsia. PLoS One 8(5):e64351. https://doi.org/10.1371/journal.pone.0064351

Chapter 23

Co-culture of H295R Adrenocortical Carcinoma and BeWo Choriocarcinoma Cells to Study Feto-placental Interactions: Focus on Estrogen Biosynthesis

Andrée-Anne Hudon Thibeault, J. Thomas Sanderson, and Cathy Vaillancourt

Abstract

Estrogens are produced in large amounts during pregnancy, as a result of a tightly regulated cooperation between the maternal and fetal adrenal cortex, which produce androgen precursors, and the placental villous trophoblast, which transforms these precursors into estrogens. These estrogens play an important role in proper placental function, in adaptation of the mother to pregnancy, as well as in adequate fetal development. Disruption of estrogen production is associated with poor pregnancy outcomes and fetal malformation or altered fetal programming. Pregnant women may be exposed to endocrine disruptors from environmental sources or medications, and it is crucial to study the effects of such compounds on feto-placental steroidogenesis. The H295R/BeWo co-culture model offers the opportunity to study these interactions, by making it possible to evaluate the effects of chemical exposures on androgen and estrogen biosynthesis, as well as on various other aspects of feto-placental communication.

Key words Steroidogenesis, Feto-placental unit, Estrogen, Co-culture, Trophoblast, Fetal adrenocortical

1 Introduction

In the human placenta, the villous trophoblast produces large amount of estrogens, including pregnancy-specific estriol. This synthesis is dependent on precursors produced by the adrenal cortex of the mother and that of the developing fetus. We have previously shown that the H295R/BeWo co-culture is a relevant model to study estrogen biosynthesis and fulfills an essential need as research tool considering the lack of suitable in vivo or ex vivo human models. In the co-culture model, H295R cells possess fetal adrenocortical characteristics, including the ability to synthetize

J. Thomas Sanderson and Cathy Vaillancourt share joint senior authorship and contributed equally to this work.

Padma Murthi and Cathy Vaillancourt (eds.), *Preeclampsia: Methods and Protocols*, Methods in Molecular Biology, vol. 1710,
https://doi.org/10.1007/978-1-4939-7498-6_23, © Springer Science+Business Media LLC 2018

16-α-hydroxylated androgens [1]. BeWo cells are used as a villous trophoblast model since they possess high aromatase (CYP19) activity, which confer them the capacity of transforming androgens to estrogens in great amounts.

The H295R/BeWo co-culture model was first characterized for its capacity to reproduce the feto-placental estrogen biosynthetic profile with interactions between the two cell types occurring in real time. Moreover, culturing BeWo cells on porous inserts allows the cell to adopt a polarized phenotype with differential expression of proteins on the fetal membrane and maternal membrane [2–4], which opens up the possibility of studying feto-placental transport. The co-culture model also offers the possibility to study several other feto-placental interactions (stress hormones, IGF axis, drug metabolism, etc.) as summarized in Table 1.

Table 1
Major human feto-placental interactions

Placenta hormone/factor	Effect on fetal compartment	Reference
Placental growth hormone (pGH) or human placenta lactogen (hPL)	Stimulation of insulin-like growth factor (IGF) axis, which stimulates growth of the fetal adrenal cortex	[6]
Estradiol, progesterone, and prostaglandins	Regulation of the expression of the enzyme 11β-hydroxysteroid dehydrogenase type 2 (HSD11B2) which oxidizes cortisol to cortisone, a major regulator of fetal organ maturation	[6–9]
Estradiol and β-human chorionic gonadotropin (β-hCG)	Regulation of DHEA sulfate synthesis, a precursor for estrogen production, in the H295R cells (REF)	[7, 8]
Estrogens	Development and maturation of fetal adrenal gland (expression of steroidogenesis enzymes) Sexual differentiation Fetal growth	[9–19]
Corticotropin-releasing hormone (CRH)	Stimulation of cortisol and DHEA production	[20–22]
Epidermal growth factor (EGF)	Stimulation of fetal adrenal cell proliferation	[23]

Fetal adrenocortical hormone	Effects on placental compartment	Reference
Aldosterone	Stimulation of proliferation of trophoblast	[24]
Cortisol	Inhibition proliferation of trophoblast	[24]
Dehydroepiandrosterone (DHEA)	Regulation of implantation (mouse)	[25]

2 Materials

2.1 Cell Culture

1. H295R medium: Dulbecco's Modified Eagle's Medium (DMEM)/F12 without phenol red supplemented with 1.2 g/L sodium bicarbonate ($NaHCO_3$), 2 mg/L pyridoxine·HCl, 2.5% Nu-serum, 1% insulin, transferrin, selenium (ITS) + premix.
2. BeWo medium: Dulbecco's Modified Eagle's Medium (DMEM)/F12 without phenol red supplemented with 0.6 g/L sodium bicarbonate ($NaHCO_3$) and 10% fetal bovine serum (FBS).
3. Co-culture medium: Dulbecco's Modified Eagle's Medium (DMEM)/F12 without phenol red supplemented with 1.2 g/L sodium bicarbonate ($NaHCO_3$), 2 mg/L pyridoxine·HCl, 2.5% Nu-serum, 1% insulin, transferrin, selenium (ITS) + premix, and 1% stripped FBS.
4. 24-well cell culture plate and polycarbonate transwell permeable support with 0.4 M pores.
5. Phosphate-buffered saline (PBS).
6. TrypLE Express.

2.2 Real-Time Monitoring of Cell Proliferation

1. The xCELLigence Real-Time Cell Analyser Single Plate (RTCA-SP, *see* **Note 1**) (ACEA Biosciences).
2. Eplate and Eplate inserts (ACEA).

2.3 Aromatase Catalytic Activity

1. Dulbecco's Modified Eagle's Medium (DMEM)/F12 without phenol red supplemented with 54 nM [1β-3H(N)] androst-4-ene-3,17-dione.
2. 12-well plate.
3. Chloroform.
4. Dextran-coated charcoal (5% charcoal + 0.5% dextran (w/v)) (*see* **Note 2**).
5. Scintiverse BD scintillation cocktail.
6. MicroBeta TriLux liquid scintillation counter.
7. Liquid scintillation counting flexible microplates in 96-well and 24-well format.
8. Plate seal.
9. Uncompleted culture medium: Dulbecco's Modified Eagle's Medium (DMEM)/F12 without phenol red.
10. Radioimmunoprecipitation assay buffer (RIPA): 150 mM NaCl, 50 mM Tris–HCl PH 7.1, 1 mM ethylenediaminetetraacetic acid (EDTA), 1% Triton X-100, 1% sodium deoxycholate, 0.1% sodium dodecyl sulfate.
11. Pierce BCA Protein Assay.

12. Powder weighing spatula (for cell scraping).
13. 70% ethanol.

2.4 Hormone Assay

Commercial enzyme-linked immunosorbent assays (ELISA) kits for β-hCG, dehydroepiandrosterone, androstenedione, estrone, estradiol, estriol, and progesterone.

2.5 Transepithelial Resistance

1. Epithelial voltohmmeter (World Precision Instruments).
2. Bleach.
3. 1.5 M KCl solution.

3 Methods

3.1 Cell Co-culture (See Note 3)

1. Use 90% confluent 75 cm^2 flasks of BeWo and H295R cells. Proceed one cell line at a time.
2. Discard the culture medium and rinse with 5 mL of PBS.
3. Trypsinize with 2 mL of TrypLE, until cells are detached.
4. Complete with 8 mL of regular culture medium for each cell type, respectively.
5. Mix by pipetting up and down and determine cell concentration.
6. Seed H295R cells in a 24-well plate at 25,000 cells/well density, 1 mL/well.
7. In another plate, seed BeWo cells in transwell inserts at 12,500 cells/well density, 0.2 mL/insert. Add 0.8 mL culture medium to the wells underneath the inserts.
8. Incubate at 37 °C for 24 h for cell adhesion.
9. Remove BeWo culture medium from the transwell inserts and wells and rinse cells twice with co-culture medium to remove FBS (*see* **Note 4**).
10. Remove H295R culture medium from the wells containing H295R cells. Rinsing is not necessary since H295R medium does not contain FBS.
11. Assemble the co-culture: 0.8 mL of co-culture medium in the wells and 0.2 mL in the transwell inserts (*see* **Note 5**).
12. Incubate at 37 °C for 24 h or longer according to the type of experiment (*see* **Note 6**).

3.2 Real-Time Monitoring of Cell Proliferation

1. Set the xCELLigence software schedule in two steps: **step 1**, background measurement (default), and **step 2**, 10 min sweeps for at least 96 h.
2. Add 50 μL of regular culture medium/well in an Eplate (96 well for SP instrument) and measure background (**step 1**).

3. To the wells of the Eplate, add 100 μL of either BeWo (10,000 cells/well) or H295R (20,000 cells/well) cells.
4. Let the cells settle for 30 min at room temperature.
5. To the Eplate inserts, add 50 μL of BeWo (10,000 cells/insert) or H295R (20,000 cells/insert) cells. Add 130 μL of culture medium to the receiver plate.
6. Monitor cell proliferation in the Eplate (**step 2**) and incubate the receiver plate with the inserts containing cells for 24 h at 37 °C.
7. Pause **step 2** and remove the Eplate from the instrument.
8. Rinse wells and inserts containing BeWo medium twice with co-culture medium, before adding the co-culture medium containing the test compound.
9. Assemble the co-culture by placing the inserts containing BeWo cells above the H295R cells in wells or vice versa.
10. Continue monitoring cell proliferation (resume **step 2**).

3.3 Aromatase Catalytic Activity (Tritiated Water-Release Assay)

1. After the treatment period (*see* **Note 7**), remove co-culture medium from the co-culture (*see* **Note 8**).
2. Place the inserts in a 12-well plate so that the bottom of the insert is in direct contact with the well.
3. Rinse inserts and wells twice with PBS.
4. Add 50 μL/insert or 250 μL/well of 54 nM [1β-3H(N)] androst-4-ene-3,17-dione in uncompleted culture medium (Table 2).
5. Incubate 1.5 h at 37 °C.

Table 2
Comparison of the protocol for inserts and wells

	Insert		Well	
	Volume	Dilution factor	Volume	Dilution factor
Working solution of [1β-3H(N)] androst-4-ene-3,17-dione (54 nM)	50 μL	50/40	250 μL	250/200
Volume of supernatant + chloroform	40 μL + 100 μL	100/40	200 μL + 500 μL	500/200
Volume of supernatant + dextran-coated charcoal	20 μL + 20 μL	40/20	100 μL + 100 μL	200/100
Volume of supernatant + scintillation cocktail	20 μL + 100 μL	120/20	100 μL + 1000 μL	1100/100
Counting microplate	96 well		24 well	
Final dilution factor		37.5		68.75

6. Take 40 μL/insert or 200 μL/well of supernatant and place in a microtube containing 100 μL or 500 μL chloroform, respectively (Table 2).
7. Vortex and centrifuge at 12,000 × *g* for 5 min.
8. Take 20 μL/insert or 100 μL/well of supernatant and place in microtubes containing 20 μL or 100 μL dextran-coated charcoal, respectively (Table 2).
9. Vortex and incubate 5 min at room temperature and centrifuge at 12,000 × *g* for 15 min.
10. Take 20 μL/insert or 100 μL/well of supernatant and place in a 96-well or 24-well liquid scintillation counting microplate, respectively (Table 2).
11. Add 10 μL of 54 nM [1β-3H(N)]androst-4-ene-3,17-dione in uncompleted culture medium in a well of the liquid scintillation counting microplate to determine the specific activity in the co-culture medium (Table 2).
12. Add 100 μL/insert or 1000 μL/well of liquid Scintiverse BD scintillation cocktail.
13. Count each well for 2 min in a MicroBeta TriLux liquid scintillation counter.
14. To assess protein content, rinse cells in the wells and inserts twice with cold PBS. Scrape cells in the wells and inserts (50 μL of RIPA/well) with powder weighing spatulas. Wash spatulas with 70% ethanol between samples. Vortex every 5 min during 30 min. Centrifuge 10 min at 21,000 × *g*. Use the supernatant for protein quantification following manufacturer's instruction (Pierce BCA Protein Assay).
15. Results are either expressed as percentage of control or in pmoles of androstenedione converted/hour (Fig. 1). This expression can be normalized to mg protein content of the well or cell number.

3.4 Hormone Assay

1. Use the supernatant from the co-cultures and monocultures (*see* **Note 9**).
2. Keep the supernatants at −80 °C until use in the commercial kits, following manufacturer's instructions (*see* **Note 10**).

3.5 Transepithelial Resistance

1. Rinse the electrodes with 70% ethanol in a 15 mL tube for 10 min.
2. Remove the electrodes from the ethanol and let dry for 15 s.
3. Place the electrodes in tubes containing pre-warmed (37 °C) culture medium for at least 5 min.
4. Remove the BeWo culture medium and change to co-culture medium in the co-culture and BeWo monoculture, and place

i) Conversion of count per minute (CPM) to disintegration per minute (DPM)

$$Considering\ a\ quenching\ of\ 15\%, \quad DPM = CPM\ x\ 1.15$$

ii) Conversion of DPM to pmol

This conversion will depend on the specific activity of your [1β-3H(N)] androst-4-ene-3,17-dione.

Example of conversion of [1β-3H(N)] androst-4-ene-3,17-dione at 26.3 Ci/mmol to DPM/mmol

$$\frac{26.3\ Ci}{mmol}\ x\ \frac{3.7\ x\ 10^{10}\ Disintegration\ per\ second\ (DPS)}{Ci}\ x\ \frac{60\ sec}{min}\ x\ \frac{1\ mmol}{10^9\ pmol} = \frac{58\ 386\ DPM}{pmol}$$

$$\frac{DPM}{\frac{58\ 386DPM}{pmol}} = pmol$$

iii) Expression considering the 3H position on androst-4-ene-3,17-dione

74.2% of tritiated-hydrogen (3H) is situated in β position in the substrate [1β-3H(N)] androst-4-ene-3,17-dione, which will lead to tritiated water release when converted.

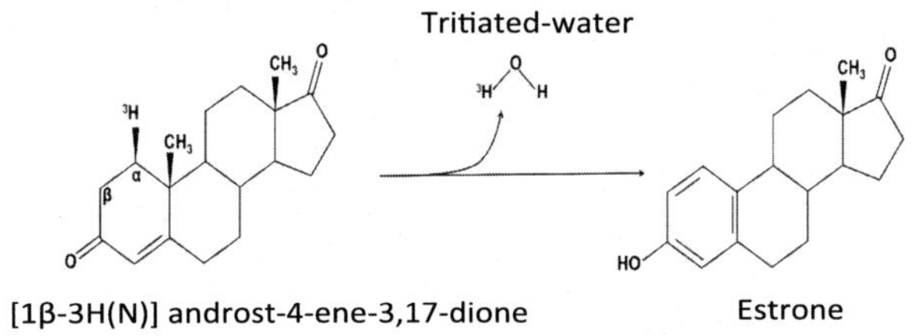

$$\frac{pmol}{0.742} = pmol_{corrected}$$

iv) Dilution factor during the extraction

The dilution factors are presented in table 1.

$$For\ inserts, pmol_{corrected}\ x\ 37.5$$

$$For\ wells, pmol_{corrected}\ x\ 68.75$$

v) Correction for time of incubation with substrate [1β-3H(N)] androst-4-ene-3,17-dione

$$\frac{pmol_{corrected}}{1.5\ hour} = pmol_{corrected}/hour$$

vi) Correction for protein content of the well or number of cells

$$\frac{pmol_{corrected}/hour}{Cell\ number\ or\ protein\ content} = pmol/hour/cell\ number\ or\ pmol/hour/\ mg\ protein$$

Fig. 1 Conversion of CYP19 activity in count per minute (CPM) to pmol of androstenedione converted/hour

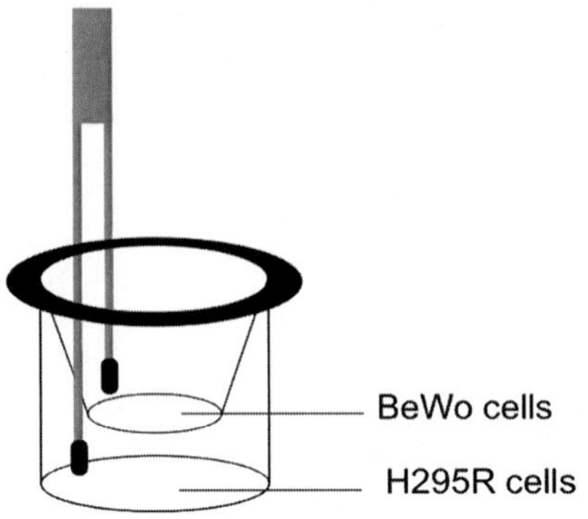

Fig. 2 Measuring transepithelial resistance in the co-culture with a voltmeter (epithelial voltohmmeter—World Precision Instruments)

the electrodes in the well and insert. The longest electrode has to touch the bottom of the well, passing through the side hole of the insert. The electrodes should stay immobile during the measurement (Fig. 2).

5. Measure 4 h after seeding the cells, directly after assembling the co-culture and every 24 h after assembly (*see* **Note 11**).
6. Place the electrode in co-culture medium between each measurement. At the end, place the electrodes in bleach for 3 min.
7. Rinse with water.
8. Between experiments, leave the electrodes in a KCl solution.

4 Notes

1. The instrument RTCA dual plate (DP) could also be used with the Eplate16. The well formats are identical, but with the DP instrument, there are only 16 wells/plate instead of 96 wells/plate with the SP.
2. Prepare and mix the solution overnight on a magnetic stir plate and mix by inverting the bottle five times before using.
3. We recommend comparing the responses of the co-culture with those of BeWo and H295R cells in monoculture.
4. To rinse the inserts, prepare wells with 0.8 mL of co-culture medium. Remove the medium from each insert as well as under the insert, where a droplet often forms, and place it in the well containing co-culture medium. Add co-culture medium to the insert and repeat.
5. In order to have an even exposure of the cells to the test compound, it should be dissolved in culture medium before treatment instead of adding the compound directly to the culture medium in the well and insert.

6. We recommend a 24-h incubation of the co-culture, since a decrease in H295R cell proliferation is observed after 24 h under untreated circumstances [5].
7. To determine specificity of the tritiated water-release assay for aromatization, an irreversible inhibitor of the catalytic activity of aromatase, formestane (4-hydroxyandrostenedione), (1 μM) should be used. Positive controls (CYP19 inducers), such as forskolin (10 μM) or phorbol-12-myristate-13-acetate (1 μM), should also be included to determine the responsiveness of the cells.
8. The culture medium from the insert and well can be placed in microtubes at −80 °C for later hormone assay. Medium from the insert and well may be mixed together (total volume of 1 mL) or harvested separately, depending on the experimental requirements.
9. If too much cell debris is present, the culture medium may be centrifuged for 5 min at 10,000 × *g*.
10. Estrogen production by the untreated co-culture should be determined as a quality control. A synergistic production of estrogens and the presence of estriol should be observed in the co-culture compared to BeWo and H295R cells in monoculture.
11. Measurements will vary depending on the experiment. Values should always be compared within the same experiment. We consider that cells form a confluent monolayer when transepithelial resistance reaches a plateau.

Acknowledgments

This work was financially supported by the Réseau de recherche en santé environnementale as part of the Fonds de recherche du Québec (FRQ)-Santé (C.V., J.T.S.), the Natural Sciences and Engineering Research Council of Canada (NSERC) grants 313312-2012 (J.T.S.) and 262011-2009 (C.V.), the March of Dimes Foundation (C.V.), as well as studentship awards to A.A.H.T. from NSERC, FRQ-Nature et Technologies, FRQ-Santé, and Canadian Institutes of Health Research.

References

1. Gazdar AF, Oie HK, Shackleton CH, Chen TR, Triche TJ, Myers CE, Chrousos GP, Brennan MF, Stein CA, Larocca RV (1990) Establishment and characterization of a human adrenocortical carcinoma cell-line that expresses multiple pathways of steroid-biosynthesis. Cancer Res 50:5488–5496
2. Poulsen MS, Rytting E, Mose T, Knudsen LE (2009) Modeling placental transport: correlation of in vitro BeWo cell permeability and

ex vivo human placental perfusion. Toxicol In Vitro 23:1380–1386

3. Prouillac C, Lecoeur S (2010) The role of the placenta in fetal exposure to xenobiotics: importance of membrane transporters and human models for transfer studies. Drug Metab Dispos 10:1623–1235
4. Audus KL (1999) Controlling drug delivery across the placenta. Eur J Pharm Sci 8:161–165
5. Hudon Thibeault AA, Deroy K, Vaillancourt C, Sanderson JT (2014) A unique co-culture model for fundamental and applied studies of human fetoplacental steroidogenesis and interference by environmental chemicals. Environ Health Perspect 122:371–377
6. Myatt L, Sun K (2010) Role of fetal membranes in signaling of fetal maturation and parturition. Int J Dev Biol 54:545–553
7. Gell JS, Oh J, Rainey WE, Carr BR (1998) Effect of estradiol on DHEAS production in the human adrenocortical cell line, H295R. J Soc Gynecol Invest 5:144–148
8. Rao CV, Zhou XL, Lei ZM (2004) Functional luteinizing hormone/chorioninc gonadotropin receptors in human adrenal cortical H295R cells. Biol Reprod 71:579–587
9. Kaludjerovic J, Ward WE (2012) The interplay between estrogen and fetal adrenal cortex. J Nutr Metab 2012:1–12
10. Mastorakos G, Ilias I (2003) Maternal and fetal hypothalamic-pituitary-adrenal axes during pregnancy and postpartum. Ann N Y Acad Sci 997:136–149
11. Tsatsaris V, Malassiné A, Fournier T, Handschuh K, Schaaps J-P, Foidart J-M, Evain-Brion D (2006) Placenta humain. Gynécol Obstétr 42:1–23
12. Albrecht ED, Aberdeen GW, Pepe GJ (2005) Estrogen elicits cortical zone-specific effects on development of the primate fetal adrenal gland. Endocrinology 146:1737–1744
13. Lash GE, Ansari T, Bischof P, Burton GJ, Chamley L, Crocker I, Dantzer V, Desoye G, Drewlo S, Fazleabas A, Jansson T, Keating S, Kliman HJ, Lang I, Mayhew T, Meiri H, Miller RK, Nelson DM, Pfarrer C, Roberts C, Sammar M, Sharma S, Shiverick K, Strunk D, Turner MA, Huppertz B (2009) IFPA meeting 2008 workshops report. Placenta 30:S4–S14
14. Jeschke U, Richter D-U, Möbius B-M, Briese V, Myolonas I, Friese K (2007) Stimulation of progesterone, estradiol and cortisol in trophoblast tumor BeWo cells by glycodelin A N-glycans. Anticancer Res 27:2101–2108
15. Albrecht ED, Bonagura TW, Burleigh DW, Enders AC, Aberdeen GW, Pepe GJ (2006) Suppression of extravillous trophoblast invasion of uterine spiral arteries by estrogen during early baboon pregnancy. Placenta 27:483–490
16. Gambino YP, Maymo JL, Perez Perez A, Calvo JC, Sanchez-Margalet V, Varone CL (2012) Elsevier Trophoblast Research Award lecture: molecular mechanisms underlying estrogen functions in trophoblastic cells – focus on leptin expression. Placenta 33:S63–S70
17. Olwenn MV, Shialis T, Lester JN, Scrimshaw MD, Boobis AR, Voulvoulis N (2008) Testicular dysgenesis syndrome and the estrogen hypothesis: a quantitative meta-analysis. Environ Health Perspect 116:149–157
18. Toppari J, Virtanen HE, Main KM, Skakkebaek NE (2010) Cryptorchidism and hypospadias as a sign of testicular dysgenesis syndrome (TDS): Environmental connection. Birth Defects Res A Clin Mol Teratol 88:910–919
19. Dumitrescu A, Aberdeen GW, Pepe GJ, Albrecht ED (2014) Placental estrogen suppresses cyclin D1 expression in the nonhuman primate fetal adrenal cortex. Endocrinology 155:4774–4784
20. Sirianni R, Rehman KS, Carr BR, Parker CR, Rainey WE (2005) Corticotropin-releasing hormone directly stimulates cortisol and the cortisol biosynthetic pathway in human fetal adrenal cells. J Clin Endocrinol Metabol 90:279–285
21. Sirianni R, Mayhew BA, Carr BR, Parker CR, Rainey WE (2005) Corticotropin-releasing hormone (CRH) and urocortin act through type 1 CRH receptors to stimulate dehydroepiandrosterone sulfate production in human fetal adrenal cells. J Clin Endocrinol Metabol 90:5393–5400
22. Smith R, Mesiano S, Chan E-C, Brown S, Jaffe RB (1998) Corticotropin-releasing hormone directly and preferentially stimulates dehydroepiandrosterone sulfate secretion by human fetal adrenal cortical cells. J Clin Endocrinol Metabol 83:2916–2920
23. Riopel L, Branchaud CL, Goodyer CG, Zweig M, Lipowski L, Adkar V, Lefebvre Y (1989) Effect of placental factors on growth and function of the human fetal adrenal in vitro. Biol Reprod 41:779–789
24. Gennari-Moser C, Khankin EV, Schuller S, Escher G, Frey BM, Portmann CB, Baumann MU, Lehmann AD, Surbek D, Karumanchi SA, Frey FJ, Mohaupt MG (2011) Regulation of placental growth by aldosterone and cortisol. Endocrinology 152:263–271
25. Frolova AI, O'Neill K, Moley KH (2011) Dehydroepiandrosterone inhibits glucose flux through the pentose phosphate pathway in human and mouse endometrial stromal cells, preventing decidualization and implantation. Mol Endocrinol 25:1444–1455

Chapter 24

Placental Lipid Transport

Evemie Dubé, Guillaume Desparois, and Julie Lafond

Abstract

The human placenta is responsible for the adequate supply of nutrients essential for proper embryonic and fetal development such as glucose, amino acids, and lipids. Processes involved in the placental transport of these nutrients are complex and tightly regulated and involve many transporters, receptors, and regulators. In this chapter, we describe the current methods to study the impact of maternal metabolic disorders on key players of human placental transfer of nutrients.

Key words Placenta, Lipids, Fatty acids, Cholesterol, Transport

1 Introduction

Fetal development and growth depend on the supply of nutrients from the maternal circulation through the placenta [1]. Numerous studies have shown that the deficiency of nutrients in the mother induces alterations in placental transport of nutrients during pregnancy and health problems in the offspring at birth but also during childhood and adulthood [2, 3]. Multiple factors can influence proper placental transport of nutrients including blood flow, placental size and morphology, and transporter abundance. Fatty acids and cholesterol are among the nutrients that are essential for fetal growth and development. The syncytiotrophoblast, which is the functional unit of the placenta, plays an important role in the exchange of these nutrients between the maternal and fetal circulation. It expresses several proteins involved in the placental transport of fatty acids and cholesterol. In the maternal circulation, fatty acids are found as free fatty acids or incorporated into lipoproteins. Fatty acids can be dissociated from lipoproteins by lipases present on the surface of trophoblasts and internalized through different transport proteins such as CD36 (also known as FAT), placental plasma membrane FA-binding protein (FABPpm), members of solute carrier family 27 (SLC27As, also known as FA transport proteins [FATPs]), and intracellular FA-binding proteins (FABPs). Cholesterol, which is also incorporated into

Padma Murthi and Cathy Vaillancourt (eds.), *Preeclampsia: Methods and Protocols*, Methods in Molecular Biology, vol. 1710,
https://doi.org/10.1007/978-1-4939-7498-6_24,

lipoproteins, is taken up by the placenta in the maternal circulation through receptor-dependent or receptor-independent transport involving among others the low-density lipoprotein receptor (LDLR), the very low-density lipoprotein/apolipoprotein (apo) E receptor (VLDLR), and the scavenger receptor class B type I (SRBI) [1]. Cholesterol can then be transported toward the maternal or fetal circulation by different ATP-binding cassette transporters such as ABCA1 and ABCG1 [4]. Our laboratory studies the impact of maternal metabolic disorders on the placental expression, function, and regulation of these different key players [5–9].

2 Materials

2.1 General

1. Tissue grinder with a pestle.
2. 96-well microtest flat bottom plates.
3. Sterile nuclease-free microcentrifuge tubes.
4. Liquid nitrogen.
5. Tissue homogenizer.
6. Spectrophotometer.

2.2 Tissue Sampling

1. Dulbecco's Modified Eagle's Medium (DMEM) containing antibiotics (0.12 mg/mL penicillin, 5 μg/mL amphotericin, 50 μg/mL gentamicin) and $NaHCO_3$ (90 mg/mL).
2. Sterile Pyrex dish for placental dissection (21 × 30 cm).
3. Sterile scissors (14 cm).
4. 10% formalin.

2.3 Quantitative Real-Time Reverse Transcription Polymerase Chain Reaction (qRT-PCR)

1. Nuclease-free sterile water.
2. High Pure Tissue RNA Kit (Roche Applied Science) to extract total RNA from tissues.
3. High Pure RNA Isolation Kit (Roche Applied Science) to extract total RNA from cultured cells.
4. iScript™ Reverse Transcription Supermix for RT-qPCR (BioRad).
5. Primers designed with Primer Blast (http://www.ncbi.nlm.nih.gov) and synthesized as desalted oligonucleotides.
6. LightCycler 480 SYBR Green I Master kit (Roche Diagnostics).
7. PCR amplification and detection instrument.
8. qPCR plates and sealing films.

2.4 Western Blot

1. Homogenization buffer: 125 mM Tris–HCl, 2 mM $CaCl_2$, 1.4% [v/v] Triton X-100, pH 8.0.
2. EDTA-free antiprotease cocktail.

3. BCA protein assay kit.
4. Sample dilution buffer 6×: 0.3 M Tris, pH 6.8, 12% SDS, 30% glycerol, 0.6% bromophenol blue.
5. Electrophoresis chamber.
6. Running buffer: 25 mM Tris, 190 mM glycine, 0.1% SDS, pH 8.3.
7. Towbin transfer buffer: 25 mM Tris, 190 mM glycine, 20% methanol, pH 8.3.
8. Polyvinylidene difluoride (PVDF) membrane.
9. Extra thick blot papers.
10. Semidry transfer apparatus.
11. Ponceau S staining solution: 0.5% Ponceau S, 1% acetic acid.
12. TBST: 50 mM Tris–HCl, pH 7.4, 150 mM NaCl, 0.1% Tween 20.
13. Blocking solution: TBST with 5% skimmed milk.
14. Primary antibody solution in TBST (Table 1).

Table 1
Primary antibodies, host species, recommended dilution, and supplier for Western blot analysis

Antibody	Host	Dilution	Furnisher
Anti-LDLR	Rabbit	1:500	Fitzgerald
Anti-SRBI	Rabbit	1:2500	Novus Biological
Anti-ABCG1	Goat	1:1000	Santa Cruz Biotechnology
Anti-VLDLR	Mouse	1:125	Santa Cruz Biotechnology
Anti-ABCA1	Mouse	1:1000	Santa Cruz Biotechnology
Anti-PCSK9	Goat	1:2500	Novus Biological
Anti-PPARα	Rabbit	1:1000	Santa Cruz Biotechnology
Anti-PPARγ	Mouse	1:1000	Santa Cruz Biotechnology
Anti-LXRα	Rabbit	1:1000	Sigma Aldrich
Anti-LXRβ	Rabbit	1:1000	Sigma Aldrich
Anti-FAT/CD36	Mouse	1:250	Abcam
Anti-FATP4	Mouse	1:1000	Abnova Corporation
Anti-LPL	Mouse	1:1000	Abcam
Anti-ABCB1	Rabbit	1:1000	LifeSpan BioSciences
Anti-ABCB4	Rabbit	1:500	LifeSpan BioSciences
Anti-ABCG1	Goat	1:1000	Santa Cruz Biotechnology
Anti-ABCG2	Rabbit	1:1000	LifeSpan BioSciences

15. Horseradish peroxidase-conjugated antibody solution (anti-rabbit, anti-goat, or anti-mouse): 1:10,000 in blocking solution.
16. Western HRP substrate.

2.5 Cholesterol Quantitation

1. BeWo cells cultured in Ham's F-12 media supplemented with 10% fetal bovine serum.
2. 7 mL flat bottom tubes.
3. PrestoBlue cell viability reagent.
4. Sterile 1× PBS.
5. Cell scrapers.
6. Sonic dismembrator.
7. Chloroform/methanol solution (2:1).
8. 1 mM $CaCl_2$.
9. 10% Triton X-100 in isopropanol.
10. Cholesterol/Cholesteryl Ester Quantification Kit (BioVision).

2.6 Activity of Lipoprotein Lipase (LPL)

1. Homogenization buffer: 150 mM NaCl, 10 mM Tris, 2 mM EDTA, pH 7.4.
2. Roar LPL Activity Assay Kit.

3 Methods

3.1 Tissue Sampling

1. Collect and immediately immerse the tissue in ice-cold DMEM supplemented with antibiotics. Keep the tissue on ice and process it within 1 h of delivery.
2. Collect morphological information (weight, size, color, membrane integrity, umbilical cord, and any pathological signs such as calcification or lipid steatosis).
3. Place the tissue on a Pyrex dish with the maternal face side up. With sterile scissors, cut a piece of tissue containing the insertion of the umbilical cord from maternal to fetal side, and store it in formalin for the pathology department of the hospital.
4. Remove the amnion, chorion, and decidual layers.
5. Collect small pieces of tissue from five to ten cotyledons to have representative samples of the total placenta. Freeze pieces of tissue in liquid nitrogen, transfer them into several sterile nuclease-free tubes (*see* **Note 1**), and store them at −80 °C until further use.

3.2 RNA Extraction

3.2.1 For Tissues

1. Transfer 25 mg of frozen tissue into a 1.5 mL microcentrifuge nuclease-free tube.

2. Add the appropriate amount of lysis buffer of the High Pure Tissue RNA Kit and homogenize the tissue on ice with a tissue grinder.
3. Extract total RNA with the High Pure Tissue RNA Kit according to the manufacturer's instructions.

3.2.2 For Cells

1. Plate 80,000 cells per well in a 6-well plate.
2. Change medium every 24 h for optimal growth.
3. Once cells become 85% confluent, remove the growth medium and rinse cells twice with 1× PBS.
4. Add 100 μL of ice-cold 1× PBS and 200 μL of lysis buffer per well. Mix well.
5. Using a cell scraper, scrape the cells off the bottom of the well. Verify with a microscope that all cells have come off.
6. Recover the cell lysate and extract total RNA as described by the manufacturer using the High Pure RNA Isolation Kit.

3.3 Quantitative Real-Time Reverse Transcription Polymerase Chain Reaction (qRT-PCR)

1. Quantify the amounts and purity of the extracted total RNA by measuring the absorbance at 260 nm (A260) and 280 nm (A280). The RNA yield (μg/μL) can be determined as follows: A260 × 0.04 μg RNA/μL × dilution factor. The ratios A260/A280 and A260/230 provide an estimate of the purity of RNA and the presence of contaminants such as protein or phenol. Ratios should be between 1.8 and 2. The RNA integrity should also be checked with a gel (*see* **Note 2**) or a bioanalyzer chip to ensure it is not degraded.
2. Synthesize cDNA from 0.5 to 1 μg of total RNA using the iScript™ Reverse Transcription Supermix for RT-qPCR (*see* **Note 3**).
3. Use cDNA to amplify genes of interest and housekeeping genes on the PCR amplification and detection instrument using specific primers (0.5 μM; Table 2) and the LightCycler 480 SYBR Green I Master kit (*see* **Note 4**).

3.4 Western Blot Analysis

3.4.1 Protein Extraction, Dosage, and Migration

1. Homogenize 800 mg of placental tissue on ice using the tissue homogenizer in ice-cold homogenization buffer supplemented with the EDTA-free antiprotease cocktail.
2. Incubate the homogenates on ice for 30 min.
3. Centrifuge the homogenates at 10,000 × *g* for 25 min at 4 °C.
4. Collect, aliquot, and store the supernatants at −80 °C until further use (*see* **Note 1**).
5. Keep an aliquot to evaluate the protein content of the samples with the BCA protein assay kit according to the manufacturer's instructions.

Table 2
Description of the primers used for real-time RT-PCR in order to detect genes involved in placental lipid homeostasis

Gene	Sequence (5′–3′) Forward	Reverse	Product size (bp)	Reference
FAT/CD36	cgaaagtcactgcgacatga	ccttggatggaagaacgaatc	179	[6]
FATP4	tggacccctcgctcagcctc	cagccctgtggtgccggatg	176	[6]
LDLR	gcagtgggcgacagatgcga	gcacgtcttgggggagcacg	141	[5]
VLDR	tacgctgttgtggaaatgtgat	attcagcacacgtcttctttaca	86	[5]
SRBI	cggctcggagagcgactac	gggcttattctccatgatcacc	76	[5]
ABCA1	acccaccctatgaacaacatga	gagtcgggtaacggaaacagg	123	[5]
ABCG1	caggaagattagacactgtgg	gaaaggggaatggagagaaga	177	[5]
LPL	atggctggacggtaacagga	gcggacactgggtaatgctc	136	[6]
PCSK9	gtctctagcagcatgatctcgatagt	tcgacgtcgctgcggaaacc	78	[5]
PPARA	agctttggctttacggaatacca	ccacaggataagtcaccgagga	115	[5]
PPARG	tcagggctgccagtttcg	ccctcggatatgagaaccc	187	[5]
LXRA	agggctgcaagggattcttcc	tctgacagcacacactcctccc	166	[5]
LXRB	ggagctggccatcatctca	gtctctagcagcatgatctcgatagt	132	[5]
ABCB1	cccatcattgcaatagcagg	gttcaaacttctgctcctga	157	
ABCB4	tttttactttcttccttcagggtttc	taaaagccattgaccgcagtct	81	
ABCG2	agatgggtttccaagcgttcat	ccagtcccagtacgactgtgaca	91	
PPIA	gtttgcagacaaggtccca	acccgtatgctttaggatg	211	[10]
HPRT1	gaccagtcaacaggggacataa	aagcttgcgaccttgacc	167	[10]
TOP1	ggcagagtgaatctaagg	cttaaagggtacaggaatg	90	[10]
GAPDH	gaaggtgaaggtcggagtcaa	ggaagatggtgatgggatttc	227	[6]

6. Prepare a resolving gel of the appropriate concentration depending on the size of the protein as described in Table 3 (*see* **Notes 5** and **6**). The recipe is for one gel (8 mL).
7. Once the resolving gel is polymerized, prepare a 4% stacking gel (*see* **Notes 5** and **6**) as described in Table 4. The recipe is for one gel (5 mL).
8. Once the stacking gel is polymerized, assemble the gel unit and add the appropriate amount of running buffer. Carefully remove the comb and gently rinse the wells by injecting running buffer with a pipette.

Table 3
Recipe for resolving gels with different acrylamide concentrations according to the size of the protein

Percentage of acrylamide	6%	8%	10%	12%	15%
Size of the protein (kDa)	60–210	40–100	20–70	20–60	10–40
Water (mL)	4.6	4.2	3.8	3.4	3
Acrylamide 40% (mL)	1.2	1.6	2	2.4	2.8
1.5 M Tris pH 8.8 (mL)	2	2	2	2	2
10% SDS (μL)	80	80	80	80	80
10% APS (μL)	80	80	80	80	80
TEMED (μL)	8	8	8	8	8

Table 4
Recipe for 4% stacking gel

Water (mL)	3.1
40% acrylamide (mL)	0.5
0.5 M Tris pH 6.8 (mL)	1.25
10% SDS (μL)	50
10% APS (μL)	50
TEMED (μL)	5

9. Dilute 50 μg of proteins in sample dilution buffer and boil the samples for 5 min at 95 °C.
10. Load an equal amount of each sample in the wells and 10 μL of prestained molecular weight standards.
11. Run the gel at 100 V.
12. At the end of the migration, disassemble the unit, remove the stacking gel, and immerse the resolving gel in transfer buffer for 15 min.

3.4.2 Protein Transfer

1. Rehydrate a piece of PVDF membrane (~8 × 10 cm) in methanol, rinse in water, and immerse in transfer buffer for 15 min.
2. Presoak blotting paper in transfer buffer for 5 min.

3. Assemble the transfer sandwich (anode/blotting paper/membrane/gel/blotting paper/cathode), and carefully remove any air bubble between the membrane and the gel.
4. Transfer for 60 min at room temperature at 0.8 mA per 1 cm^2 of gel area and maximum 15 V.
5. Rinse the membrane with water and verify the transfer efficiency with Ponceau S.
6. Wash with water to remove Ponceau S.

3.4.3 Membrane Blocking, Incubation with Antibodies, and Revelation

1. Immerse membranes in blocking buffer for 1 h at room temperature.
2. Incubate with primary antibodies overnight at 4 °C.
3. Wash membranes three times 10 min at room temperature with TBST.
4. Incubate membranes with the appropriate horseradish peroxidase-conjugated antibody for 1 h at room temperature.
5. Wash membranes three times 10 min at room temperature with TBST.
6. Incubate membranes for 5 min with Western HRP substrate, wrapped in plastic layer and exposed on an autoradiography film.

3.5 Preparation of Material for Cholesterol Quantitation

3.5.1 For Tissues

1. Transfer 100 mg of frozen tissue (*see* Subheading 3.1) into an ice-cold 7 mL flat bottom tube.
2. Under a chemical hood (*see* **Note** 7), add 2 mL of chloroform/methanol to the tissue. The solution should be well mixed before using it.
3. Homogenize the mixture with the tissue homogenizer (1 min at speed 12 if using a Polytron PT 3000).
4. Transfer the homogenate to a 2 mL microcentrifuge tube. Complete to maximal volume (~2.4 mL) with 1 mM $CaCl_2$ and vortex 10 s at maximal speed.

3.5.2 For Cells

1. Plate 80,000 cells per well in a 6-well plate.
2. Change medium every 24 h for optimal growth.
3. Once cells become 85% confluent, add the PrestoBlue cell viability reagent according to the manufacturer's instructions (*see* **Note 8**).
4. Remove the medium and wash the cells several times with 1× PBS.
5. Remove the 1× PBS and add 500 μL of 1 mM $CaCl_2$ per well.
6. Remove the cells using a cell scraper and transfer the lysate to a microcentrifuge tube.

7. Under a chemical hood (*see* **Note 7**), add 1 mL of chloroform/methanol (*see* **Note 9**) to the lysate. The solution should be well mixed before using it.
8. Vortex 10 s at maximal speed.
9. Sonicate the lysate (5 s at power 3 if using the 550 Sonic Dismembrator).
10. Vortex 5 s at maximal speed.

3.6 Cholesterol Quantitation in Placental Tissues and Cells

1. Centrifuge 10 min at 21,000 × *g* at room temperature to separate the mixture into three layers: the upper layer is the aqueous fraction, the bottom layer is the organic fraction, and the thin layer found between the aqueous and organic fractions contains cellular debris.
2. Remove the upper layer and the layer of cellular debris.
3. Recover and evaporate the bottom layer overnight under the hood (*see* **Note 10**).
4. Resuspend the resulting dried fraction in 200 μL of isopropanol containing 10% Triton X-100. This step takes time (~5–10 min) and requires vortexing the sample.
5. Quantify the amount of free and total cholesterol with the Cholesterol/Cholesteryl Ester Quantification Kit according to the manufacturer's instructions. Determine the cholesterol ester fraction by subtracting the amount of free cholesterol to the amount of total cholesterol (*see* **Note 11**). Incubate the plate for a maximum of 15 min at 37 °C. Shake slightly and protect from the light.
6. Normalize results on the amount of tissue extracted or on the number of cells measured with the PrestoBlue reagent as described previously (*see* Subheading 3.5.2).

3.7 Activity of Lipoprotein Lipase (LPL)

1. Homogenize placental tissues (20–100 mg) in 400 μL of ice-cold homogenization buffer.
2. Centrifuge 30 min at 10,000 × *g* at 4 °C. Recover and aliquot the supernatant. Keep an aliquot to quantify total proteins as described in Subheading 3.4.1.
3. Quantify the activity of LPL with the Roar LPL Activity Assay Kit according to the manufacturer's instructions.
4. Normalize the results on the amount of proteins.

4 Notes

1. For each tissue, several samples should be prepared in individual tubes. Once frozen, samples should remain frozen to avoid RNA and protein degradation caused by repeated freeze-thaw cycles.

Table 5
Standard guidelines for qPCR experiments

Category	Item to check	Quality criteria
Primer design	Optimal length of the primers	18–22 bp
	Optimal primer melting temperature (Tm)	55–58 °C (the difference of Tm between primers should be within 1 °C)
	GC content	50–60%
	Repeats of a single base longer than four bases	To avoid
	Primer and template secondary structures	To avoid
	3′ end of primers	Should contain Gs or Cs but no more than three in the last five bases
	Exon-exon junctions	To have in the target sequence to avoid amplification from contaminating genomic DNA
	Specificity of the target sequence	Sequences of primers should be blasted
	Amplicon size	75–200 bp
Negative controls	No-template negative control	Detects any contamination in the SYBR Green I Master mix
	No reverse transcriptase negative control	Detects any contamination with genomic DNA. This step is not necessary if primers have been designed to span exon-exon junctions
Specificity of the assay	Melting/dissociation curve	Perform at the end of each run to ensure the specificity of the assay. A single peak should be detected
Analysis of data	Normalization of gene of interest expression	Use appropriate housekeeping genes [10]

2. RNA integrity can be evaluated on gel using an inexpensive and safe technique based on bleach [11].
3. Negative controls should be performed with the mix that doesn't contain any reverse transcriptase included in the kit to ensure that the sample of total RNA is free of genomic DNA. This step is not necessary if primers have been designed to span exon-exon junctions.
4. The experiment should follow standard PCR guidelines described in Table 5. Conditions of amplification should be optimized for each gene and samples should be done in triplicates.

5. Acrylamide and bisacrylamide should be handled with extreme care because these chemicals are highly neurotoxic.
6. APS and TEMED are responsible of gel polymerization and should be added just before pouring the gels.
7. Chloroform is a volatile and possibly carcinogenic compound that may be harmful if inhaled, swallowed, or in contact with the skin. Exposure to chloroform may have adverse effects on the respiratory tract, gastrointestinal tract, kidneys, liver, and central nervous system.
8. PrestoBlue reagent should also be added to an empty well with only growth medium. This will constitute the blank. Take a sample, if necessary at multiple time points, to read fluorescence or absorbance in triplicate according to the manufacturer's instructions.
9. Do not add the mix of chloroform/methanol directly into the 6-well plate. Most plastics are weakened and can even be dissolved by chloroform.
10. This process can be accelerated using compressed nitrogen (Product grade 4.8, Praxair). Evaporation should occur in 5–10 min.
11. A blank sample of isopropanol with 10% Triton X-100 should be included for the reading of the plate.

Acknowledgments

ED is the recipient of postdoctoral fellowships from the *Fonds de Recherche du Québec en Santé* (FRQS) and L'Oréal Canada in collaboration with UNESCO for Women in Science. This work was funded by a Natural Sciences and Engineering Research Council of Canada (NSERC) grant to J.L.

References

1. Lager S, Powell TL (2012) Regulation of nutrient transport across the placenta. J Pregnancy 2012:179827
2. Gil-Sanchez A, Koletzko B, Larque E (2012) Current understanding of placental fatty acid transport. Curr Opin Clin Nutr Metab Care 15:265–272
3. Baardman ME, Kerstjens-Frederikse WS, Berger RM, Bakker MK, Hofstra RM, Plosch T (2013) The role of maternal-fetal cholesterol transport in early fetal life: current insights. Biol Reprod 88:24
4. Aye IL, Keelan JA (2013) Placental ABC transporters, cellular toxicity and stress in pregnancy. Chem Biol Interact 203:456–466
5. Dube E, Ethier-Chiasson M, Lafond J (2013) Modulation of cholesterol transport by insulin-treated gestational diabetes mellitus in human full-term placenta. Biol Reprod 88:16
6. Dube E, Gravel A, Martin C, Desparois G, Moussa I, Ethier-Chiasson M, Forest JC, Giguere Y, Masse A, Lafond J (2012) Modulation of fatty acid transport and metabolism by mater-

nal obesity in the human full-term placenta. Biol Reprod 87(14):11–11

7. Ethier-Chiasson M, Duchesne A, Forest JC, Giguere Y, Masse A, Mounier C, Lafond J (2007) Influence of maternal lipid profile on placental protein expression of LDLr and SR-BI. Biochem Biophys Res Commun 359:8–14
8. Ethier-Chiasson M, Forest JC, Giguere Y, Masse A, Marseille-Tremblay C, Levy E, Lafond J (2008) Modulation of placental protein expression of OLR1: implication in pregnancy-related disorders or pathologies. Reproduction 136:491–502
9. Marseille-Tremblay C, Ethier-Chiasson M, Forest JC, Giguere Y, Masse A, Mounier C, Lafond J (2008) Impact of maternal circulating cholesterol and gestational diabetes mellitus on lipid metabolism in human term placenta. Mol Reprod Dev 75:1054–1062
10. Lanoix D, Lacasse AA, St-Pierre J, Taylor SC, Ethier-Chiasson M, Lafond J, Vaillancourt C (2012) Quantitative PCR pitfalls: the case of the human placenta. Mol Biotechnol 52:234–243
11. Aranda PS, LaJoie DM, Jorcyk CL (2012) Bleach gel: a simple agarose gel for analyzing RNA quality. Electrophoresis 33:366–369

Chapter 25

EG-VEGF Maintenance Over Early Gestation to Develop a Pregnancy-Induced Hypertensive Animal Model

Déborah Reynaud, Frédéric Sergent, Roland Abi Nahed, Sophie Brouillet, Mohamed Benharouga, and Nadia Alfaidy

Abstract

During the last decade, multiple animal models have been developed to mimic hallmarks of pregnancy-induced hypertension (PIH) diseases, which include gestational hypertension, preeclampsia (PE), or eclampsia. Converging in vitro, ex vivo, and clinical studies from our group strongly suggested the potential involvement of the new angiogenic factor EG-VEGF (endocrine gland-derived-VEGF) in the development of PIH. Here, we described the protocol that served to demonstrate that maintenance of EG-VEGF production over 11.5 days post coitus (dpc) in the gravid mice caused the development of PIH. The developed model exhibited most hallmarks of preeclampsia.

Key words Animal model, Preeclampsia, Pregnancy, EG-VEGF, Placenta, Hypertension, Glomerulosclerosis, Invasion

1 Introduction

One of the major contributing factors to the development of PIH is the failure of the extravillous trophoblast cell (EVT) to invade deep into the maternal decidua, compromising the normal establishment of the feto-maternal circulation [1]. Failure in the invasion process results in reduced placental perfusion [2], increased trophoblast apoptosis [3], and abnormal production of anti-angiogenic factors such as soluble fms-like tyrosine kinase 1 (sFlt1) and soluble endoglin (sEng) by the placenta [4]. These two anti-angiogenic factors are known to directly affect kidney function as well as maternal vascular system [4]. Anti-angiogenic factors are proposed to diagnose preeclampsia (PE) onset by mid second trimester of pregnancy [4, 5]. Nevertheless, early biomarkers of PE diagnosis are still to be identified.

Endocrine gland-derived VEGF (EG-VEGF) is an angiogenic factor secreted by the placenta during the first trimester of human pregnancy [6–8]. We have recently demonstrated that EG-VEGF

Padma Murthi and Cathy Vaillancourt (eds.), *Preeclampsia: Methods and Protocols*, Methods in Molecular Biology, vol. 1710, https://doi.org/10.1007/978-1-4939-7498-6_25,

controls trophoblast invasion, is upregulated by hypoxia, and is abnormally elevated in pathological pregnancies complicated with PE and IUGR (intrauterine growth restriction) [6–10].

EG-VEGF circulating levels are around 50 pg/mL in the serum of nonpregnant women and increase fivefold during the first trimester of pregnancy (≈250 pg/mL) [7, 10]. In relation to pregnancy PE and IUGR, circulating EG-VEGF levels are significantly increased during the third trimester, suggesting that sustained EG-VEGF levels beyond the first trimester of pregnancy may contribute to the development of pregnancy pathologies including PIH and that elevated EG-VEGF levels might constitute a potential biomarker for PE development. To test this hypothesis, we developed an animal model by implanting subcutaneously osmotic pumps delivering EG-VEGF into gravid OF1 mice on 11.5 days post coitus (dpc), which is equivalent to the end of the first trimester of human pregnancy. Mice were sacrificed at 15.5 and 18.5 dpc to assess (1) litter size and placental and fetal weight, (2) placental histology and function, (3) maternal blood pressure, (4) renal histology and function, and (5) circulating sFlt1 and sEng. Another group of mice was treated at 7.5 dpc and sacrificed at 12.5 dpc to assess trophoblast invasion within the maternal decidua.

Increased EG-VEGF levels caused significant defects in placental organization and function since 12.5 dpc. Both increased hypoxia and decreased trophoblast invasion were observed. Treated mice had elevated circulating sFlt1 and sEng and developed gestational hypertension with dysregulated maternal kidney function. EG-VEGF effect on the kidney function was secondary to its effects on the placenta, as similarly treated male mice had normal kidney functions. Altogether, this model provides a strong evidence to confirm that sustained EG-VEGF beyond the first trimester of pregnancy contributes to the development of PIH.

PE is generally described as a disease of two stages. Stage 1 occurs during trophoblast invasion, and stage 2 consists of the clinical manifestations. The great majority of animal models aim to mimic the second stage. We believe that the developed model mimics more stage 1 than stage 2 of the disease. While the present model does not recapitulate full symptoms of a typical PE observed in women and to certain extent in strong models such as the RUPP, sFlt-1, and sEng animal models [4, 11, 12], it does bring strong information about the mechanism of stage 1 development of PIH.

2 Materials

2.1 Mice and Chemicals

1. Female mice nulliparous around 8–12 weeks of age.
2. Male mice (used as control).
3. Osmotic pumps: delivery 0.5 μL/h for 5–7 days.

4. Recombinant human EG-VEGF.
5. Vehicle: 0.9% NaCl solution.
6. Surgical kit (clamps, scissors, and surgical suture).
7. General anesthesia device based on isoflurane.
8. Chemical anesthesia: ketamine/xylazine mix (1 mL ketamine +0.5 mL xylazine +8.5 mL 0.9% NaCl).

2.2 Characterization of the PIH Model

1. Noninvasive computerized tail-off system: CODA8 system.
2. 25 G needle.
3. 1 mL syringes.
4. EDTA.
5. 1.5 mL blood collection tubes containing heparin.
6. Metabolic chambers that allow the separation of urine and feces.
7. Tissue fixation: 4% paraformaldehyde (PFA); free formalin fixative (FFF).
8. Human EG-VEGF ELISA assay kit.
9. Murine sFLT1 ELISA assay kit.
10. Murine sEndoglin ELISA assay kit.
11. Hematoxylin.
12. Eosin.
13. Antibodies used for placental characterization: CD31 (marker of trophoblast vascularization), carbonic anhydrase IX (CA9; marker of hypoxia), cytokeratin 7 (trophoblast marker), and PCNA (proliferating cell marker).
14. Image J software to measure placental zones.

3 Methods

3.1 Assessment of Stage 1 of PIH: Trophoblast Invasion

Group 1 of animals ($n = 20$) was used to assess the degree of trophoblast invasion and hence stage 1 of preeclampsia development. Group 1 was treated at 7.5 dpc after the observation of the plug at 0.5 dpc (*see* **Note 1**). During their gestation and before the delivery of the treatment, all mice were adapted to the blood pressure device (*see* **Notes 2** and **3**). These mice were randomly assigned to receive an osmotic pump delivering either recombinant human EG-VEGF (4 μg; 0.5 μL/h for 5 days) or saline (Fig. 1) (*see* **Notes 4** and **5**). During this procedure mice were under isoflurane anesthesia (*see* **Notes 6** and **7**).

At 12.5 dpc, control and treated mice were euthanized. Chemical anesthesia was induced by intraperitoneal injection of ketamine/xylazine mixture (100 μL per 10 g of weight). After anesthesia, blood was collected by intracardiac puncture performed

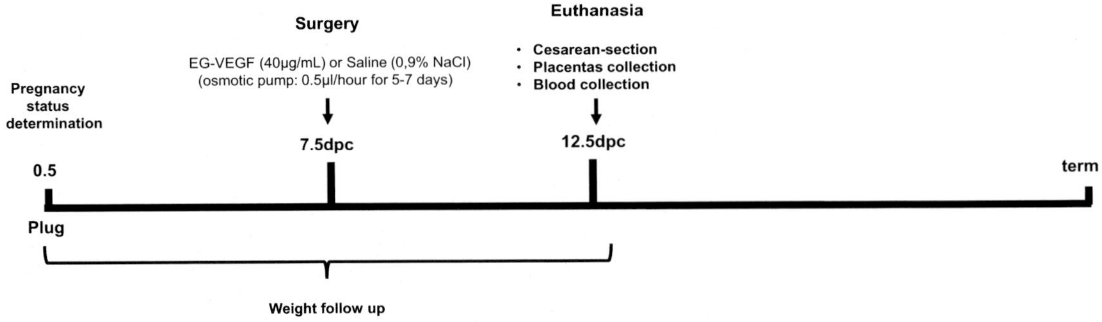

Fig. 1 Experimental procedures for group 1 of gravid mice. The flowchart shows the experimental procedures performed during the first study. The gravid mice were randomly assigned to receive at 7.5 either osmotic pump containing recombinant EG-VEGF or saline. Gravid mice were sacrificed at 12.5 dpc (n = 20 mice). At 12.5 dpc, placenta and maternal blood were collected

with 25 G needle mounted on 1 mL syringes damped with EDTA. After exsanguination, the heart was removed to ensure the death and cesarean section was performed.

Placentas and fetuses were collected and weighed. Placental tissues were fixed in 4% PFA and FFF for histological characterization or frozen at −80 °C for RNA or protein analysis.

Blood collection tubes were centrifuged at 1200 × g for 10 min; plasma was collected and stored at −20 °C.

3.2 Assessment of Stage 2 of PIH: Development of PIH Symptoms

Group 2 of animal (n = 41) was used to assess stage 2 of pre-eclampsia development and hence clinical manifestations of the disease. This group was treated at 11.5 dpc after the observation of the plug at 0.5 dpc. These mice were randomly assigned to receive an osmotic pump delivering either recombinant human EG-VEGF (4 µg, 0.5 µL/h for 5–7 days) or saline (Fig. 2). A subgroup of ten mice was sacrificed at 15.5 dpc, and the second subgroup of ten mice was sacrificed at 18.5 dpc.

3.2.1 From 0.5 to 7.5 dpc

OF1 mice were housed under controlled illumination (12:12, light: dark cycle) and feed ad libitum. Two- to three-month-old mice were mated and used to generate gravid mice. The date of the presence of the vaginal plug was taken at 0.5 dpc.

Plugged mice were weighed every day, and blood pressure was measured using noninvasive computerized tail-off system. It consists of 7-day adaptation in order to reduce the stress during the experimentation.

At 7.5 dpc, blood pressure was taken and mice were housed for 24 h in metabolic chambers in order to collect urine and feces separately. Urine was stored at −20 °C until the test.

3.2.2 From 8.5 to 12.5 dpc

Mice were weighed every 2 days (9.5 and 11.5 dpc) and mean arterial pressure was taken at 11.5 dpc just before the surgery. Mice were randomly assigned to receive an EG-VEGF (40 µg/mL)

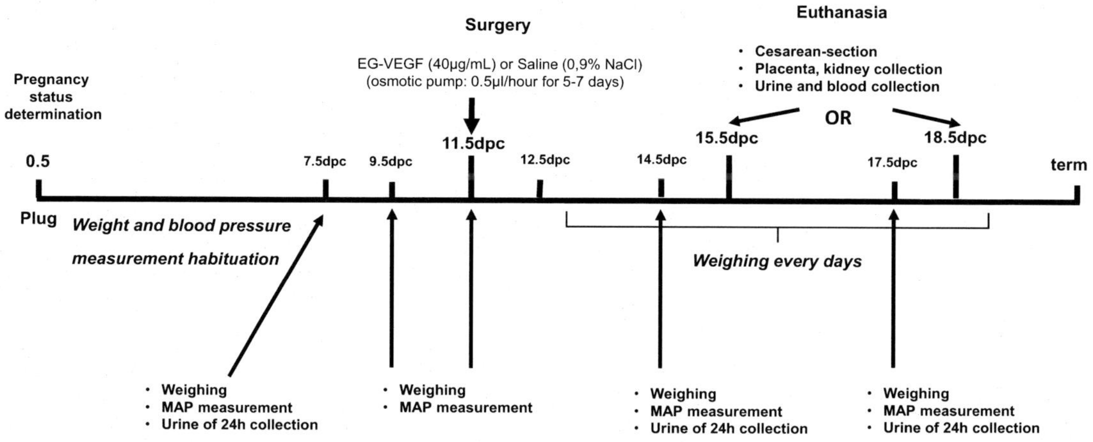

Fig. 2 Experimental procedures for group 2 of gravid mice. The flowchart shows the experimental procedures performed during the second study. The gravid mice were randomly assigned to receive at 11.5 dpc either osmotic pump containing recombinant EG-VEGF or saline. Gravid mice treated at 11.5 dpc were sacrificed at 15.5 dpc ($n = 21$ mice) or 18.5 dpc ($n = 20$ mice). At 15.5 dpc and 18.5 dpc placenta, maternal kidney, urine, and blood were also collected. Blood pressure was measured at 15.5 dpc and 18.5 dpc

osmotic pump ($n = 20$) or saline osmotic pump ($n = 20$). Anesthesia induction was performed by 4% isoflurane in the box. Then mice were placed on hot plate and anesthesia was maintained at 1.5% isoflurane in the mask.

At 11.5 dpc, mice skin was shaved at the abdomen level and opened of about 2 cm; the osmotic pump was loaded with 100 µL of EG-VEGF (4 µg) or saline and placed in the peritoneal cavity at the left flank.

Surgical incision was closed in two steps, peritoneum and muscles were sewn up with surgical wire and four to five staples were placed to reattach the skin. The closed wound was sanitized with betadine before mice replacement in the cage.

3.2.3 From 13.5 to 15.5 dpc

After surgery, mice were weighed every day. At 14.5 dpc, mean arterial pressure was measured and mice were placed in metabolic chambers for 24 h; collected urine was frozen at −20 °C. At 15.5 dpc, ten mice of EG-VEGF treated and of control group were randomly euthanized. Chemical anesthesia was induced by intraperitoneal injection of ketamine/xylazine mixture (100 µL/10 g of weight). After anesthesia, blood was collected by intracardiac puncture performed with 25 G needle mounted on 1 mL syringes soaked with EDTA. After exsanguination, the heart was removed to ensure the death.

Placentas and fetuses were weighed. Placental tissues, kidneys, and all other organs of interest were fixed in 4% PFA and FFF for histological characterization or frozen at −80 °C for RNA or protein analysis.

Blood collection tubes were centrifuged at 1200 × *g* for 10 min; plasmas were collected and stored at −20 °C.

3.2.4 From 16.5 to 18.5 dpc

At 17.5 dpc, the 20 mice remaining were weighed and mean arterial pressure measured. Then the mice were housed in metabolic chambers for 24 h; collected urines were frozen at −20 °C.

At 18.5 dpc, mice were euthanized and blood and tissues collected. Placentas and fetuses were weighed. Placental tissues, kidneys, and all other organs of interest were fixed in 4% PFA and FFF for histological characterization or frozen at −80 °C for RNA or protein analysis.

Blood collection tubes were centrifuged at 1200 × *g* for 10 min; plasmas were collected and stored at −20 °C.

3.2.5 Validation of the Pregnancy-Induced Hypertension Model

Gravid mice treatment with EG-VEGF caused a significant increase in the maternal circulating levels of EG-VEGF. These levels reached 2.5 times the normal levels (*see* **Note 8**).

At day 15.5 dpc, there was a significant increase in the maternal arterial pressure (20% increase).

Compared to saline mice, EG-VEGF-treated mice exhibited a significant increase in the anti-angiogenic factor, sFlt-1. An average of 20% increase was observed both at 12.5 and 15.5 dpc. One hundred microliter of plasma was used to assess sFlt-1 levels using the ELISA kit from Ray Biotech Company. Significant increase in sEndoglin circulating levels was also observed in EG-VEGF-treated mice at 15.5 and at18.5 dpc. One hundred microliter of plasma was used to assess sEndoglin in the ELISA kit from R&D System.

Deleterious effects were also observed in the maternal renal function of EG-VEGF-treated mice. There was a significant increase in the albumin to creatinine ratio. Renal histology showed an increase in the number of abnormal glomeruli compared to the kidneys of saline-treated mice. Abnormal glomeruli corresponded to renal glomerulosclerosis instead of endotheliosis, as observed in full PE models (Fig. 3).

4 Notes

The present protocol was set up to assess stage 1 and stage 2 of the development of preeclampsia in relation to a deregulation of a given factor, in our case EG-VEGF. This protocol could be applied to any study that aims at assessing the effect of a circulating factor on the development of preeclampsia at both stages of its development and manifestation. Nevertheless, this protocol was subjected to strict follow-ups that generated the following difficulties.

1. Plugs needed to be verified early in the morning, as total liquefaction occurs 12–14 h after coitus.

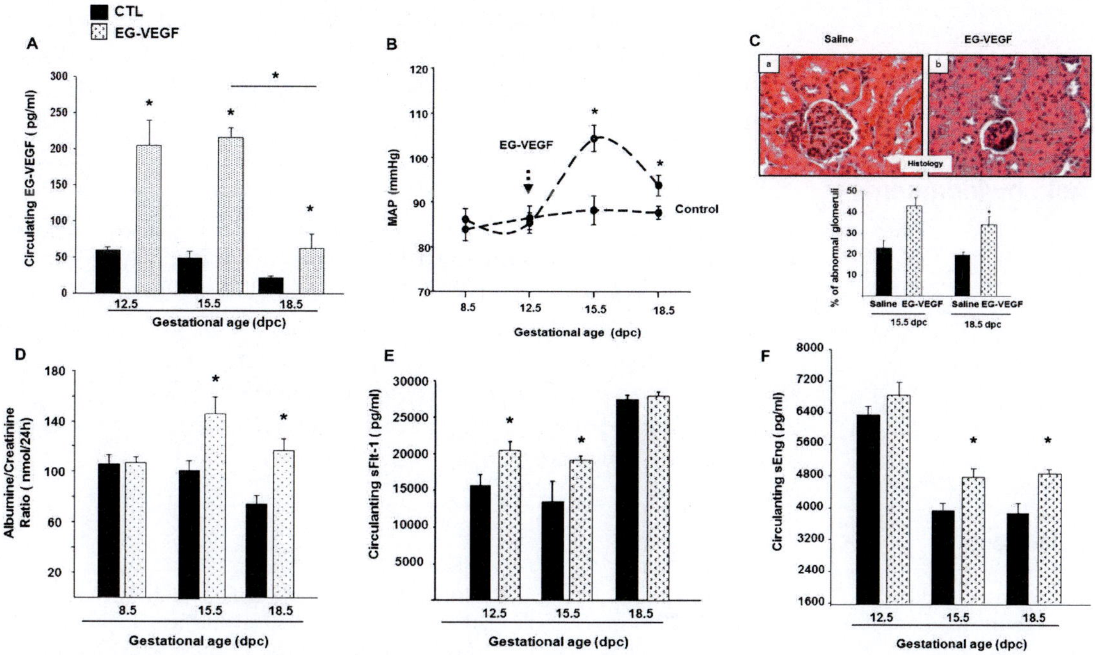

Fig. 3 (**a**) Reports EG-VEGF serum levels in gravid mice treated with EG-VEGF. A total of 65 serum samples were analyzed. Data are presented as bar graphs (* $P < 0.05$). (**b**) Reports summary of MAP recorded longitudinally before and during EG-VEGF treatment (arrow). Data are expressed as mean ± SEM (*$P < 0.05$). (**c**) Shows representative photomicrographs of hematoxylin-eosin-stained kidney sections from gravid saline and EG-VEGF-treated mice at 15.5 dpc of gestation. (**d**) Reports percentage of abnormal glomeruli in control and treated mice at 15.5 and 18.5 dpc. Data are expressed as mean ± SEM (* $P < 0.05$). (**e**) Reports summary of 24 h urinary albumin/creatinine ratio at days 8.5, 15.5, and 18.5 of gestation. Data are expressed as mean ± SEM (* $P < 0.05$). (**f**). EG-VEGF treatment increased circulating sFlt-1 (* $P < 0.05$). (**G**) EG-VEGF treatment increased circulating sEng. Data are expressed as mean ± SEM (* $P < 0.05$)

2. Adaptation of mice to the blood pressure device was crucial for the good practice of this assessment and to get reliable results.
3. Because of their gain of weight during gestation, blood pressure measurements had to be adapted by using larger tubes, such as those conceived to assess blood pressure in rats. This problem starts after 12.5 dpc of gestation.
4. In the absence of ultrasound analysis, mice gestation should be verified before inserting the osmotic pump. This should be performed with delicacy in order to not disrupt the progress of gestation.
5. Pump should be introduced gently with the drain device down.
6. Animals should not suffer during experimentation. During surgery, isoflurane anesthesia should be controlled until the end.
7. If animals show any pain signs (e.g., loss of 10% of weight, prostration, facial mimics, spiky hairs), they must be excluded of the experiment and euthanized.

8. The 2.5 fold eleveted concentration was chosen because we previousely demonstrated that EG-VEGF levels were 2.5 higher in PE women compared to age-matched control women.

Acknowledgments

We thank Dr. J. Boutonnat and Dr. A. Florin for their help for the histological assessment of kidney sections. We acknowledge the following sources of funding: *Institut National de la Santé et de la Recherche Médicale* (U1036), the University Grenoble-Alpes, *Commissariat à l'Energie Atomique* (DSV/iRTSV/BCI), the *Région Rhône-Alpes*, the *Ligue Nationale contre le Cancer*, and the *Ligue Départementale (Isère) contre le Cancer.*

References

1. Sibai B, Dekker G, Kupferminc M (2005) Pre-eclampsia. Lancet 365(9461):785–799
2. Backes CH et al (2011) Maternal preeclampsia and neonatal outcomes. J Pregnancy 2011: 214365
3. Carty DM, Delles C, Dominiczak AF (2010) Preeclampsia and future maternal health. J Hypertens 28(7):1349–1355
4. Maynard SE, Karumanchi SA (2011) Angiogenic factors and preeclampsia. Semin Nephrol 31(1):33–46
5. Zeisler H et al (2016) Predictive Value of the sFlt-1:PlGF Ratio in Women with Suspected Preeclampsia. N Engl J Med 374(1):13–22
6. Brouillet S et al (2012) EG-VEGF: a key endocrine factor in placental development. Trends Endocrinol Metab 23(10):501–508
7. Hoffmann P, Feige JJ, Alfaidy N (2006) Expression and oxygen regulation of endocrine gland-derived vascular endothelial growth factor/prokineticin-1 and its receptors in human placenta during early pregnancy. Endocrinology 147(4):1675–1684
8. Hoffmann P, Feige JJ, Alfaidy N (2007) Placental expression of EG-VEGF and its receptors PKR1 (prokineticin receptor-1) and PKR2 throughout mouse gestation. Placenta 28(10):1049–1058
9. Brouillet S et al (2010) Molecular characterization of EG-VEGF-mediated angiogenesis: differential effects on microvascular and macrovascular endothelial cells. Mol Biol Cell 21(16):2832–2843
10. Hoffmann P et al (2009) Role of EG-VEGF in human placentation: Physiological and pathological implications. J Cell Mol Med 13(8B): 2224–2235
11. Gilbert JS, Babcock SA, Granger JP (2007) Hypertension produced by reduced uterine perfusion in pregnant rats is associated with increased soluble fms-like tyrosine kinase-1 expression. Hypertension 50(6):1142–1147
12. Granger JP et al (2006) Reduced uterine perfusion pressure (RUPP) model for studying cardiovascular-renal dysfunction in response to placental ischemia. Methods Mol Med 122: 383–392

Chapter 26

Real-Time Blood Pressure Recording Using Radiotelemetry in a Rat Model of Preeclampsia

Bryan Leaw, Seshini Gurusinghe, Rebecca Lim, and Euan M. Wallace

Abstract

Radiotelemetry is increasingly being recognized not just as the gold standard but a necessity for validation of gestational hypertension seen in preeclampsia. Here we describe radiotelemetry probe implantation into the descending aorta of Sprague-Dawley rats to allow real-time blood pressure recording over the entire gestational period. This is a valuable tool to be able to track changes in maternal blood pressure throughout gestation and the efficacy of novel therapeutic agents in controlling hypertension.

Key words Preeclampsia, Radiotelemetry, Blood pressure, Hypertension, Rat model

1 Introduction

Radiotelemetry is a high fidelity state-of-the-art method [1, 2] which allows real-time recording of arterial pressure, venous pressure, kidney pressure, ECG, EMG, EEG, glucose, temperature, activity, and numerous other parameters in small or large animals [3]. Current technology is now sufficiently developed to allow high fidelity blood pressure recordings over several months with little or no drift. This is of particular interest for preeclampsia (PE) research, as real-time recording of blood pressure over gestation would allow better elucidation of novel therapies that can both target the underlying endothelial dysfunction and also manage the clinical hypertension. More generally, radiotelemetry can also be applied by researchers working with other disease models seeking to predict the effectiveness and safety of new therapeutic compounds prior to clinical trials.

Here, we describe the application of radiotelemetry technology to a rat model of PE. Soluble fms-like tyrosine kinase 1 (sFlt1) has been shown to contribute to endothelial dysfunction, and increased circulating sFlt1 levels have been touted as a potential early marker of PE [4]. In seminal work by Venkatesha et al., soluble endoglin (sEng) was shown to act in concert with sFlt1 in pregnant rats, amplifying typical PE symptoms into severe PE,

Padma Murthi and Cathy Vaillancourt (eds.), *Preeclampsia: Methods and Protocols*, Methods in Molecular Biology, vol. 1710, https://doi.org/10.1007/978-1-4939-7498-6_26,

including HELLP syndrome (hemolysis, elevated liver enzymes, low platelets) as well as restriction of fetal growth [5]. We first implanted the radiotelemetry probes into 12- to 13-week-old female Sprague-Dawley rats to collect baseline measurements and mated and confirmed pregnancy, and then using adenovirus-associated vectors (AAVs), we overexpressed sFlt1 and sEng on day 8 of gestation (0.4 term). This results in the clinical features of preeclampsia, such as increased proteinuria and gestational hypertension, which resolves upon delivery. Importantly we show here the workflow needed to record high-quality blood pressure data as well as the steps required to verify the clinical validity of the model.

Figure 1 presents results that can be expected following stable and reliable telemetry recordings. It is thus important to monitor the changes in blood pressure during normal circadian rhythm, to be able to differentiate between intrinsic and pathogenic fluctuations in blood pressure. Five days following sFlt1 and sEng adenoviral delivery, we observe that blood pressure begins to increase up to a maximum of 10–15% of baseline (Fig. 1, left panel). There is also notable proteinuria, as evidenced by an increase in albumin/creatinine ratio in the urine of the rats over pregnancy (Fig. 1, right panel). These features support the claim that upregulation of sFlt1

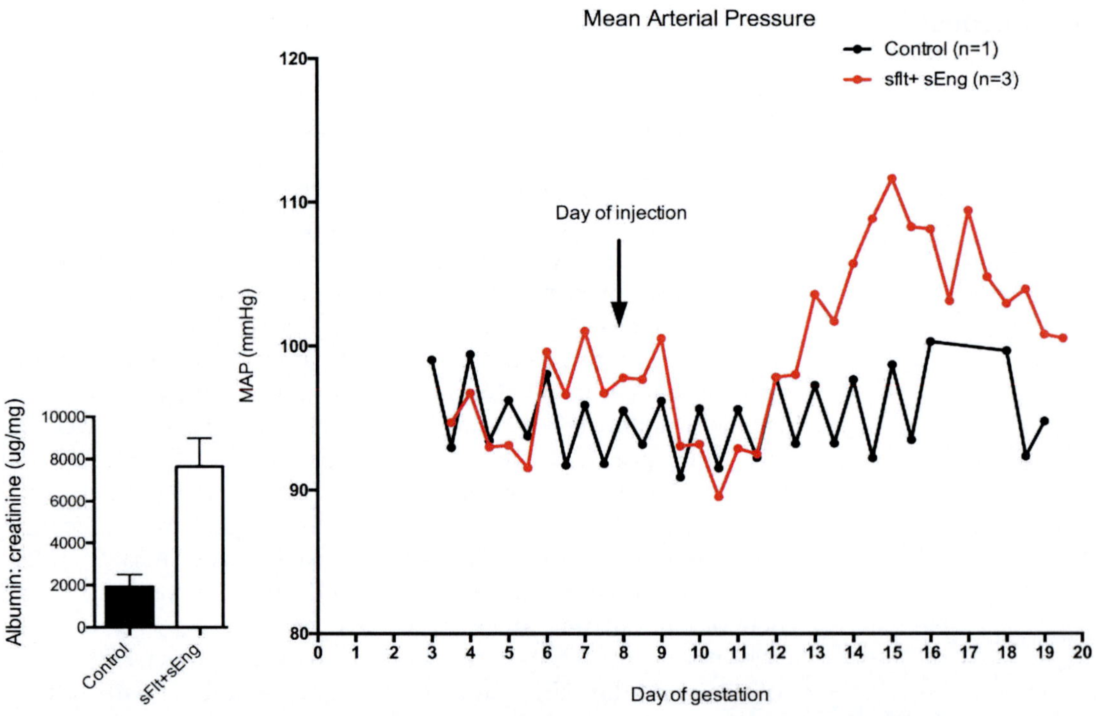

Fig. 1 Expected results after viral-mediated overexpression of sFlt and sEng in a pregnant rat. *Left*: increased albumin/creatine ratio in the preeclamptic rats. *Right*: example blood pressure trace showing increase in mean arterial pressure (MAP) commencing at approximately day 13 of gestation and resolving upon delivery

and sEng is sufficient to create the clinical hallmarks of preeclampsia and lend weight to the use of this model to study novel therapeutic interventions.

2 Materials

2.1 Drugs

1. 5 mg/mL dose of carprofen.
2. Tribactral/Baytril.

2.2 Surgical Equipment

1. Blunt curved forceps.
2. Graefe Iris Forceps (straight and curved).
3. High precision titanium Dumont Tweezers (style 5).
4. Tissue forceps.
5. Dressing scissors (sharp/blunt).
6. Iris scissors (straight).
7. Special purpose tip tweezers (cannula holders).
8. Hemostatic forceps (Spencer Wells, straight).
9. Scalpel handle and blades.
10. Self-retaining abdominal retractor.
11. Motic® SMZ-168 Stereo Zoom Microscope.
12. OXD301 halogen cold, high-intensity fiber light source.
13. PA-C40 PhysioTel Telemetry probes (DSI).
14. Radiotelemetry recording plate.
15. Cellulose patch (5 cm × 5 cm, DSI).
16. Heating pad.
17. Inhalation anesthetic system.
18. Isoflurane.
19. Stereo radio.
20. Industrial-strength magnets.
21. Veterinary shaver for rodents.

2.3 Miscellaneous Surgical Consumables

1. 0.9% saline.
2. Betadine.
3. Sterile gauze.
4. 3 M Vetbond veterinary glue.
5. Cidex.
6. Re-gel syringes to refill catheters (DSI).
7. Nonabsorbable sutures (PDS, 4–0, C-14, reverse cutting).
8. Absorbable sutures (catgut, 4–0, C-14, cutting).

9. Cotton tip applicators.
10. Sterile drapes.
11. 70% ethanol.

3 Methods

3.1 Selection of Experimental Area

Preferably, identify an experimental housing room where the animals are to be housed for the duration of the radiotelemetry recording. Traffic in this area should be kept to a minimum, and preferably only investigators should be allowed access to this area. The room should have sufficient ventilation to maintain appropriate housing conditions, ambient temperature, moisture, and noise which should be monitored and should also have an automatic day/night switching system.

3.2 Animal Housing and Handling

1. House rats in filter-top cages or if possible individually ventilated cages.
2. Prior to surgery, rats can be housed in pairs to avoid isolation-related stress. However, following probe implantation, rats should be housed individually to avoid rats manipulating wound stitches or sutures.
3. Rats should be kept on a 12 h day/night cycle, and when lights are off, investigators should be cautious not to use the room lighting so as not to disturb natural circadian rhythm.
4. Rats should be allowed to acclimatize for 1 week in the experimental holding area before surgery commences. By the end of the acclimatization period, rats should be 12–13 weeks of age, with a body weight of 260 g or more to maximize postsurgical recovery times.

3.3 Preparation Before Surgery

Radiotelemetry probes (PA-40, DSI) require an offset to be measured prior to implantation.

3.3.1 2 Days Prior to Surgery

1. Assign a probe to each animal to be implanted.
2. Ensure that the tip of the catheter (the pressure-sensing end) is sufficiently gelled to improve recording fidelity, if probes have been explanted previously (*see* **Note 1**).
3. Assign each probe to a radiotelemetry recording plate. Place the probe on the plate and turn them on (*see* **Note 2**). Record the pre-offset value on the acquisition software.
4. Set the appropriate calibration values (provided by the manufacturer on the original packaging of the probes) on the receivers attached to each telemetry plate.
5. Cut out a trouser-shaped cellulose patch (approx. 6 mm across), used to wrap around the aorta at the cannulation point (Fig. 2). Dip cellulose patch in Cidex and allow to dry overnight.

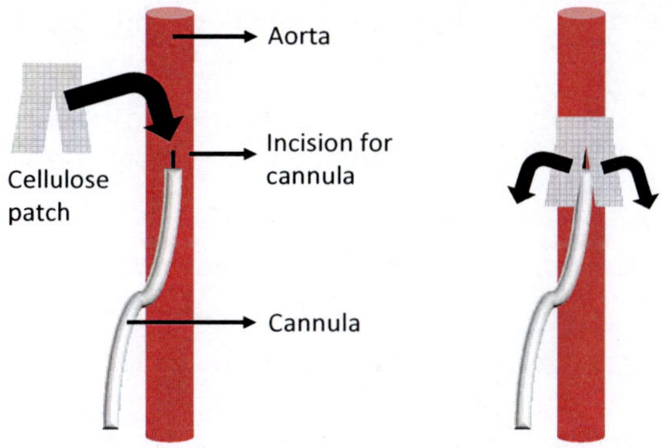

Fig. 2 Schematic showing the appropriate shape of cellulose patch and position after cannulation. After placing the cellulose patch over the incision point, both "legs" of the patch should be pressed down and sealed along the sides of the aorta

3.3.2 1 Day Prior to Surgery

1. Transmitter probes are provided sterile from the manufacturer (*see* **Note 3**).
2. During this time, autoclave surgical instruments (including gauze, applicator sticks, and sterile drapes).
3. Place the trouser-shaped cellulose patch in UV light for 20 min.
4. After 10–12 h, remove probes from Cidex and wash probes thoroughly in running water for 2–3 min. Immerse them in a sterile container until surgery.

3.3.3 Day of the Surgery

1. Pre-warm heating pad, ensuring that dissecting microscope, light source, radio, shaver, and instruments are prepared on the bench.
2. Warm saline and betadine in kidney trays on the heating pad.
3. Prepare drugs for administration—carprofen, Tribactral, and saline in syringes. Weigh rats at this point to prepare the appropriate dosage.

3.4 Surgery

3.4.1 Induction of Anesthesia

The levels of isoflurane required vary from animal to animal, based on genetics, background, age, and sex. The levels provided here are intended as a general guide only.

1. Place the rat in the induction chamber of the AAS Stinger Anesthesia machine, set the isoflurane vaporizer to 4–5%, and maintain a flow rate of 2 L/min.
2. After noting a lack of tail pinch reflex and righting response, move the rat onto the silicone breathing cone, making sure to change the isoflurane to a level of 1.5–3% and oxygen to 0.5 L/min.
3. Carefully monitor the respiration rate of the rat (ideally this should be ~100 breaths per minute). If respiration slows down dramatically, temporarily reduce isoflurane to 1–1.5%.

3.4.2 Preparation for Surgery

Having a surgical microscope and cold light source is highly recommended before commencing the surgical procedure.

1. Apply a petroleum-based ointment to the rat's eyes to prevent damage to the cornea during the surgical procedure.
2. Using the veterinary shaver, clip the fur over the abdominal area.
3. Apply betadine over the shaved surface using sterile gauze, and wipe away with 70% ethanol (*see* **Note 4**).
4. Place a sterile drape over the rat, precutting a window which will lie over the exposed abdominal area, approximately 5 cm × 5 cm.
5. Ensure that hind limbs and other areas with unclipped fur are covered to create a sterile field. This will also assist with maintaining the rat's core body temperature during the surgical procedure.

3.4.3 Surgical Procedure

1. Using a scalpel, make a skin incision approximately 1 cm below the sternum. Make the muscle incision using tissue forceps and dressing scissors.
2. Using sterile cotton-tipped applicator sticks, move the intestines, colon, kidney, spleen, and stomach aside to expose the descending aorta. The ideal positioning of the cannula is such that the aortic clip should be placed just below the left renal branch. This allows sufficient clearance for the aortic clip, sutures, and cannula incision.
3. Use sterile gauze dipped in warm saline, wrap the internal organs, and tuck the gauze under the muscle on each side of the incision to hold them in place and reduce moisture loss.
4. Place a self-retaining tissue retractor, ensuring the teeth are placed on the sterile gauze and not underlying organs to prevent damaging them.
5. Using the curved blunt forceps, isolate the aorta by separating the connective tissue between the aorta and vena cava, directly below the left renal branch point (Fig. 3).
6. Pull through a ~20 cm silk suture, clamp with a hemostat, and pull upward to restrict the blood flow through the aorta.
7. Isolate the vena cava and aorta just above the aortic bifurcation (*see* **Note 5**).
8. Pull through a ~20 cm silk suture, clamp with a hemostat, and pull downward to restrict the backflow of blood through the aorta.
9. Prepare for aortic occlusion; ensure that your cannula, cannula holder, and bent 23-G syringe needle (*see* **Note 6**) are placed within reach.
10. The order of occlusion is important. Firstly, ensure the bottom suture is retracted sufficiently. This will allow the aorta to fill with blood and assist with cannula insertion.

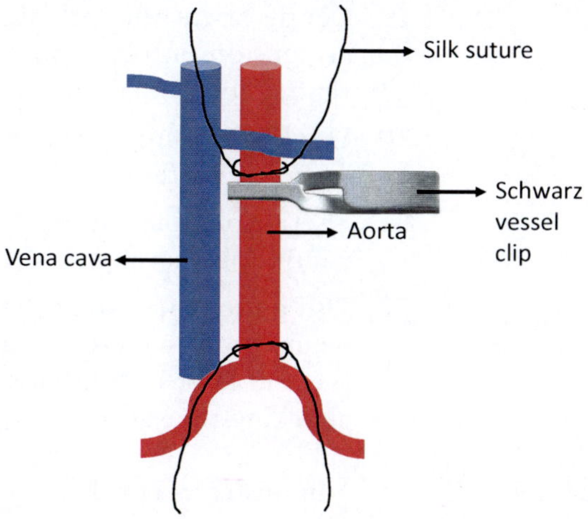

Fig. 3 Schematic showing the relative positions for silk sutures as well as Schwarz vessel clip placement on the aorta. The clip should be placed as high as possible near the bifurcation of the vena cava to the renal artery

11. Place the top aortic clip. Blood flow should now be absent from this segment of the aorta.
12. Make an incision on the aorta in the middle of the isolated aortic segment using the bent 23-G needle. While keeping the needle tip in place, slide the cannula of the telemetry probe underneath. Slowly advance the cannula while retracting the needle tip, pulling the needle upward if necessary.
13. Advance the cannula until it lies just below the Schwarz clip. Dab the incision point with gauze to prepare the surface for the cellulose patch.
14. Place the cellulose patch (as described in Fig. 2), pressing down the "legs" of the trouser-shaped patch so that it wraps around the aorta. Apply 1–2 drops of Vetbond onto the cellulose patch (*see* **Note 7**).
15. Once the Vetbond is completely dry, release the bottom hemostat and the Schwarz clip (*see* **Note 8**).
16. Remove the silk ligatures by cutting the knot near the vessel surface. This reduces the dragging distance and minimizes damage to the aorta.
17. Remove the saline-soaked gauze pieces and self-retaining retractor.
18. Ensure the intestines fall back into place smoothly by flooding the abdominal cavity with 2 mL of saline with Tribactral. Carefully massage the organs back into place, making sure not to entangle the probe catheter in the rat's organs.

19. Gently orient the catheter in the abdominal cavity so there is no tension on the cannula, and insert the probe close to the ventral abdominal region.
20. Use PDS sutures to secure the probe to the abdominal muscle layer (*see* **Note 9**).
21. Use absorbable sutures to secure the muscle incision with a continuous horizontal suture, burying the suture ends.
22. Using the same suture thread, perform a subcuticular stitch to secure the skin incision, ending with an Aberdeen knot. Ensure the end knot is well buried to minimize the chance of the rat attacking the sutures.

3.4.4 Postoperative Care and Monitoring (See Note 10)

1. Administer 3 mg/kg carprofen in 0.1 mL via subcutaneous injection.
2. Administer 1 mL saline subcutaneously, place Baytril in drinking water, and monitor post-recovery until the rat regains consciousness.
3. Once the rat has awakened, carefully monitor any change from normal behavior (e.g., grooming, walking). In particular, watch for any potential hind limb movement impairment, which could indicate damage to the femoral nerve bundles.
4. For postoperative pain management, administer carprofen every 12–24 h for the next 3 days.
5. Monitor feeding and drinking behavior carefully for the next 24–48 h (*see* **Note 11**).

3.4.5 Induction of Preeclampsia

1. After mating, check and confirm pregnancy daily via positive vaginal plug (or vaginal swab).
2. On day 8 of pregnancy, administer the appropriate dose of AAV to overexpress sFlt1 and sEng in the pregnant rat (*see* **Note 12**). A detailed example experimental protocol has been included with this study (Fig. 4).

4 Notes

1. If reusing a transmitter probe, cannulas at the pressure-sensing region (which is inserted into the aorta) might require re-gelling. Failure to properly maintain this region of the cannula will result in blood pressure drift over time and prevent proper interpretation of data. Carefully refill the tip using the re-gel syringe purchased from DSI, or follow the manufacturer's instructions.

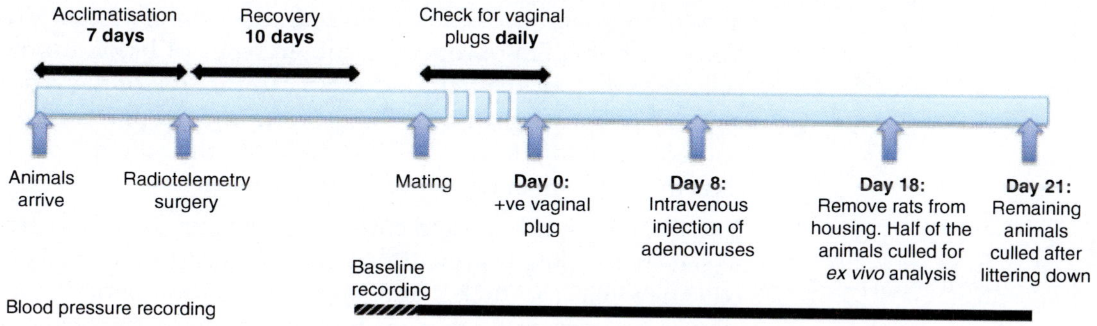

Fig. 4 Schematic showing the experimental timeline used in this study

2. The PA-40 probes come with an additional feature, which emits a radio-frequency noise when turned on. To detect this, tune into a quiet AM channel, and after the probes are turned on, distinct interference noise can be heard from the radio.
3. If transmitter probes are being reused, it is important to re-sterilize transmitter probes before use. Place probes in sterile containers filled with sufficient Cidex for full immersion in the morning (minimum 10 h, maximum 12 h). Improper sterilization procedures could result in severe infection of the rat and severe distress. If unsure, follow the manufacturer's instructions for the re-sterilization process.
4. When sterilizing, always wipe from the inside-out of the exposed skin surface in concentric circles, to ensure that the gauze is wiping from a more sterile area to a less sterile area. Wiping across the exposed skin merely spreads bacteria and dirt from the unclipped fur on the edge of the exposed skin, reducing the sterility of the surgical site.
5. When isolating just above the lower aortic bifurcation, be wary of the nerve bundles lying alongside the vessels. Damaging these nerves could impair proper hind limb movement. To do so, carefully separate the nerve bundles from the aorta using fine blunt forceps or cotton applicator sticks. Ensure the surface is moist to prevent abrasive injury.
6. For our surgeries, we use a 23-gauge syringe needle, bent 90° approximately 3–4 mm from the tip. We have found that this gives us the best success for cannula insertion, as careful use of the 23-G needle is better at preventing inadvertent tearing of the incision site. Alternatively, use a Vanna's type microscissors and an introducer or fine forceps to pick up the vessel flap.
7. It is critical that the Vetbond-coated cellulose patch is completely dry before proceeding. Failure to properly seal the cannula incision could result in the rat bleeding out once the aortic clips are released or fluctuations in blood pressure read-

ings over gestation. We have found that common cause of Vetbond not sealing properly is the presence of blood on the cellulose patch or the Vetbond sliding to the side of the vessel and drying rather than over the incision site. To prevent this, consider dabbing the drop of Vetbond onto the cellulose patch directly, rather than dropping from a height.

8. Initially, loosen the clip and ensure that the incision is properly sealed. If bleeding is present, dry the incision site using sterile cotton applicator sticks, and apply more Vetbond, before allowing to dry. If there is no bleeding, remove the Schwarz clip entirely and proceed.
9. When securing the transmitter probe, use individual sutures through each suture tab. Ensure stitches are ~3 cm away from and parallel to the incision site to reduce the risk of tearing. Properly securing the probe will prevent tension on the cannula at the incision point, which would otherwise result in the cannula being pulled off entirely and the rat bleeding out.
10. Typically, allow 10–14 days for recovery before proceeding with the next phase. This will allow stabilization of the blood pressure trace and establish the baseline recording period.
11. Typically rats will have an increased water intake during this time, so ensure there is sufficient water available.
12. We use a CMV-based vector at a dosage of 1×10^9 PFU for sFlt1 and sEng, respectively, in 0.2 mL saline, delivered via intravenous tail vein injection. As controls, we administer an equivalent PFU of mock virus (expressing galactosidase)—2×10^9 PFU total. The exact dose depends on the type of vector used and will require prior optimization.

References

1. Brockway BP, Mills PA, Azar SH (1991) A new method for continuous chronic measurement and recording of blood pressure, heart rate and activity in the rat via radiotelemetry. Clin Exp Hypertens A 13(5):885–895
2. Kadam SD et al (2010) Continuous electroencephalographic monitoring with radio-telemetry in a rat model of perinatal hypoxia–ischemia reveals progressive post-stroke epilepsy. J Neurosci 30(1):404–415
3. Kramer K, Kinter LB (2003) Evaluation and applications of radiotelemetry in small laboratory animals. Physiol Genomics 13(3):197–205
4. Maynard SE et al (2003) Excess placental soluble fms-like tyrosine kinase 1 (sFlt1) may contribute to endothelial dysfunction, hypertension, and proteinuria in preeclampsia. J Clin Invest 111(5):649–658
5. Venkatesha S et al (2006) Soluble endoglin contributes to the pathogenesis of preeclampsia. Nat Med 12(6):642–649

Chapter 27

Phase I Pilot Clinical Trial of Antenatal Maternally Administered Melatonin to Decrease the Level of Oxidative Stress in Human Pregnancies Affected by Preeclampsia

Sebastian R. Hobson, Rebecca Lim, and Euan M. Wallace

Abstract

This chapter describes the methodologies which may be used in the development of a phase I clinical trial investigating a therapy of choice in treating preeclampsia.

Key words Preeclampsia, Melatonin, Clinical trial, Oxidative stress

1 Introduction

Preeclampsia is a multi-organ syndrome of pregnancy that manifests after 20 weeks' gestation with new-onset hypertension alongside maternal end-organ dysfunction and/or intrauterine fetal growth restriction [1]. It affects between 3% and 7% of all pregnancies and is associated with substantial maternal and perinatal morbidity and mortality, with a significant proportion of fetal complications due to prematurity [2]. To date, the exact pathophysiology of preeclampsia is unknown, but early placental dysfunction plays a central role in all leading hypotheses [3, 4]. This placental dysfunction is thought to result in a local and systemic cascade of increasing oxidative stress in the mother, leading to endothelial dysfunction and subsequent end-organ consequences.

Placental hypoxia and reperfusion, as a consequence of abnormal placentation, result in oxidative stress leading to apoptotic and necrotic disruption of the syncytial structure [5]. This disruption then results in the release of various factors and compounds from the intervillous space into the maternal circulation that stimulate the production of pro-inflammatory cytokines, such as tumor necrosis factor alpha (TNF-α), interleukin (IL)-6, and anti-angiogenic factors such as soluble fms-like tyrosine kinase 1 (sFlt1) and soluble endoglin (sEng) [4]. The resultant effect involves

Padma Murthi and Cathy Vaillancourt (eds.), *Preeclampsia: Methods and Protocols*, Methods in Molecular Biology, vol. 1710, https://doi.org/10.1007/978-1-4939-7498-6_27,

potentially widespread increased oxidative stress with anti-angiogenic compromise to the maternal vasculature.

Melatonin (5-methoxy-N-acetyltryptamine) is an endogenous lipid-soluble antioxidant hormone produced primarily by the pineal gland in humans, providing circadian and seasonal timing cues. In addition, melatonin is also a powerful antioxidant, acting both as a direct scavenger of oxygen free radicals, especially the highly-damaging hydroxyl radical, and indirectly via upregulation of other antioxidant enzymes including GSHPx, GSH reductase, superoxide dismutase, and catalase [6, 7].

Melatonin has several characteristics that make it an appealing treatment for use in pregnancy. Melatonin freely crosses the placenta [8] and blood-brain barrier [9] and has an excellent safety profile with no known adverse effects [10, 11]. Reduced levels of melatonin are found in pregnant women with preeclampsia [12]. Placentae express receptors for melatonin [13], and thus melatonin may protect against oxidative stress generated by the dysfunctional organ, thereby inhibiting the release of vasoactive factors responsible for the clinical syndrome of preeclampsia.

Our group has previously shown that in an animal model of fetal growth restriction (FGR), melatonin administration reduced fetal hypoxia, improved neurodevelopment, and decreased brain injury and oxidative stress in newborn lambs [14]. In another published experiment, we administered melatonin shortly before and during a short period of severe fetal asphyxia induced by umbilical cord occlusion at late gestation. Melatonin prevented the formation of free radicals (hydroxyl radical) within the fetal brains and decreased lipid peroxidation and brain cell death [8]. The protective effects of melatonin on ischemia-reperfusion-induced oxidative damage to mitochondria in the rat placenta have also been published [15]. Melatonin treatment improves placental function (fetal/placental weight ratio), improves birth weight, and induces antioxidant enzymes in a rat model of maternal undernourishment, known to promote oxidative stress [16].

Melatonin has been studied in several clinical trials in humans at varying gestations and for different purposes. Melatonin has been assessed in assisted reproductive technology where the quality of oocytes is important for the success of in vitro fertilization (IVF). Melatonin is a key compound found in the follicular fluid that has been shown to be important for oocyte maturation and quality and has been suggested to improve pregnancy outcomes with IVF [17–19]. To date, no babies born from melatonin-treated pregnancies have been shown to have any increase in abnormalities [20]. Melatonin has also been shown to upregulate antioxidant enzymes in human pregnancies leading to the conclusion that melatonin might provide an indirect protection against injury caused by reactive oxygen species as seen in preeclampsia, FGR, and fetal hypoxia [21].

Melatonin does not have any acute pharmacological effects in the nervous or vascular systems, apart from its benign but active effect on sleep mechanisms [22]. Mice that have received extremely high doses of up to 800 mg/kg melatonin did not have increased mortality, and as such the median lethal dose could not be established [22]. In humans, a phase II clinical trial conducted in the Netherlands administered 75 mg melatonin nightly to 1400 women over 4 years, with no serious side effects reported [23]. The maternal no-adverse-effect level (NOAEL) for melatonin has been found to be 100 mg/kg/day with the fetal NOAEL established at ≥200 mg/kg/day when administered to the mother. The maternal lowest-observed-adverse-effect level (LOAEL) toxicity was 200 mg/kg/day [24].

1.1 Rationale

Preeclampsia is a life-threatening condition for both mother and baby affecting up to 7% of pregnancies [2]. Despite ongoing advancements in perinatal care, preeclampsia remains an incurable disease. Extensive animal studies demonstrate that the use of melatonin as an antioxidant in high-risk pregnancies is very promising. Melatonin readily crosses the placenta and does not harm the developing fetus, not even when administered in extremely high doses [22]. This study aims to be the first human trial to assess the potential clinical and biochemical effects of melatonin in pregnancies complicated by preterm preeclampsia.

1.2 Aims

The aim of the trial is to establish whether melatonin will afford a clinical or biochemical benefit in women with early-onset preeclampsia. To test the hypothesis, we will pose the following research aims:

1. To determine the effect of daily maternal oral treatment with melatonin on the clinical outcomes of pregnancies affected by preterm preeclampsia
2. To determine the effect of daily maternal oral treatment with melatonin on the oxidative stress response in the maternal, placental, and fetal circulation in pregnancies affected by preterm preeclampsia
3. To determine the effect of daily maternal oral treatment with melatonin on the clinical and biochemical measures of vascular function in the mother and fetus in pregnancies affected by preterm preeclampsia

2 Methods

2.1 Clinical Trial Methods

The phase I trial is an exploratory prospective trial to establish proof of principle of melatonin as an antioxidant treatment in pregnancies affected by preterm preeclampsia. The conduct of the trial was in accordance with the Therapeutic Goods Administration guide to the International standards of Good Clinical Practice (GCP). A flowchart is included below depicting the five phases of the trial (Fig. 1).

2.2 Identification and Recruitment of Participants

2.2.1 Source of Potential Participants

Potential participants for the trial will be more than 24^{+0} weeks' and below 35^{+6} weeks' gestation, as determined by either the first day of the last menstrual period (LMP) or following determination from first trimester ultrasound scan.

Women with preeclampsia will be identified from routine antenatal clinics, pregnancy assessment units, and labor ward admissions. The clinician or midwife will measure blood pressure and test the urine for proteinuria, initially with a dipstick. Women eligible for inclusion in the trial will have clearly diagnosed preeclampsia as judged by the principal investigator (PI) who is experienced in the management of preeclampsia. The following SOMANZ criteria [25] outline the minimum criteria for the diagnosis of preeclampsia: (1) hypertension arising after 20 weeks' gestation and (2) accompanied by one or more of the following—renal involvement, hematological involvement, liver involvement, neurological involvement, pulmonary edema, fetal growth restriction, and/or placental abruption.

In women who have preexisting hypertension, preeclampsia is diagnosed when there is rapidly increasing blood pressure, thrombocytopenia, liver transaminitis, the presence of new-onset proteinuria (defined above), and/or a sudden increase in proteinuria in those who have preexisting proteinuria.

Normal clinical care in these circumstances would be followed, with a blood sample taken to measure full blood count, renal and liver function testing, uric acid, and coagulation studies along with a spot urine protein-creatinine ratio. A fetal assessment will also be made with cardiotocograph (CTG, if $>28^{+0}$ weeks) and ultrasound assessment. Women with preeclampsia between 24^{+0} and 35^{+6} weeks will be either admitted to the hospital or managed as an outpatient if deemed suitable by the attending clinician for ongoing routine clinical management. The attending clinician should notify the PI and/or the research midwife by telephone of a potential participant.

2.2.2 Inclusion Criteria

To be eligible for the trial, the women must:

1. Be at least 18 years of age.
2. Be between 24^{+0} weeks' and 35^{+6} weeks' gestation.
3. Have a singleton pregnancy.
4. Have a diagnosis of preeclampsia.
5. Be considered capable of safely continuing the pregnancy for 48 h or more, as determined by the attending clinician.

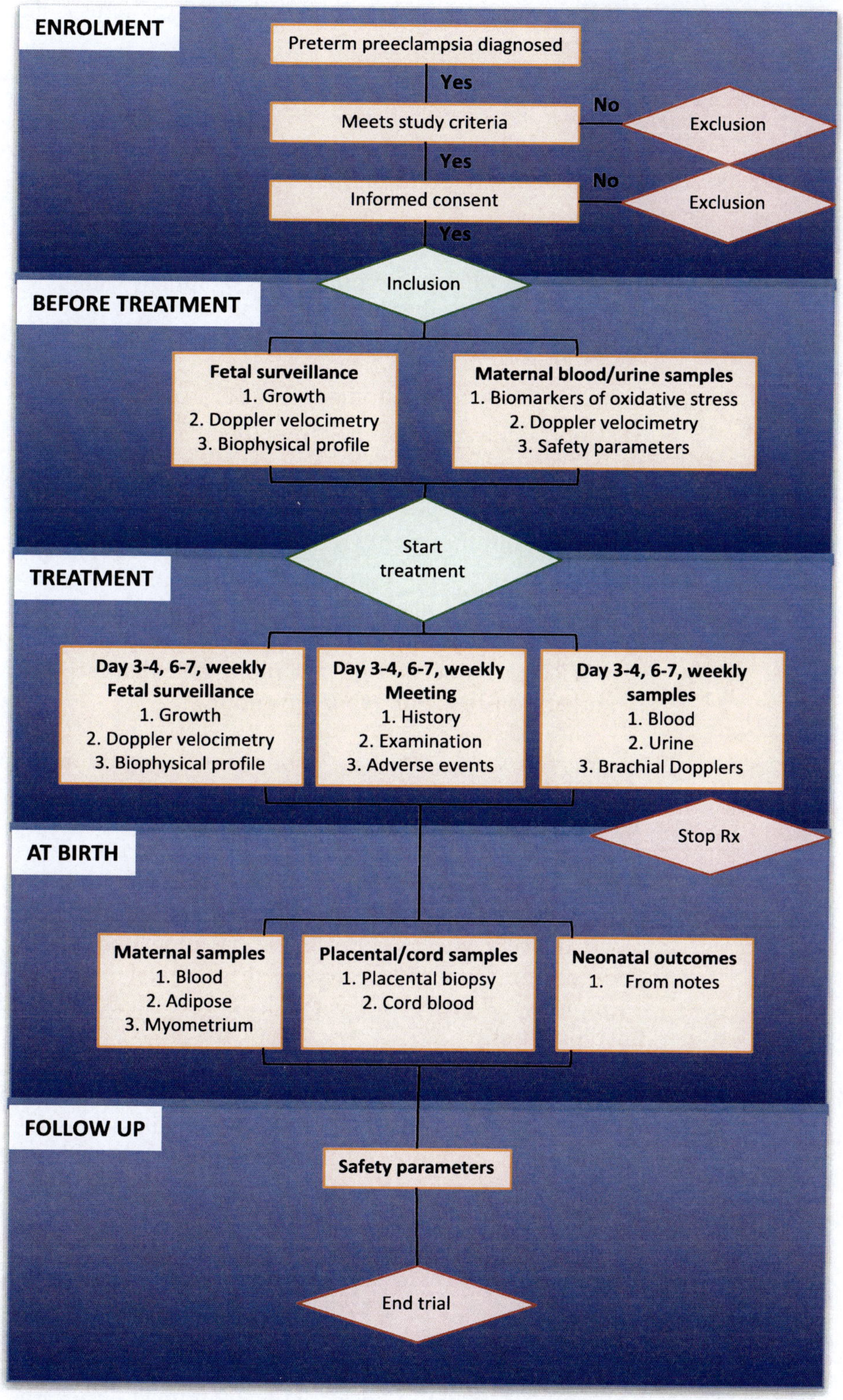

Fig. 1 Flowchart representing the five phases of trial participation

6. Obstetrician and neonatologist believe the fetus is likely to be viable.
7. No major anomalies evident on the mid-trimester morphology scan.
8. Be capable of understanding the information provided, with the use of an interpreter if required.
9. Give written informed consent.

2.2.3 Exclusion Criteria

Any women, who at the point of recruitment exhibit any of the following, are not eligible for the trial:

1. Eclampsia.
2. Current use of melatonin.
3. Contraindications to melatonin use.
4. Imminent transfer to a non-trial center due to unavailability of neonatal beds.
5. Significant uncertainty regarding gestational age.
6. Use of any of the following medications: fluvoxamine, 5- or 8-methoxypsoralen, cimetidine, quinolones, and other CYP1A2 inhibitors; carbamazepine, rifampicin, and other CYP1A2 inducers; and zaleplon, zolpidem, zopiclone, and other non-benzodiazepine hypnotics.

2.2.4 Control Group

During this study, the main cohort and outcome measures were derived from one group of participants as described previously. They acted as their own internal controls comparing pretreatment to posttreatment with melatonin.

For certain aspects of the trial, such as the collection of clinical characteristics including blood pressure and interval from diagnosis to delivery, a retrospective cohort of matched controls was derived from patients treated at the hospital over the previous 24 months. All groups will carry the same exclusion criteria as outlined previously.

2.3 Treatment

2.3.1 Supply and Formulation of Melatonin

The trial drug is supplied as 10 mg melatonin sustained release tablets, containing melatonin 10 mg, vitamin B6 (as 10 mg pyridoxine HCl), cellulose, dibasic calcium phosphate, hypromellose, magnesium stearate, stearic acid, silica, methylcellulose, and glycerin.

The drug did not contain yeast, wheat, corn, milk, egg, soy, artificial colors or flavors, added sugar, or preservatives.

2.3.2 Route of Administration, Dosage, Dosage Regimen, and Treatment Period

At recruitment, a trial number is allocated to each participant, and the pharmacist on duty will receive notification of the name and trial number of the recruited woman and will ensure the ward or patient has adequately dispensed quantities of the medication available.

One 10 mg melatonin tablet must be taken three times daily (at 8 h intervals), orally with or without food. On the day of recruitment, the first dose should be given as soon as possible after baseline measurements and samples have been taken. Treatment should continue t.d.s. until the pregnancy is ended.

The pharmacist should keep accurate records of trial drugs dispensed using a pharmacy log provided by the Trial Office. The attending clinician administering the treatment will also be required to record each dose on the trial drug chart, or if treated as an outpatient, the patient will keep a log of compliance. Trial drugs must be kept in the packaging supplied and under no circumstances used for other participants or nonparticipants.

2.3.3 Compliance Monitoring

The daily dispensing of the trial drug will be recorded on the patient's usual drug chart, with any deviations from the daily schedule noted on the chart. The research midwife or PI will periodically monitor the trial drug chart to verify that the dispensing system is being followed, and the PI will address any problems or deviations. Participants treated as outpatients will complete a medication compliance log which will be monitored by the treating clinician and PI.

2.4 Outcome Measures

This study will seek to determine appreciable changes in both clinically relevant outcomes and biomarkers in pregnancies affected by preterm preeclampsia treated with melatonin. The most significant factor in the increased burden of disease in preterm preeclampsia is preterm delivery, and pregnancies affected with preeclampsia are only expected to continue for an average of 11.5 days. This justifies why the authors have selected the interval from diagnosis to delivery as the primary outcome measure, as compared to gestational age-matched women with preterm preeclampsia not treated with melatonin. Secondary outcome measures after treatment will be compared to those measured before treatment. They will also be compared to the end points determined in healthy pregnancies, established in local tissue banks. Maternal blood, tissues, and other recordings will be collected, along with placental tissue, and umbilical cord bloods collected at the time of birth. Where the study participants receiving melatonin cannot act as their own controls, samples from gestational age-matched controls will be obtained from the existing tissue bank.

2.4.1 Primary Outcome Measures

1. The time interval from diagnosis with preeclampsia to delivery.
2. Maternal and fetal safety data, including serious adverse events and reactions.

2.4.2 Secondary Outcome Measures

1. Biomarkers of oxidative stress assessed through commercially available assay kits including 8-isoprostane, total antioxidant capacity, melatonin, and prostaglandin E2.
2. Biomarkers of preeclampsia assessed through commercially available assay kits including soluble fms-like tyrosine kinase-1 (sFlt-1), soluble endoglin (sEng), activin A, and placental growth factor (PlGF).
3. Severity of preeclampsia more than 48 h after recruitment as indicated by maternal blood pressure, level of proteinuria, hemoglobin and platelet count, liver transaminases, renal function, fetal ultrasound Doppler flow (see below), and composite of preeclamptic symptoms: edema, headache, visual disturbance, and epigastric or left upper quadrant pain.
4. Maternal morbidity more than 48 h after recruitment as indicated by serum creatinine ≥120 μmol/L, proteinuria ≥5 g/24 h, signs of left ventricular failure (pulmonary edema, oxygen sats <95%), hypertension ≥170/110 mmHg despite antihypertensive treatment, disseminated intravascular coagulation and/or platelets $<50 \times 10^9$, eclampsia, cerebrovascular event, and liver transaminase ≥500 IU/L.
5. Maternal brachial artery Doppler studies.
6. Maternal uterine artery Doppler studies.
7. Pregnancy end points including gestation at birth; mode of birth; placental histology; cord lactates, artery and vein; and abnormal cardiotocogram (CTG).
8. Fetal end points on ultrasound including amniotic fluid indices (AFI); fetal characteristics, heart rate, tone, breathing, and movements; and Doppler velocimetry, umbilical artery, middle cerebral artery, and ductus venosus.
9. Neonatal outcomes: neonatal Apgar score at 1, 5, and 10 min; weight at birth; and composite neonatal outcome (admission to NICU, duration of admission, need and duration of respiratory support, intraventricular hemorrhage, necrotizing enterocolitis, abnormal neurology, mortality prior to discharge).
10. Use of antenatal antihypertensives.
11. Use of antenatal magnesium sulfate.
12. Level of melatonin in the cord blood at delivery relative to maternal levels.
13. Maternal Karolinska sleepiness scale on melatonin.

2.4.3 Karolinska Sleepiness Scale (KSS)

The KSS measures the subjective level of sleepiness at a particular time during the day [26]. On this scale, subjects indicate which level best reflects the psychophysical state experienced in the last 10 min. The KSS is a measure of situational sleepiness and is sensitive to fluctuations. In a study conducted by Kaida et al. [27], the authors investigated the validity of the KSS and found that it was highly correlated to electroencephalography (EEG) and behavioral variables and also demonstrated that KSS has a high validity.

Participants of the trial will have their KSS measured through baseline pretreatment questionnaire and then twice a week during treatment and at delivery. The questionnaire will be filled out at the same time on each day of completion to minimize inter-result variables.

2.4.4 Proposed Analyses

The length of gestation post recruitment will be analyzed using a *t*-test. The biomarkers will be analyzed using a repeated measure analysis, including the baseline value as a covariate. For the primary analysis, the treatment effect will be considered constant over time; secondary analyses will examine the possibility of a trend over time. Plots of mean score over time will be shown for clarification. Initially, the treatment effect will be assumed to be constant over time, but if time by treatment interaction is shown to be important by including this parameter in the model (the conventional level of $p = 0.05$ will be used here), then further investigation into effects at differing time points will be made by analyzing the least square means as above. Plots of mean score over time will be shown for clarification.

All other continuous measures (e.g., clinical measures) will be considered in the same manner as above (adjusting by baseline value if available). Dichotomous outcomes (e.g., mortality) will be presented as risk ratios, with a corresponding chi-squared test performed.

Apart from baseline value, no adjustments for covariates will be made in the first instance in any of the investigations. Treatment estimates will only be adjusted when subgroups are explored. Interaction between treatment and subgroup variables will be examined in a similar fashion as above by including the relevant parameters in the model. This will be done in turn for each subgroup variable and adjusted estimates presented.

All tests are two-sided and results will be presented as a point estimate along with 95% confidence intervals.

2.4.5 Adverse Events

Participants will usually be inpatients for the duration of the trial. As such, a senior obstetric clinician who will be in ongoing communication with the research team will see them daily. The PI of the trial will be contactable by telephone at all times in the case of an adverse event. Any serious adverse events that occur after joining the trial will be reported in detail in the participant's medical notes, followed up until resolution of the event and reported to the Local Site's Human Research Ethics Committee, Therapeutics Committee, and Therapeutic Goods Administration immediately or within 24–72 h.

2.4.6 Trial Discontinuation or Modification

Participants will be withdrawn from the trial at participant request or if they or their fetus suffer an unexpected serious adverse event as noted above. Worsening preeclampsia is within the natural history of the disease and as such will not be part of discontinuation criteria. There will be no allowance for modification of the trial intervention.

References

1. Lowe SA, Brown MA, Dekker GA, Gatt S, McLintock CK, McMahon LP, Mangos G, Moore MP, Muller P, Paech M, Walters B, Society of Obstetric Medicine of A, New Z (2009) Guidelines for the management of hypertensive disorders of pregnancy 2008. Aust N Z J Obstet Gynaecol 49(3):242–246. https://doi.org/10.1111/j.1479-828X.2009.01003.x
2. Payne B, Magee LA, von Dadelszen P (2011) Assessment, surveillance and prognosis in preeclampsia. Best Pract Res Clin Obstet Gynaecol 25(4):449–462. https://doi.org/10.1016/j.bpobgyn.2011.02.003
3. Roberts JM, Gammill HS (2005) Preeclampsia: recent insights. Hypertension 46(6):1243–1249. https://doi.org/10.1161/01.HYP.0000188408.49896.c5
4. Steegers EA, von Dadelszen P, Duvekot JJ, Pijnenborg R (2010) Pre-eclampsia. Lancet 376(9741):631–644. https://doi.org/10.1016/S0140-6736(10)60279-6
5. Burton GJ, Jauniaux E (2011) Oxidative stress. Best Pract Res Clin Obstet Gynaecol 25(3):287–299. https://doi.org/10.1016/j.bpobgyn.2010.10.016
6. Reiter RJ, Tan DX (2003) Melatonin: a novel protective agent against oxidative injury of the ischemic/reperfused heart. Cardiovasc Res 58(1):10–19
7. Reiter RJ, Tan DX, Osuna C, Gitto E (2000) Actions of melatonin in the reduction of oxidative stress. A review. J Biomed Sci 7(6): 444–458
8. Miller SL, Yan EB, Castillo-Melendez M, Jenkin G, Walker DW (2005) Melatonin provides neuroprotection in the late-gestation fetal sheep brain in response to umbilical cord occlusion. Dev Neurosci 27(2-4):200–210. https://doi.org/10.1159/000085993
9. Welin AK, Svedin P, Lapatto R, Sultan B, Hagberg H, Gressens P, Kjellmer I, Mallard C (2007) Melatonin reduces inflammation and cell death in white matter in the mid-gestation fetal sheep following umbilical cord occlusion. Pediatr Res 61(2):153–158. https://doi.org/10.1203/01.pdr.0000252546.20451.1a
10. Gitto E, Pellegrino S, Gitto P, Barberi I, Reiter RJ (2009) Oxidative stress of the newborn in the pre- and postnatal period and the clinical utility of melatonin. J Pineal Res 46(2):128–139. https://doi.org/10.1111/j.1600-079X.2008.00649.x
11. Fulia F, Gitto E, Cuzzocrea S, Reiter RJ, Dugo L, Gitto P, Barberi S, Cordaro S, Barberi I (2001) Increased levels of malondialdehyde and nitrite/nitrate in the blood of asphyxiated newborns: reduction by melatonin. J Pineal Res 31(4):343–349
12. Lanoix D, Guerin P, Vaillancourt C (2012) Placental melatonin production and melatonin receptor expression are altered in preeclampsia: new insights into the role of this hormone in pregnancy. J Pineal Res 53(4):417–425. https://doi.org/10.1111/j.1600-079X.2012.01012.x
13. Lanoix D, Beghdadi H, Lafond J, Vaillancourt C (2008) Human placental trophoblasts synthesize melatonin and express its receptors. J Pineal Res 45(1):50–60. https://doi.org/10.1111/j.1600-079X.2008.00555.x
14. Miller SL, Wallace EM, Walker DW (2012) Antioxidant therapies: a potential role in perinatal medicine. Neuroendocrinology 96(1):13–23. https://doi.org/10.1159/000336378
15. Okatani Y, Wakatsuki A, Shinohara K, Taniguchi K, Fukaya T (2001) Melatonin protects against oxidative mitochondrial damage induced in rat placenta by ischemia and reperfusion. J Pineal Res 31(2):173–178
16. Richter HG, Hansell JA, Raut S, Giussani DA (2009) Melatonin improves placental efficiency and birth weight and increases the placental expression of antioxidant enzymes in undernourished pregnancy. J Pineal Res 46(4):357–364. https://doi.org/10.1111/j.1600-079X.2009.00671.x
17. Tamura H, Nakamura Y, Terron MP, Flores LJ, Manchester LC, Tan DX, Sugino N, Reiter RJ (2008) Melatonin and pregnancy in the human. Reprod Toxicol 25(3):291–303. https://doi.org/10.1016/j.reprotox.2008.03.005

18. Rizzo P, Raffone E, Benedetto V (2010) Effect of the treatment with myo-inositol plus folic acid plus melatonin in comparison with a treatment with myo-inositol plus folic acid on oocyte quality and pregnancy outcome in IVF cycles. A prospective, clinical trial. Eur Rev Med Pharmacol Sci 14(6):555–561
19. Unfer V, Raffone E, Rizzo P, Buffo S (2011) Effect of a supplementation with myo-inositol plus melatonin on oocyte quality in women who failed to conceive in previous in vitro fertilization cycles for poor oocyte quality: a prospective, longitudinal, cohort study. Gynecol Endocrinol 27(11):857–861. https://doi.org/10.3109/09513590.2011.564687
20. Unfer V (2012) Personal communication via email
21. Okatani Y, Okamoto K, Hayashi K, Wakatsuki A, Tamura S, Sagara Y (1998) Maternal-fetal transfer of melatonin in pregnant women near term. J Pineal Res 25(3):129–134
22. Barchas J, DaCosta F, Spector S (1967) Acute pharmacology of melatonin. Nature 214 (5091):919–920
23. Silman RE (1993) Melatonin: a contraceptive for the nineties. Eur J Obstet Gynecol Reprod Biol 49(1-2):3–9
24. Jahnke G, Marr M, Myers C, Wilson R, Travlos G, Price C (1999) Maternal and developmental toxicity evaluation of melatonin administered orally to pregnant Sprague-Dawley rats. Toxicol Sci 50(2):271–279
25. Lowe SA, Brown MA, Dekker G, Gatt S, McLintock C, McMahon L, Mangos G, Moore MP, Muller P, Paech M, Walters B (2009) Guidelines for the management of hypertensive disorders of pregnancy. Aust N Z J Obstet Gynaecol 49(3):242–246
26. Shahid A, Wilkinson K, Marcu S, Shapiro CM (2011) Karolinska Sleepiness Scale (KSS). Springer, New York, NY, pp 209–210. https://doi.org/10.1007/978-1-4419-9893-4_47
27. Kaida K, Takahashi M, Akerstedt T, Nakata A, Otsuka Y, Haratani T, Fukasawa K (2006) Validation of the Karolinska sleepiness scale against performance and EEG variables. Clin Neurophysiol 117(7):1574–1581. https://doi.org/10.1016/j.clinph.2006.03.011

Chapter 28

A Randomized Double-Blinded Placebo-Controlled Intervention Trial of Melatonin for the Prevention of Preeclampsia in Moderate- and High-Risk Women: The MELPOP Trial

Sebastian R. Hobson, Euan M. Wallace, John C. Kingdom, and Ryan J. Hodges

Abstract

This chapter describes the methodologies which may be used in the development of a randomized controlled trial investigating a therapy of choice in preventing preeclampsia.

Key words Preeclampsia, Melatonin, Prevention, Clinical trial, Oxidative stress

1 Introduction

Preeclampsia, one of the hypertensive disorders of pregnancy, remains a leading cause of maternal death worldwide, with the majority of deaths occurring in developing countries [1]. Preeclampsia is a multi-organ syndrome of pregnancy that manifests after 20 weeks' gestation with new-onset hypertension alongside maternal end-organ dysfunction and/or fetal growth restriction [2]. Importantly, preeclampsia poses serious health risks for the baby, implicated in 12% of cases of fetal growth restriction, and is a known antecedent in up to 19% of preterm births [3]. There is currently no effective treatment for preeclampsia except delivery of baby, and as such it remains a significant burden of disease for both mothers and their babies worldwide.

Screening for women at risk of preeclampsia is an important part of antenatal care. Once women are identified as high risk, they can be targeted for more intensive antenatal surveillance and prophylactic interventions. Most current strategies for risk assessment are based on the obstetric and medical history and clinical

Padma Murthi and Cathy Vaillancourt (eds.), *Preeclampsia: Methods and Protocols*, Methods in Molecular Biology, vol. 1710, https://doi.org/10.1007/978-1-4939-7498-6_28,

examination. However, there is surprisingly little reliable evidence on the actual risk associated with individual factors and how they might interact.

Risk factors with a particularly high association with preeclampsia (more than one in ten risks) include maternal diabetes [4, 5], chronic hypertension [4–6], and renal disease [7]. Thrombophilia and autoimmune disease have a strong association with severe early-onset preeclampsia [8]. Obstetric factors associated with high risk are multiple pregnancy [5, 9], history of preeclampsia in a previous pregnancy especially if severe or early onset [4, 10, 11], and a current hydropic pregnancy [12]. Other factors linked with preeclampsia but associated with a somewhat lower risk include first pregnancies [5, 13], age less than 20 or more than 35 years [5], a family history of preeclampsia [14], and obesity [5, 15, 16].

Routine screening for preeclampsia is based on measurement of blood pressure and urinalysis for proteinuria. Overall, 15–25% of women with gestational hypertension progress to preeclampsia [17]. Although various physiologic and biochemical screening tests have also been developed, so far none have proved to be of good predictive value and few are used in clinical practice. Doppler ultrasound looking for increased resistance of the uterine arteries is a noninvasive imaging test to assess for abnormal blood flow to the placenta and at present holds more promise [18]. As the cause of preeclampsia is not well understood, and screening tests remain unreliable, it is difficult to develop appropriate strategies for prevention of preeclampsia. Current strategies for prevention focus on antenatal surveillance, modification of lifestyle, nutritional supplementation, and pharmacological therapy [19].

Supplementing women with melatonin (5-methoxy-N-acetyltryptamine), a potent antioxidant, may increase their resistance to oxidative stress and subsequently limit the systemic and uteroplacental endothelial damage that is observed in preeclampsia [20].

The exact pathogenesis of preeclampsia is unknown but it is likely that its evolution is multifactorial involving a complex interplay between the mother, the fetus, and the placenta (*see* Chapter 27). With the previously described initial abnormal placentation of preeclampsia, it is now widely accepted that resultant placental hypoperfusion can induce a state of oxidative stress [21]. Oxidative stress, coupled with an exaggerated inflammatory response, may cause the release of maternal factors that result in inappropriate endothelial cell activation and dysfunction culminating in the clinical manifestations of the disease. So while the exact pathogenesis of preeclampsia is not entirely known, it has been shown that oxidative stress is key to the origins and sequelae of the disease [22].

As described in Chapter 27, melatonin is an endogenous antioxidant hormone which has been proposed as a suitably safe and potentially effective drug to ameliorate the placental and/or endothelial oxidative stress response in preeclampsia. Furthermore, it may have more beneficial effects when used as a preventative therapy prior to diagnosis with preeclampsia, as opposed to an adjunct treatment in those with established disease. Following promising results from in vitro and early phase clinical trials, a randomized controlled trial would be a suitable study design to answer this research question.

2 Method

2.1 Study Design

This is a randomized double-blinded placebo-controlled intervention trial investigating preeclampsia, defined according to the Society of Obstetric Medicine of Australia and New Zealand (SOMANZ) [2]. The population of interest involves women attending the study hospital for antenatal care and delivery. The intervention involves randomization to oral melatonin tablets 10 mg nocte or identical placebo tablet from recruitment until delivery. Randomization is achieved using computational random allocation, and both participants and researchers will be blinded to the intervention given. Calculation of the sample size takes into account that the incidence of preeclampsia is 5% in the population of interest. In order to detect a 50% reduction in incidence (with 80% power, two-sided $p < 0.05$), 984 women are required in each group with a 1:1 ratio.

2.2 Participant Inclusion Criteria

1. Age 16 years or more.
2. Pregnant women presenting prior to 17^{+0} weeks' gestation.
3. Moderate to high risk of preeclampsia. One or more of the following: previous history of preeclampsia, antiphospholipid antibodies, pre-existing diabetes, pre-existing hypertension, pre-existing renal disease, autoimmune disease, nulliparity, family history of preeclampsia, elevated BMI > 25, and maternal age <20 or >35.
4. Give written informed consent.

2.3 Participant Exclusion Criteria

1. Multiple pregnancies.
2. Current or previous melatonin ingestion within the last 6 weeks.
3. Melatonin sensitivity.
4. Use of any of the following medications which can interfere with melatonin metabolism and/or elimination: fluvoxamine, 5- or 8-methoxypsoralen, cimetidine, quinolones, and other CYP1A2 inhibitors; carbamazepine, rifampicin, and other CYP1A2 inducers; and zaleplon, zolpidem, zopiclone, and other non-benzodiazepine hypnotics.

2.3.1 Primary Outcome Measure(s)

Incidence of preeclampsia determined after delivery.

2.4 Secondary Outcome Measure(s)

2.4.1 For the Woman

1. Death: during pregnancy or up to 42 days after end of pregnancy.
2. Severe morbidity including eclampsia, liver or renal failure, hemolysis, elevated liver enzymes and low platelets syndrome (HELLP), disseminated intravascular coagulation (DIC), stroke, and pulmonary edema.
3. Gestational hypertension: defined where possible as hypertension (blood pressure ≥140 mmHg systolic or ≥90 mmHg diastolic) after 20^{+0} weeks' gestation.
4. Abruption of the placenta or antepartum hemorrhage.
5. Elective delivery: induction of labor or caesarean section.
6. Caesarean section: emergency and elective.
7. Postpartum hemorrhage: defined as blood loss of 500 mL or more.
8. Side effects: any side effects or adverse events related to the intervention, intervention stopped due to side effects.

2.4.2 For the Child

1. Death, classified by timing of death: miscarriage (fetal loss up to 19 completed weeks' gestation), stillbirth (death in utero at or after 20^{+0} weeks' gestation), perinatal death (stillbirth or death in the first 7 days of life), neonatal death (death in the first 28 days after birth), and infant death (death in the first year of life).
2. Preterm birth: $<37^{+0}$ weeks' gestation.
3. Small for gestational age: defined as growth below the 10th centile or lowest centile reported.
4. Apgar score at 5 min: low (less than 7) and very low (less than 4) or lowest reported.
5. Endotracheal intubation or use of mechanical ventilation.
6. Neonatal morbidity: respiratory distress syndrome, chronic lung disease, sepsis, necrotizing enterocolitis, retinopathy of prematurity, and intraventricular hemorrhage.
7. Side effects associated with the intervention.
8. Use of hospital resources: admission to neonatal intensive care unit and duration of hospital stay after delivery.

2.5 Statistical Analysis

All analyses are by intention to treat and performed with a computational statistics program such as SPSS, Stata, or GraphPad Prism. Summary data is presented by group as number (%) or mean (±SD) as appropriate. Analyses of the primary outcome (occurrence of preeclampsia) and maternal/child secondary endpoints are expressed as simple risk ratios with 95% CIs. Continuous outcome measures are analyzed by linear regression with robust standard errors. Subgroups can be analyzed with the same approach used for the main analysis. Where necessary to achieve convergence, odds ratios may be considered rather than risk ratios.

References

1. Lo JO, Mission JF, Caughey AB (2013) Hypertensive disease of pregnancy and maternal mortality. Curr Opin Obstet Gynecol 25(2):124–132. https://doi.org/10.1097/GCO.0b013e32835e0ef5
2. Lowe SA, Bower L, Lust K, McMahon LP, Morton MR, North RA, Paech M, Said JM, Society of Obstetric Medicine of A, New Z (2014) Guidelines for the management of hypertensive disorders of pregnancy 2014. Aust N Z J Obstet Gynaecol 49(3):242–246. https://doi.org/10.1111/j.1479-828X.2009.01003.x
3. Kramer MS, Seguin L, Lydon J, Goulet L (2000) Socio-economic disparities in pregnancy outcome: why do the poor fare so poorly? Paediatr Perinat Epidemiol 14(3):194–210
4. Caritis S, Sibai B, Hauth J, Lindheimer M, VanDorsten P, Klebanoff M, Thom E, Landon M, Paul R, Miodovnik M, Meis P, Thurnau G, Dombrowski M, McNellis D, Roberts J (1998) Predictors of pre-eclampsia in women at high risk. National Institute of Child Health and Human Development Network of Maternal-Fetal Medicine Units. Am J Obstet Gynecol 179(4):946–951
5. Conde-Agudelo A, Belizan JM (2000) Risk factors for pre-eclampsia in a large cohort of Latin American and Caribbean women. BJOG 107(1):75–83
6. Rey E, Couturier A (1994) The prognosis of pregnancy in women with chronic hypertension. Am J Obstet Gynecol 171(2):410–416
7. Cunningham FG, Cox SM, Harstad TW, Mason RA, Pritchard JA (1990) Chronic renal disease and pregnancy outcome. Am J Obstet Gynecol 163(2):453–459
8. Dekker GA, de Vries JI, Doelitzsch PM, Huijgens PC, von Blomberg BM, Jakobs C, van Geijn HP (1995) Underlying disorders associated with severe early-onset preeclampsia. Am J Obstet Gynecol 173(4):1042–1048
9. Long PA, Oats JN (1987) Preeclampsia in twin pregnancy—severity and pathogenesis. Aust N Z J Obstet Gynaecol 27(1):1–5
10. Hnat MD, Sibai BM, Caritis S, Hauth J, Lindheimer MD, MacPherson C, Van Dorsten JP, Landon M, Miodovnik M, Paul R, Meis P, Thurnau G, Dombrowski M, National Institute of Child H, Human Development Network of Maternal-Fetal M-U (2002) Perinatal outcome in women with recurrent preeclampsia compared with women who develop preeclampsia as nulliparas. Am J Obstet Gynecol 186(3):422–426
11. Sibai BM, Mercer B, Sarinoglu C (1991) Severe preeclampsia in the second trimester: recurrence risk and long-term prognosis. Am J Obstet Gynecol 165(5 Pt 1):1408–1412
12. Scott JS (1958) Pregnancy toxaemia associated with hydrops foetalis, hydatidiform mole and hydramnios. J Obstet Gynaecol Br Emp 65(5):689–701
13. Brown MA, Hague WM, Higgins J, Lowe S, McCowan L, Oats J, Peek MJ, Rowan JA, Walters BN, Australasian Society for the Study of Hypertension in P (2000) The detection, investigation and management of hypertension in pregnancy: executive summary. Aust N Z J Obstet Gynaecol 40(2):133–138
14. Chesley LC, Annitto JE, Cosgrove RA (1968) The familial factor in toxemia of pregnancy. Obstet Gynecol 32(3):303–311
15. Baeten JM, Bukusi EA, Lambe M (2001) Pregnancy complications and outcomes among overweight and obese nulliparous women. Am J Public Health 91(3):436–440
16. Sebire NJ, Jolly M, Harris JP, Wadsworth J, Joffe M, Beard RW, Regan L, Robinson S (2001) Maternal obesity and pregnancy outcome: a study of 287,213 pregnancies in London. Int J Obes Relat Metab Disord 25(8):1175–1182. https://doi.org/10.1038/sj.ijo.0801670
17. Saudan P, Brown MA, Buddle ML, Jones M (1998) Does gestational hypertension become pre-eclampsia? Br J Obstet Gynaecol 105(11):1177–1184
18. Papageorghiou AT, Yu CK, Nicolaides KH (2004) The role of uterine artery Doppler in predicting adverse pregnancy outcome. Best Pract Res Clin Obstet Gynaecol 18(3):383–396. https://doi.org/10.1016/j.bpobgyn.2004.02.003

19. Meher S, Duley L (2007) Nitric oxide for preventing pre-eclampsia and its complications. Cochrane Database Syst Rev 2:CD006490. https://doi.org/10.1002/14651858.CD006490
20. Hobson SR, Lim R, Gardiner EE, Alers NO, Wallace EM (2013) Phase I pilot clinical trial of antenatal maternally administered melatonin to decrease the level of oxidative stress in human pregnancies affected by pre-eclampsia (PAMPR): study protocol. BMJ Open 3(9):e003788. https://doi.org/10.1136/bmjopen-2013-003788
21. Hubel CA (1999) Oxidative stress in the pathogenesis of preeclampsia. Proc Soc Exp Biol Med 222(3):222–235
22. Iliadis S, Papageorgiou G (2012) Oxidative stress, preeclampsia and cardiovascular disease. Curr Hypertens Rev 8(2):130–135

INDEX

Padma Murthi and Cathy Vaillancourt (eds.), *Preeclampsia: Methods and Protocols*, Methods in Molecular Biology, vol. 1710, https://doi.org/10.1007/978-1-4939-7498-6, © Springer Science+Business Media LLC 2018

T

U

V

X

MIX
Papier aus verantwortungsvollen Quellen
Paper from responsible sources
FSC® C105338

Printed by Books on Demand, Germany